# Welcome To KATIE'S BRAIN

*A Brain Cancer Survivor's Story*

KATIE KAISER SMITH

outskirts
press

Welcome To Katie's Brain
A Brain Cancer Survivor's Story
All Rights Reserved.
Copyright © 2024 Katie Kaiser Smith
v5.0

The opinions expressed in this manuscript are solely the opinions of the author and do not represent the opinions or thoughts of the publisher. The author has represented and warranted full ownership and/or legal right to publish all the materials in this book.

This book may not be reproduced, transmitted, or stored in whole or in part by any means, including graphic, electronic, or mechanical without the express written consent of the publisher except in the case of brief quotations embodied in critical articles and reviews.

Outskirts Press, Inc.
http://www.outskirtspress.com

Paperback ISBN: 978-1-9772-6710-8
Hardback ISBN: 978-1-9772-6711-5

Cover Photo © 2024 www.gettyimages.com. All rights reserved - used with permission.

Outskirts Press and the "OP" logo are trademarks belonging to Outskirts Press, Inc.

PRINTED IN THE UNITED STATES OF AMERICA

*This book is dedicated to
Micah, Lucky and Haven,
My reasons for living.*

"Katie Smith takes us on her daily journey with brain cancer. We get a front row view as to the impact this disease has on her, her family and loved ones. Katie's book taught me much about the struggles, joys and most importantly, bravery in patients who battle with brain cancer. Thank you for this rare and poignant gift."

Timothy Cloughesy, MD
Neuro oncologist and distinguished
Professor of Neurology at UCLA Medical Center

When my husband was first diagnosed with Brain Cancer, someone we knew immediately phoned Katie to contact us. We met and realized what an angel she was. She gave us important information that no one else could've even begin to know. Her outlook and perspective was invaluable and I'm so glad she's put all that knowledge into her new book. It will outline clearly what you need to do to keep going. It will also make you smile, laugh, but mostly inspired. You'll be glad to have read her story and thankful for her insight.

Maria Quiban
Morning Meteorologist/Author
Fox 11 KTTV News Los Angeles
Author of "You Can't Do It Alone"

How I first came to meet Katie Smith in 2012. I received a phone call from her one afternoon. She needed someone to talk to because she had been diagnosed with a brain tumor. I was familiar with this because our daughter had been diagnosed as well. She just wanted some reassurance about surgery, treatment, surgeons. I was able to personally meet her a few months later at a school function. She showed so much strength. You could see that she had every intention of beating this. Fast forward 11yrs later. Katie has beaten the odds. She is stronger and she wants to share her journey and help inspire hope. She is a wife, mother, friend and a SURVIVOR!

Rebecca Neidorf
President, Heart Of The Brain Foundation

# Introduction

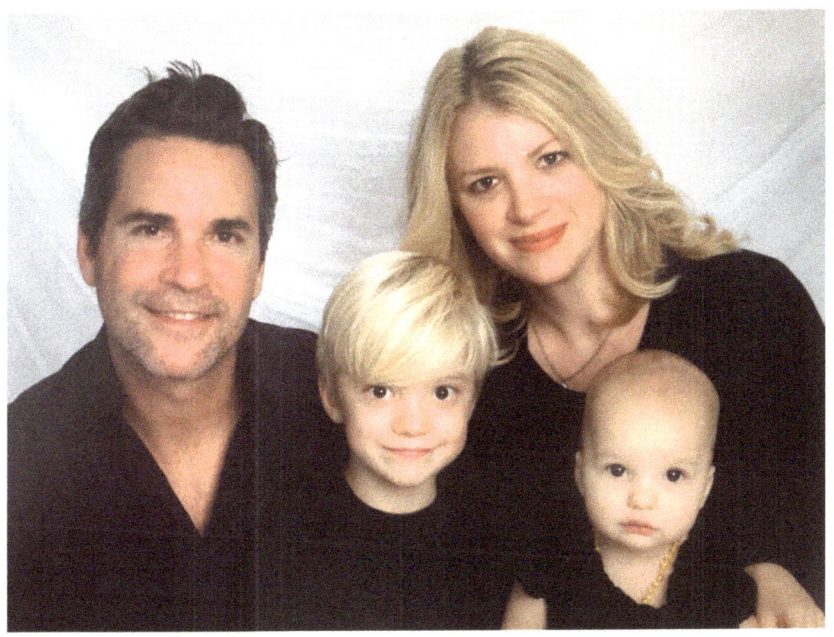

A few months prior to being diagnosed

Dear Reader,

10 years ago, I was diagnosed with a brain tumor at the age of forty-two. This book is a series of blog posts that I wrote during my struggle through diagnosis, treatment, and eventual recovery, a process that spanned the length of four years and still continues today. I blogged about it so that my friends and family could stay up to date

with my situation. They then shared it with their friends, and after a while, it became obvious that it served a much deeper purpose for both me and the readers, including many people I had never even met.

The following pages contain all of the details of that time, including very personal, raw, heartfelt, terrified, and vulnerable feelings and words. This is a story of fear, hope, humor, strength, discovery, and transformation.

The posts are the innermost thoughts that I went through in real time, and I am sharing them with you in the hopes that if you or someone you know is going through an illness, this will help inspire you to never give up and to know that anything is possible. Sadly, everything in this book really happened, and nothing has been added for dramatic or comedic effect.

As you will see, finding the funny, the silly, and the ridiculous whenever we could was important in getting me, my family, and my friends through the darkest of times. I hope that you get a chuckle out of some of these posts!

Welcome to my brain.

# In The Beginning

The most common thing I get asked is, "How did you know something was wrong?" or "How did you first find out?" So here it is:

It started in the fall of 2011 with a strange tingling in the fingertips of my left hand, very subtle and intermittent as I would brush my hand against my leg or across the steering wheel. I didn't pay much attention to it but did take note of it. As anyone would, I figured I was developing magic powers!

Out of the blue one day my husband said that my eyes looked different, that one of them was more open than the other, but I just brushed it off because I always knew that my face wasn't symmetrical.

About six months later I noticed my left hand began feeling weaker than my right and would tire easily. Holding my hairdryer became a chore; my arm would feel heavy and tired. Then, one night while on the couch watching television with my husband, Micah, I casually tested the things I could do with my right hand compared with my left. I tried to do the Star Trek Vulcan hand signal; then I tried to just rub my fingers together quickly but realized I couldn't even hold my fingers straight. I tried things like holding up three fingers or snapping my fingers and found that my left hand was not the same as the right. Everything was a struggle. *Oh God, this isn't good.* My heart sank.

I had been having a lot of back problems since giving birth to my one-year-old daughter, Haven, carrying her everywhere, along with a full diaper bag and my purse, all with my left arm. I assumed and hoped my hand issue could be related to my back and neck pain, so I consulted a chiropractor. He said I most definitely had the type of problem he could fix, and my weakness was most likely a result of my neck and back problems. After I'd seen him for two weeks, my back felt great, but my hand had not improved at all. In fact, it slowly seemed to be getting worse. I started talking with my friends about it. One friend, Lisbet, whose husband was a neurology resident at UCLA Medical Center, asked if I wanted to talk with him about my situation, and the next thing I knew, Dan was at my house. He did some basic tests to check whatever neurologists check for, and when he did my reflexes, he said I had a bit of "hyperreflexia." Well, I knew what hyper meant, but I could only guess what reflexia meant. He said it usually means something is going on in the spine or brain. When I spoke with Dan on the phone before the visit, we had been thinking it could be carpal tunnel syndrome or possibly a compressed nerve in my elbow or neck. Now he didn't think so. I was trying to hold it together and be polite, but inside all I could think was *fuck…fuck…oh my God.* When Dan left after fifteen minutes of listening to Micah make painful small talk, my handsome, but slightly dense, husband said, "Well, don't you feel better?"

I burst into tears. "Didn't you hear what he just said? He thinks there's something wrong with my spine or brain!"

"I never heard him say that," he said.

*Jesus Christ.*

In this day and age, the first thing many people do when they suspect a medical problem is Google it. This is unequivocally a huge mistake, and my Googling the terms "hand weakness" and "hyperreflexia" was no exception. Only a few results came up. Behind curtain number one was multiple sclerosis (MS). Behind curtain number two was Lou Gehrig's disease (ALS), and behind curtain number three was a brain tumor. The one I was most worried about was ALS because it's usually fatal within two to five years from the onset of symptoms. I was terrified and certain that's what I had. The symptoms of a brain tumor are dizziness, nausea, seizures, and headaches, all of which I didn't have, so it was down to ALS or MS…and there I was, rooting for MS. Go MS! Woohoo! What a sad state of affairs when you hope you have MS.

My next step was to see another neurologist. I went to someone local my internist recommended, a very upbeat and positive man. My best friend since 10th grade, Krista, came with me for moral support. The neurologist immediately told me I didn't have ALS. I asked him how he knew that, and he said, "Well, we could spend all day talking about what you don't have, or we can figure out what it is." Well, alrighty then. But because he never told me why he said that, I never fully believed him. He agreed that it could be something in my neck, so he ordered an MRI of my upper spine and brain. I was still breastfeeding my baby girl, who was 15 months old at this point, so we decided not to use the contrast dye they would normally use in the MRI because you can't nurse for 24 to 48 hours afterward. The neurologist said that if something looked suspicious then I could always go back and do it with the dye later.

I had my MRI on May 18th, 2012. That day was nerve-racking to say the least. Leading up to it I was hyper-aware of any change in my hand, and I couldn't keep myself off of the Internet. I prayed it was a pinched nerve in my neck. *Please, God, I have a one-year-old and a six-year-old to raise.*

An MRI is a unique experience. I have had CAT scans before but never an MRI. The big Russian tech asked me if I was claustrophobic, and I said, "Only in small spaces," just to lighten the mood.

I was to have two MRIs, each 30-45 minutes long. Strapped down on a gurney with my head locked in place, I was pushed into the MRI tube. I wore earplugs and headphones to protect my ears from the deafening sound the huge, doughnut-shaped magnetic machine makes. If you've never had an MRI, it sounds like you are in a *Star Wars* movie battle: PING PING PING, BONG BONG BONG, BOOM BOOM BOOM and high-pitched screeching at a decibel that could make you deaf. On top of that it shakes like there is an earthquake.

I got through the first half, which was the spine. Next was the brain scan. Halfway through, the tech came in and pulled me out of the machine. He took off my headphones, but my head was still immobile. He said to me, "We need to use the contrast dye." I told him no, and that my doctor said I did not have to use the dye because I am nursing. My nerves were on end, and I was beginning to get really frustrated with this doofus. He left the room for a moment, and upon his return he abruptly said, "The radiologist says we NEED to use the contrast dye." This is where the panic set in. Instantly, I began to cry. I knew something was very wrong. I was freaking out because my first thought was that I would not be able to nurse my baby for two days. *How could I do that to her?* And then I really freaked the fuck out because I was sure I was dying. Something was wrong with my BRAIN.

This realization sent me into full panic attack mode. I couldn't move the tiniest muscle or they would have to start over. I desperately tried to pull myself together while trying to read the faces of the techs. *What is it? MS? Tumor? ALS?* I was hysterical. They started an IV of contrast dye while the tech made small talk about his kids. Somehow I managed to make it through the rest of the test.

The original plan was to give me the MRI film, and being a Friday afternoon, I would just bring it to my doctor's appointment

Monday morning. While I sat in the waiting room waiting for the film, they called me in and then handed me the telephone.

"Your doctor's on the phone," the man said.

*Oh, my God.*

"You have a mass in your brain," my doctor informed me.

"What?" was all I could say.

"It's a four-centimeter mass."

"How big is that?"

"About two inches."

*Holy shit, that's a golf ball!*

Stunned, I didn't know what else to say or ask. *Think fast.* My doctor told me he was out of town and to bring the film to his office on Monday. The only thing I could think to ask was "Is it in an operable location?" A genius question under the circumstances I think. "Yes" was his answer.

Immediately after walking out of the office, I called Micah, who I knew was about to leave to pick up our six-year-old son, Lucky, from school and was waiting for me to come home to stay with Haven while she napped.

"It's really bad," I told him. "I have a mass in my brain."

I told him I was hurrying to come home but didn't think I'd be there in time. That's how Micah found out. He was basically stunned silent. We had no time to talk or process the information.

As I left the building holding the gigantic film, I couldn't believe I had to deal with waiting in line to prepay my parking. I just wanted to scream to the world, *"Don't you know I have a brain tumor?! Get outta my way!"* But I had to act like a normal person, someone who didn't just receive this horrible news.

I got home in time to give Micah a brief hug in the driveway as he hurried to go get Lucky. I finally got a chance to look at the film, and I was shocked.

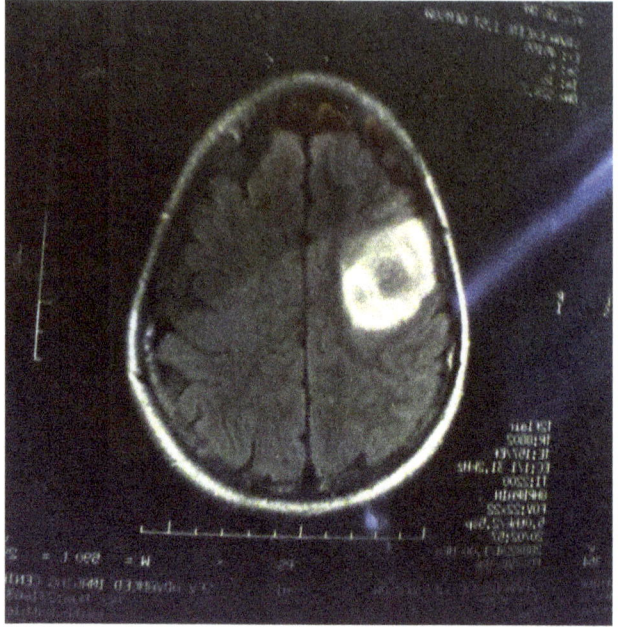

This was my first look at the tumor

The tumor was *huge*.

Micah and I didn't get a chance to talk about it until the kids were asleep. While he was picking up Lucky, I called my parents. They were appropriately shocked and horrified. Since I had very little information myself, there wasn't much to tell them. Why do things like this always happen on a Friday afternoon?

I immediately started Googling brain tumors to find out about all the different kinds. By the end of the evening, I knew what the best kinds were and what were the worst kinds. I hoped and prayed that I had the best kind, a meningioma(benign), but was terrified that it could be a glioblastoma multiforme or GBM, the worst of the worst, terminal in a short period of time, worse than ALS. I didn't think that was possible.

That next Monday, while Micah was at work, I met with the doctor and discussed the situation. By the look of it he thought it was a low-grade glioma (not cancer). Better than a glioblastoma multiforme

(GBM) but not as good as a meningioma. He referred me to a doctor at UCLA because he wasn't equipped to deal with brain tumors.

Thus began the process of interviewing doctors, getting opinions, and making decisions. I was in a state of panic I had never experienced before.

I was willing to do anything anyone suggested, and I did. It's amazing how many people prey on our fears. I was so vulnerable and bought it all, hook, line, and sinker. I also started my blog on Cedars Sinai Hospital's website "CarePages" to keep family and friends informed. Up until then I had been emailing or calling everyone. It gets exhausting trying to repeat the information over and over again, so a blog is a cancer fighter's best friend. Cedars was the hospital where one of the doctors I was to interview worked. I was required to give the blog a name, so I just decided to call it Katie's Brain, straight and to the point. Every time I logged in, it would say, "Welcome to Katie's Brain." I liked that. It had a double meaning, so I kept it.

Here are the exact entries from my blog. Sadly, I've had to leave out all the readers' comments I received because it would make this book over 1,000 pages long, but often it was the comments and support from everyone that got me through each day. A few other things had to be edited out like certain names and song lyrics for legal reasons, but they are easy to find.

Blog one:

## 5/22/12

Hi. As of today I have an appointment with a neurosurgeon at City of Hope National Medical Center in Duarte. I didn't feel like going there, but it is important to my mom that I have a consultation there. Wednesday the 30th I have an appointment with (who will be known as) Dr. X, known for being the best at removing brain tumors, at Cedars Sinai. Right now I have no real news about what kind of tumor it is. Possibly a low-grade glioma or a meningioma. I will keep you posted.

I also made an appointment today with Dr. Linda Liau at UCLA for next Tuesday the 29th. After I get my three opinions, I will decide what I'm going to do.

Xo Katie

# Candidate #1

## 5/23/12

I had my appointment today at City of Hope. I didn't get much hope from that city. The doctor never even smiled. Basically, the surgeon just confirmed what I was already told: it looks like a low-grade glioma. Gliomas are the most common type of brain tumor, and there are different grades—one, two, three, and four—with one and two being the best, and three and four being the most aggressive, malignant tumors. Even a low-grade can be malignant, just not as aggressive. There are subcategories like astrocytoma, etc. The thing about gliomas is that they are considered incurable, even if you remove the whole tumor, which he thought he could. The brain is made up of glial cells, and cancer tends to infiltrate those brain cells, so you can never really get all of it out, and it will eventually come back. How quickly depends on several factors.

So… There are other tumors that I would rather have. I am not happy about having to always worry if it's back. I was hoping to have the surgery and be done with it. He said he would probably do an "awake" surgery on me, to see if I still can move my left side when he touches certain parts of my brain. Uh, no thank you. I heard they only do that for speech anyway, and speech is on the left side of the brain, my tumor is on the right, so this guy has already lost credibility with me. I still have two more opinions to get, but I don't think they will change much, just maybe their approach. After the surgery, it's going to be about doing everything in my power—holistics, nutrition, exercise, supplements, whatever—to make sure this thing doesn't come back. At least not until they have found a cure.

Thank you for all of your messages. They lift me up :)

Xo Katie

## 5/24/12

I just want to say that I have the best friends and family EVER! I can't believe how everybody is rallying to help me in every way possible. I called a friend today because I needed to get out of the house to get my mind off this, so a group of my girlfriends took me to see a movie. It backfired because throughout the movie all I could think of when I saw a character was *You don't have a brain tumor! You are going to live! You have no problems!* I couldn't believe I was watching these people on screen with such stupid complaints when I could have brain cancer and die. Why didn't the world stop? Why wasn't everyone as miserable as I was? I had to walk out of the theater crying. My friends and I all ended up sitting outside, and they gathered around me while I cried hysterically. A friend, Lauren, who had had a benign brain tumor years before told me that there were a lot of things I could do to help myself, and there were things I could do to get super healthy and fight this thing. She told me that she would take me food shopping to use food as medicine. Taking control of my health would help me feel more in control of my situation and not just a passenger on this terrible roller coaster.

I'm starting a "cancer diet" to prevent cancer cells from growing. I'm going to be seeing Chinese herbalists, energy healers, acupuncturists, everything. Lauren is also going to help me get disability and educate me on how to live after going through this. I have friends cooking for me as I speak. My friend Joy got the number for the psychologist who works with Dr. X's patients at Cedars Sinai. My dear friend Renee is researching gliomas on the Johns Hopkins website and found some optimistic news (that it is possible to not have a glioma recur), and I am so grateful for that.

I feel so loved and held right now. I feel like such a lucky girl. Thank you. And to everyone who leaves a message and sends a prayer, I read them every day.

Xo Katie

## 5/25/12

Today I saw a Chinese medicine specialist recommended by a friend. I'm skeptical but also panic-stricken, so I will pretty much do anything at this point. It was a unique experience. After over an hour of "testing" involving lots of snapping his fingers and making clicking sounds, he said he thinks this originated from the fact that I had varicella encephalitis and meningitis at age 13 (caused by chickenpox), and he felt that I had Epstein-Barr virus as well, probably at the same time as chickenpox. This made me vulnerable to tumors/cancer. Who knows? That could be true. He wants to put me on a regimen of herbs, but only after my surgery so as to not interfere with any treatment I may get. The herbs will be to keep the tumor from coming back. In addition, he thinks I should be on a macrobiotic diet for life. Literally. No dairy at all, low animal protein, whole grains only, no white flour or sugar (no fun), very low sugar period. Lots of cooked veggies (especially broccoli and cauliflower), beans, rice, lentils, nuts, avocado, garlic, cranberries, a little fruit, and soy anything although soy is not good for cancers that are estrogen-related like breast, uterine, and ovarian. Also no raw vegetables as he said they are full of bacteria and pesticides and my body doesn't need to be fighting those off right now. It's the anti-cancer diet. Probably a good idea for everyone but hard to do without sufficient motivation. I am VERY motivated. This is my new

normal and I am going to try to convert Micah and the kids too, good luck. Too bad my favorite foods are dairy, sugar, and salad :( Of course.
Xo Katie

## 5/26/12

Today I went to Whole Foods and spent an obscene amount of money on groceries. I'm excited, though. I'm trying to cut out white sugar, carbs, and any and all artificial sweeteners (only plant-based, natural ones like Stevia and Xylitol are okay), as well as switching to a plant-based diet and lots of green juice. Only sprouted grains, whole grains, and lots of nuts, which is how I feel. Right now I am going for quick and easy. I am open to getting recipes, but it seems overwhelming. Cooking is the last thing I want to do. Changing my diet is going to be a huge change for me, a sugar and dairy addict. Ironically, I will truly be healthier than ever with a brain tumor in my head. I have an appointment on Monday with an energy healer. I'm excited about that.
Xo Katie

## 5/27/12

This tumor has no idea who it's dealing with.
Xo Katie

## 5/27/12

Everyone has been asking me what they can do for me or saying, "If you need anything, please don't hesitate to ask." Thank you! Also, many, many people are telling me they have been thinking about me a lot, or even all day. What I would like to ask is that if you are thinking about me, or if you want to do something for me, don't spend time thinking about me with sympathy, sadness, or fear. Don't approach me with a face that says, "Oh my God, you're dying," but think of me as happy and in perfect health.

P.S. Instead of asking, "Do you need anything? What can I do for you?" Just do it. If there is anything I have learned, it's that people who really need help rarely ask for it. What we appreciate is someone who calls and says, "I'm at the grocery store. What do you need?" And don't take no for an answer. My friend Cynthia did that and I really appreciated it. You can send a gift card to a favorite restaurant for Micah and the kids, or send a card that says, "I'm thinking about you."

Xo Katie

### 5/28/12

Today I saw the energy healer. What a bizarre and horrible experience. He said the tumor was caused by the four babies I lost, the sadness, trauma, etc., and get this—he said I have an energy block in my vagina, and, of course, he could clear it for me if I wanted. Oh sure, I guess I have "idiot" stamped on my head in addition to the tumor. I should have called the police. But instead, I gave him a donation! Stupid. I just couldn't wait to run out of there and take a shower. Shame on people who take advantage of someone at their weakest moment.

Xo Katie

## Candidate #2

### 5/29/12

I had my appointment with Dr. Liau at UCLA today. It was a good appointment. She said it did look like a low-grade glioma and then said, "This is my favorite kind of tumor" (woohoo!). That surprised me, but if it does turn out to be low-grade (grade two), then she felt like she could get it out no problem and we'd be done, meaning no radiation or chemo. If it's grade three, then they might do some radiation, but to her trained eye, it has all the characteristics of a grade-two. They will not know until they take it out and biopsy it. She even said it could be low-grade with a few grade-three cells in it, but hopefully not. Not only do they do a biopsy but they run DNA tests on it looking for markers that would indicate what subtype it is; that would give them an idea of how aggressive it is and what the chances are it would come back and how soon.

She also said if you have a brain tumor, then the right frontal lobe is where you want to have it (score!). It seems to be in an area right in front of the motor and sensory function, and the swelling is pushing on that area and causing the issues with my hand. It's kind of shocking that I can have a two-inch tumor in my brain and not even have so much as a headache.

Post-surgery would be one day in intensive care, three to four days in the hospital, and two weeks of lying low at home. She would not need me to be awake during surgery (thank GOD, I knew it!) and that you only need to do that when speech may be affected. (City of No Hope, and no expertise.)

Unfortunately, UCLA isn't contracted with my insurance; they are in a dispute. So this visit is just for her expert opinion. Dang. All in all a good appointment, positive and optimistic. I'm very curious about how it will go with Dr. X at Cedars tomorrow.

Xo Katie

# Candidate #3

## 5/30/12

I had my meeting with the infamous Dr. X today. His office takes up the entire fourth floor of the medical tower at Cedars Sinai. When we walked in, we were immediately greeted by the equivalent of a manservant who quickly rushed us over to the registration window, where Micah and I were met by a very bored-looking woman sitting down who asked for all my IDs and insurance info. As we waited in the hotel-esque waiting room with the requisite fish tanks, I saw a variety of people of all ages and races. I saw a four or five-year-old with half of her head shaved and a huge, obviously fresh, incision. I realized that everyone in that room had a brain tumor. I wanted to grill each and every one of them for information. I was finally called in, and we scurried nervously down a long hallway. As we walked, a very tall, immaculately dressed, handsome Black man in a black suit walked briskly by me, and we locked eyes. What was funny was the entourage of workers hurriedly following him, trying desperately to keep up and in obvious awe and fear.

We waited in an exam room, and a nurse walked in and took my blood pressure, etc., and after a few more minutes, another woman of an obviously higher rank came in and had me do a series of neurological tests that were becoming uncomfortably familiar. They never tell you if you pass the test. She left and we waited some more. My only saving grace is that I never have to change into a flimsy gown.

Despite the freezing cold temperature of the room, my hands were sweating. We waited and we waited. The first nurse came back in and made some kind of excuse, and Micah, with his constant and perfect comedic timing, said, "Does anyone ever tell Dr. X to hurry up, that people are waiting?" She got a look of horror on her face like he had pulled out a gun and said with a nervous giggle, "Oh, no!"

HE finally came in, God-like. Picture a taller, younger Morgan Freeman, only less smiley. He shook our hands and didn't sit or stand but kind of leaned on the exam table. We were sitting in chairs, so he was towering over us, which was obviously a conscious decision. He spoke. He asked me to stand and do some similar neurological tests (walk a straight line, follow his finger with just my eyes, squeeze his fingers). He said my tumor looks like a low-grade glioma, a benign tumor made up of glial cells, brain tissue. He thought it should come out; he thought he could do it but needed to do a functional MRI to be sure. A functional MRI is like a regular MRI except you move different parts of your body, and your brain lights up to show which parts control which movements. It shows him if the tumor is in my pre-motor area (function will come back) or my motor area (permanent paralysis). All of this was explained at lightning speed, and my mind went blank. I couldn't think of a single question. Before we knew it, he was gone and a nurse came back in to schedule the MRI and to set a surgery date. Whoa.

If the tumor is only pushing on the motor area, then I should get full function back after they remove it. If it has infiltrated, then he will want my input as to how aggressive he should be because it will impact my ability to use my left side. He said if I do lose function, I could get it back. It could take weeks or months with rehab, but I would probably not get back 100 percent. So how much to cut is a big decision. A lot depends on this MRI. Obviously, I don't want to be paralyzed on my left side, but of course, I want the entire tumor out.

We did set a surgery date, though, for June 21st, so at least it would be on the books. They will call me to let me know when my MRI appointment is.

Praying now that not only has the tumor shrunk but that it has not infiltrated.

Xo Katie

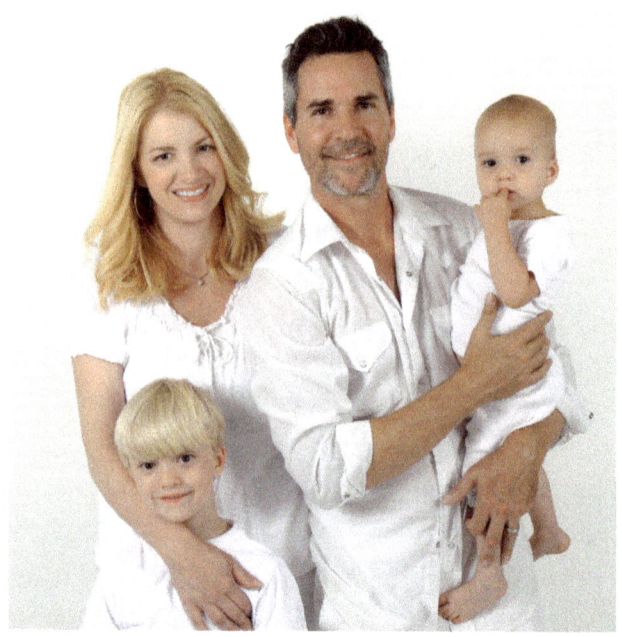

This is a photo we took just a couple of weeks before my surgery. My kids were so little!

## 5/31/12

Micah and Lucky found our old, sweet cat, Turtle, dead this morning. Not so much dead as torn in half and eviscerated in our neighbor's driveway. Not a good way to start the day, but I'm going to think of her as one more angel looking out for us.

Xo Katie

## 5/31/12

The guy who rents a room from my dad and who works as an "herbalist" or "tonic mixer" or whatever at Erewhon health food store came over today. His name is Truth (naturally). My dad wanted me to talk with him because Dad thinks he's a genius and can cure me with alternative treatments. This rumpled, greasy, foul-smelling young man came in and sat at my table for two hours, talking at high speed and furiously scribbling on a yellow legal pad. He said if he was in my position, these are the things he would do. He would definitely not have surgery, chemo, or radiation. He listed all of these tonics I needed to buy and treatments I needed to do, all of which cost thousands of dollars, of course. Granted, he didn't make any money off the stuff, but he swears by them. That's why he looks like he's on death's door.

According to Truth, I need coffee colonics five days a week. I need to drink coconut kefir water, which would give me a ton of gas, but eventually, I would get used to it (one bottle and I was curled up in the fetal position for two days). I need to buy a rebounder, which is a fancy name for a very expensive mini trampoline to help my lymphatic system. I need to spend 300 hours in a magnetic molecular energizer for only $10,000, in Arizona.

The list goes on and on: ionic foot baths, hyperbaric chambers, neurofeedback, special teas, and electro-acuscope ear clip treatments (huh?). A weird drink called Cantron that costs $200 a bottle and is the most disgusting thing I've ever had in my mouth, and that's saying something! It tastes like motor oil mixed with melted pennies. I thought I was being poisoned. In the spirit of camaraderie and support, everyone who came over had to take a sip. That was always good for a laugh. As my friends, twin brothers Warren and Kenny said, the taste just keeps on changing as time goes by, morphing into something even more disgusting!

I did end up buying some of the teas and tonics. I even did the ionic foot bath, which is the biggest bunch of malarkey ever. I met Truth at some hole-in-the-wall vitamin store that has hyperbaric chambers and ionic foot baths. The owner was short, overweight, with greasy hair and bad skin. With my feet in the gross orange water,

I felt like the world's most gullible ass. If they are so health conscious, why do they look so terrible and smell so bad?

Xo Katie

## 6/1/12

This morning around four a.m. I woke up and couldn't fall back to sleep. I started panicking. I walked into my backyard and called the only person I knew who would be awake, my friend Robyn, who lives in New York. When she answered I started bawling about how scared I was and how I didn't want to die and I didn't want to leave my children. I hadn't broken down like that yet. When I got back in bed, Micah spooned me and I heard him softly crying into my neck. That's how I knew it was bad. Micah rarely shows emotions like that. The thought of someone else raising my children, or Micah having to do it alone, is too much for me to bear. I can't believe that God would put me through all that I had to endure to have kids only to take me away from them this soon. I just can't.

I'm trying to get my affairs in order; there's so much to do. I'm overwhelmed. Making lists, instructions, appointments, advance directives, a will, etc. UGH. I don't like having to think about this stuff. I've written for each of my children what I want and hope for them in the future. Even down to the smallest things, like for Haven, "Don't wear too much makeup. Less is more." Things I would hope that I would be able to teach them, but might not be around to. I wrote Micah a private letter for my mom to give him while I'm in surgery, things I want to tell him but never really do. Facing brain surgery is very frightening. I have had to write down instructions about my funeral and what my wishes are, just in case. I hate this.

Xo Katie

### 6/2/12

Hi. I'm down eight pounds, not really a diet I would recommend, but it's doing the trick!
Xo Katie

### 6/3/12

It was a good day with Micah and the kids, making memories.
I'm loving all the food (and green juice) my dear friends are bringing me, made with such love :) I don't know what I would be doing without it, starving for sure!
We went to a birthday party today, and of course, they had the most beautiful cake ever. It was so hard not to eat it! I love birthday cake. I thought I might be spending my birthday in the hospital, but I will be home in time. My functional MRI is tomorrow morning. I won't hear the results until my meeting with Dr. X on Wednesday, but I am nervous anyway. Visualizing the tumor just pushing on the motor area and not infiltrating it.
Xo Katie

### 6/4/12

I had my functional MRI today. I was pretty stressed out and broke down right before I went into the machine. Before this, they went through with me what "tasks" they were going to have me do, like making a fist in and out, blinking my eyes hard, pumping my left foot like I was pushing on a gas pedal, touching my tongue from one side of my mouth to the other, etc. I would wear goggles that would show me their computer screen. And when the screen was green, I was to start doing a particular task. When the screen turned red, I had to stop. This would go on five times for each task. They would also talk to me through earphones, and I had a microphone to talk back.

Sometimes they would type on the computer screen things like "relax now" or "just five more minutes." It was like being inside an un-fun video game. Plus, I had to pee about halfway through it, so that was great. You can't even move to scratch an itch (so, of course, I got very itchy), and in the last 20 minutes, it felt as if something I was resting on was cutting into my head. Plus I had an IV with dye going into my body. All in all a pretty good time.

I have to say, though, that Cedars has its shit together. I didn't even get to read one page of my book, they moved me in so quickly. Also the people there were so nice. But I hate it when the staff looks at me with pity and those sad eyes and say, "Oh, I'm so sorry." It's like they think I'm dying—and I'm NOT! Don't tell me you're sorry; tell me everything's going to be okay. Hospitals need to do sensitivity training.

Xo Katie

## 6/5/12

I think my 71-in-1 superfood blend that I put in my smoothie this morning must have cocaine as one of the 71 ingredients. I've been buzzing all day! Gettin' stuff done!

Xo Katie

## 6/6/12

The appointment today didn't go as well as we had hoped. I feel like I am falling from space and waiting to hit the ground. It feels like the day when I first found out. I am lost right now.

The tumor has infiltrated my premotor area 95 percent (where movement is initiated) and, unfortunately, also my motor area five percent. What this means is that 95 percent of the tumor can be removed, and there is a 95 percent chance that I will lose some function on my left side (arm, hand for sure, maybe leg—20 percent chance, maybe face). The face will probably come back quickly, and the arm and leg, if they are affected, may take weeks or months of physical therapy to get back. I can get back anywhere from 40-90 percent, probably 85-90 percent in the doctor's opinion.

The worst news to me is that the five percent of the tumor that is in the motor area cannot be removed without permanent paralysis on the left side. So part of the tumor will not be removed.

Dr. X was sitting across from me, and he knew this was not the greatest news. He said to me, "So you have a tough decision to make." I said, "No, I don't. I have two kids. It's a no-brainer," and he smiled, finally. I wanted the entire tumor to be out so I wouldn't have to be looking over my shoulder all the time or living in fear. Usually, if they start growing, they change from a low-grade (benign) to a high- grade (malignant). A high-grade glioma, called a glioblastoma multiforme (GBM), is the most aggressive and deadly form of brain tumor.

So to keep this tumor that's left from growing back, they may give me a chemotherapy pill to take for 12-18 months, but that will only keep it at bay for a while, not destroy it. We won't really know what the treatment after surgery will be until they biopsy it. Those results will be back about four days after surgery.

I'm trying right now to hold it together until my kids are asleep because I just want to curl up in a ball and cry. Fucking tumor.

Xo Katie

## 6/7/12

Okay. I cried and cried with my good friend and neighbor, Betsy, last night. Now I'm back. I do believe in miracles, both the kind from God and the kind you make yourself. There is no other option because I will see my children grow up, graduate, and get married. I will hold my grandchildren and spoil them rotten.

Today is Micah's and my anniversary; we have been married for nine years. In that time Micah has been there for me through everything. He has seen me in a hospital bed nine times in nine years. Hmmm...maybe he's bad luck!

Just kidding. Micah is a pillar of support and always has been.

Xo Katie

## 6/9 /12

My friend Amy made me a Little Katie Kick-Ass doll with a superhero cape!

Xo Katie

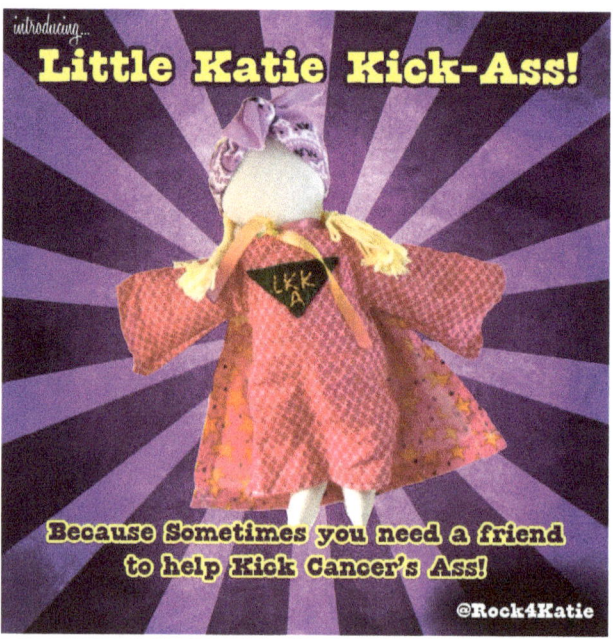

My Little Katie Kick-Ass doll!

## 6/10/12

I had a really nice day at the beach today. Haven's first time and she can already say beach! Naturally, I was busy taking care of everyone else and forgot to put sunblock on myself and got very burned :( My continuing lesson to take better care of myself.

I felt almost normal today. Getting nervous, though, about not having the use of my left arm and hand, even if it's only for weeks or months. I can't imagine how that will feel.

Xo Katie

## 6/11/12

I spent a lovely day dealing with government agencies. An hour at Social Security trying to convince them that I qualify for disability (the form I had to fill out asks, "Could this disability result in your death?" Having to answer "yes" to that was like a slap in the face. Fuck.). Tomorrow is going to be fun. I am surprising Lucky with a trip to Disneyland! Some friends got us tickets so Lucky and I can have some quality time together, just the two of us. I feel like a recipient of the Make-a-Wish Foundation!

Xo Katie

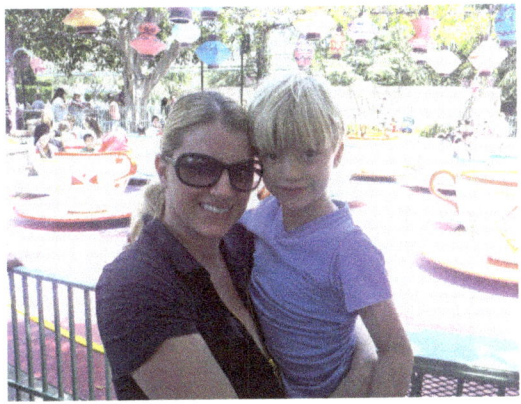

Lucky and I at Disneyland

## 6/13/12

A productive day. I went to Social Security, then went to see my therapist, who I revisit every few years when I'm in crisis. She's the best. I don't have to be strong for her or try to make her feel better about me. She lets me go to "the bad place" where all the fears live, and she doesn't try to talk me out of it. I can get mad at the unfairness of life, be scared, be vulnerable. Then I can come out the other side.

Micah's going out with some dads from school tonight—he has a playdate! He needs it. He's been holding down the fort while I've been out and about all week.

Tomorrow: two doctor's appointments. The first is with Dr. X's nurse to go over pre- and post-surgery instructions and to get the antibacterial shampoo to use the day before surgery, and then an appointment with the internist in Dr. X's practice to make sure I'm fit for surgery. I guess I hope he says yes :)
Xo Katie

## 6/14/12

An exhausting day full of blood tests, EKGs, chest X-rays, etc. So I am sitting in my little paper gown with my friend Joy, who drove me, and in walks the internist, who looks about 80 years old with a bad, black, comb-over toupee. Since he works with Dr. X's team, I assume he knows why I am there. He also appears to be carrying a chart about me. He comes in, sits down, and lets out a huge sigh. Joy and I look at each other and stifle a giggle. Again, I assume he is sighing because he knows the gravity of the situation. He says, "So, why are you here?" Huh? Joy and I almost burst out laughing at this point. I say, "I have a brain tumor." He looks at my chart and says, "So it's on your left frontal lobe?" Okay, I'm quickly losing faith in this idiot. How old *is* he? "No, it's on my right." He does his series of non-tests and asks if I need some anxiety medication. Yes, please. He prescribed some Xanax and let me go to get my chest X-ray. A strange day.

Xo Katie

## 6/15/12

A couple of things I found out yesterday at my pre-op appointment at Dr. X's office: I am having surgery at 7:15 Thursday morning, and I may be home on Saturday! That's nuts. I stayed in the hospital longer after I gave birth to Lucky. It should be a four-hour surgery, and I will eventually end up in a room in the north tower at Cedars.

Xo Katie

## 6/18/12

I'm going to tell Lucky today about my surgery. He doesn't know anything yet, and I have been dreading this day.

It has been a hard couple of weeks for him. He found his cat dead, he's leaving kindergarten and already missing it and his teacher so much that he cried about it the other night, and the other day we released a butterfly that we raised from a chrysalis, and I told him to make a wish as we let it go, and he said, "I hope you survive," just as a bird swooped down and ate that butterfly right out of the sky. WTF? This morning he asked me if I knew anybody besides people in our family who had died. UGH.

He has such a big heart and feels things very deeply. I am worried about him most of all. I can't wait until this week is over.

Xo Katie

## 6/18/12 Later...

It went really well. I took him into the backyard and I asked him to help me pull some weeds. Then I asked him what would happen if we didn't pull the weeds out, and just as I hoped, he said, "They would just keep growing bigger." I said that's right and that I had something in my body that's like a weed in our garden, and the doctor is going to take it out. I told him it was in my head, and he said, "They're going to cut your head open?" I said yes, and laughed at the absurdity of it! I told him I would be in the hospital for two to three days and that his grandparents were coming to stay and help out.

He seemed okay with everything, so I told him more about the fact that I would have a bandage on my head and about how the tumor is affecting my hand and that it might be worse after the surgery but that my brain would heal, and it would get better. He said, "Yeah, your brain will grow back, but the bad cells won't," and I said yes, but it might take some time.

I asked him if he had any questions and he said no, so I dropped it. I think he handled it really well. I know that more emotion will come later, but for now, things are as good as they can be. Saying goodbye on Thursday morning will be another story, especially for me.

Xo Katie

## 6/19/12

I'm feeling nervous about the two unknowns I am facing: what function will I have when I wake up from surgery, and what will the biopsy show? The thought of waking up and having my arm, hand, and maybe leg paralyzed, even temporarily, gives me a panicky feeling.

Also, my fears about this being a higher-grade tumor are coming to the surface.

Xo Katie

## 6/20/12

My MRI was scheduled for 6:00 p.m. tonight. I was so upset because it meant I couldn't put my kids to bed for the last time before my surgery. To make matters worse, I don't know how this happened, but my mother-in-law, bless her heart, put Haven down for her nap. I was really looking forward to that since I couldn't put her to bed. I didn't want to make her feel bad, but I burst into tears. I felt bad for making her feel bad, but I was devastated. All day I called the hospital and was finally able to move my MRI appointment today from 6:00 p.m. to 2:15 p.m., so I get to put my kids to bed tonight! I'm so happy. The morning will be hard, but at least I can put them to bed.

Xo Katie

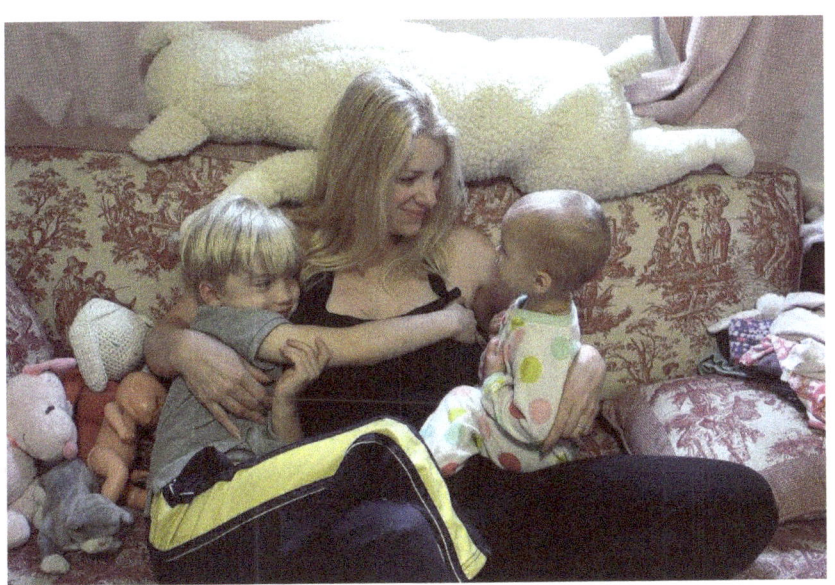

Cuddling before bed the night before surgery

## 6/21/12

Micah will be posting here as soon as surgery is finished. Stay tuned…

Xo Katie

*Welcome To* KATIE'S BRAIN

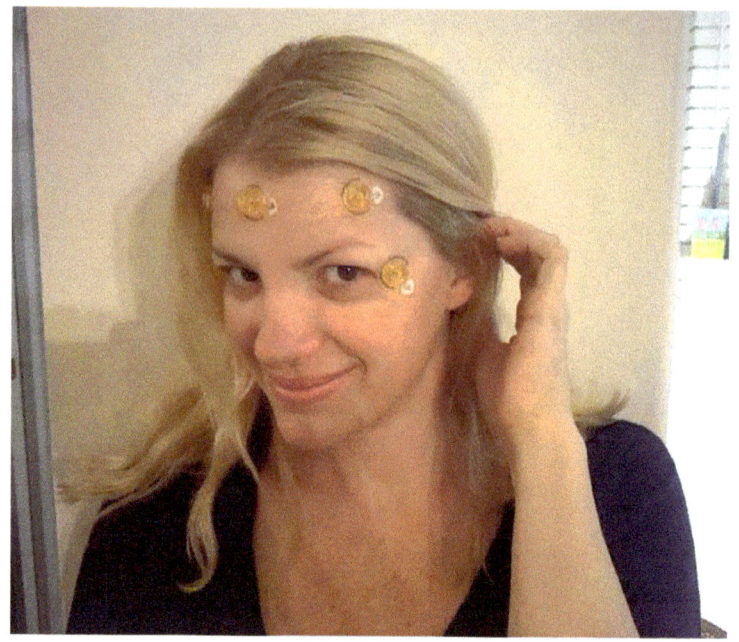

Brain mapping—done

## 6/21/12

Hello, everyone. Dr. X just came out two hours early to tell us that the tumor is 100 percent in the motor area of her brain and that he did not want to remove any of it. He did take a biopsy, and the pathology report will be back next Wednesday.

Originally, he told us that he would be able to remove 95 percent of it since he thought only five percent was in her motor. He told us to never let anyone touch this tumor. We are devastated.

Katie is in recovery now and will be awake in a few hours, and Dr. X and I will tell her the news.

For now please hold all visits for today, and I'm sure Katie will reach out to you all soon. Please keep the positive prayers flowing.

Love to all,
Micah

KATIE KAISER SMITH

## 6/21/12

Hi everyone,

Katie is lucid and fine and has some mobility in all of her limbs, hands, etc. She knows everything and has personally spoken to Dr. X. There is so much to tell and so many details that she will share when she is in her room tomorrow and out of intensive care. Thanks for all of the love and support. Have a nice evening and most likely after 9:00 a.m. to 10:00 a.m. I will have a room number for everyone, and we will have a new update after we see Dr. X in the morning.

Love to all.

Micah

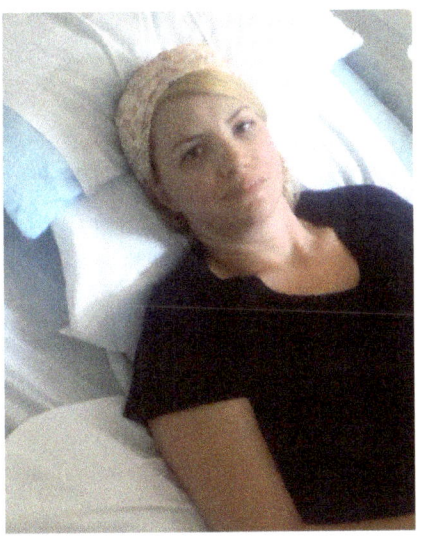

The morning after surgery

## 6/22/12

Hey guys, Katie is fine and recovering in intensive care.

We are waiting for her hospital room to become available, and they will move her there today. If all goes well, she comes home this

Saturday! She will update this page ASAP after she meets with a few more docs. Love and thanks to everyone.

Micah

## 6/22/12

So this was unexpected. One more bump in the road as I type one-handed. I awoke from surgery without the use of my left hand and still with a brain tumor.

To say we were disappointed, even devastated, would be an understatement. I have about a six-inch gash on my head and nothing to show for it.

During the surgery, they were using electrodes to stimulate different parts of my body when I started having seizures, four of them in total. So surgery was stopped. And it was discovered that the whole tumor was in my motor area. Inoperable. I met with my neuro-oncologist today. He came into my room smiling and said, "Everything's going to be great!" That was amazing. He said he is pretty sure, and the preliminary pathology reports show as well, that it is a grade-two glioma. That means it's non-aggressive, not yet cancer. Yay! We will know more by Wednesday when the final report comes in. At that time all the oncologists, neurosurgeons, and pathologists will meet to discuss my case. He thinks this has been growing for at least 10 years! He says the likely protocol will be a high-dose chemo pill to shrink the tumor. If they can shrink it, or just keep it from growing, then I just have to wait a year or two for technologies that are right around the corner. He told my dad he thought my prognosis was "very good," so don't count me out yet! Very loopy and tired from the seizure medication; must go to sleep now!

Xo Katie

## 6/23/12

I got a decent night's sleep last night, only woken by nurses four times to take my vitals, give me meds (anti-seizure, steroids), check my blood sugar, etc. The great news is I get to go home today, and I woke up to find my hand had improved some. It's true what they say about sleep being restorative. Thanks to everyone who came to visit and who sent flowers and posted messages. I can't wait to go see my babies. Cedars has been very nice to me. A lot of kind, caring people work here. I'm looking forward to enjoying our summer and getting on with living while the experts find a way to get me out of this jam. The "tumor board" meets on Wednesday, and I will see them Wednesday or Thursday to hear their plan. Not nervous about that at all :)

Xo Katie

## 6/23/12

My theme song today is "**Celebrate Me Home**" **by Kenny Loggins.** I'm just waiting for physical therapy to come to visit me to set up some home visits, then I'm outta here. I got on Skype with my kids this morning. Haven kept saying "up" like I could pick her up :(

Xo Katie

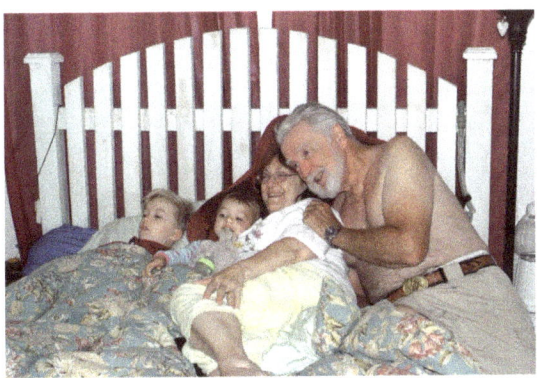

The grandparents home with the kids

## 6/23/12

I'm home, but not feeling so great. I am having a pity party and you're all invited. Here is my list of grievances in no particular order: my left hand is virtually useless, and also one giant bruise from wrist to palm from the restraints that held me down during the seizures. Both arms are covered in bruises as well as my left earlobe (what's up with that?), I have small scabs around my head from the halo that was screwed into my skull, my scalp hurts and itches, I have a six-inch incision, and I feel like Frankenstein. I have a cough and sore throat from the intubation. They had given me so many seizure drugs during surgery that after they took the breathing tube out, I wouldn't wake up, so they had to put the tube back in. I finally woke up with the tube still in, and as I was revived from the anesthesia, I felt like I was choking and drowning, and I tried desperately to pull it out. I was restrained by my dad and Micah (I didn't know it was them at the time), and I couldn't talk to tell them that I couldn't breathe. I thought I was dying and I started vomiting and gagging and panicking (my mom said she was yelling at them to take it out). I must have inhaled something because I have a bad cough as well as post-traumatic stress disorder. That was traumatizing. Then I got the great news that they didn't get out any of the tumor and that I had four seizures during surgery.

Now I am on steroids for brain swelling and anti-seizure medication that makes me feel like a zombie. I can barely keep my eyes open. I am not supposed to lift more than five pounds, which means no holding my baby, and I'm not allowed to bend forward or wash my disgusting, sticky hair. At least my drooping eye and slurred speech are better. Other than all this crap, I feel fucking great! Sorry for being a downer. I just had to vent because I'm feeling pretty sad right about now.

Xo Katie

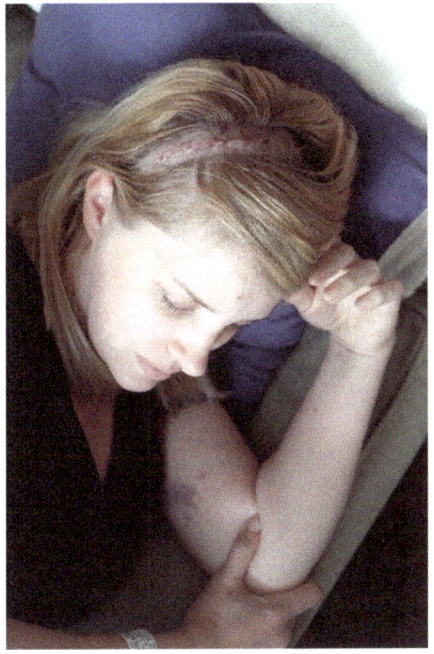

Home, battered and bruised.

## 6/24/12

It's been a rough morning. I don't really know what to expect from all of this. I woke up feeling very depressed, not much like myself. I have been crying most of the morning, and while I was eating some breakfast, my left hand started tingling, then felt dead, and then the feeling started creeping up my arm. Seems I was having a seizure. Very scary. I didn't know when it would stop or how far it would travel. I called Dr. X's assistant and she confirmed that that's probably what it was. We realized my anti-seizure medication dosage was incorrect so we increased it.

I also found out that the seizure meds, as well as the steroid, can make me depressed, irritable, and angry. Good to know! I'm definitely not feeling like myself. I'm going to try to shower now; I'm feeling gross.

Xo Katie

## 6/25/12

So, here it is. My parents, Micah, and I went to Dr. X's office today to get the results of the biopsy. The pathology report shows that it is mostly a grade-two, but it does have some grade-three cells in it. Cancer. I was in shock and my parents cried. The actual report states, "Barely meets the criteria for anaplastic astrocytoma (grade-three glioma)." But because they were only able to biopsy it and not remove it, that means they can only test that bit they took out. So, in essence, the cells they found in the biopsy that are grade-three could have been the only ones, and now they're out, or there could still be more. Because we can't know for sure, we have to treat it as if it's all grade-three, which means radiation and chemotherapy.

So...brain cancer, a very daunting diagnosis, one of the worst, but not the worst it could be. The good news is twofold: it appears to still be mostly grade-two, and also I have a particular genetic marker called IDH1 mutation that means it is less aggressive and slower growing than if I didn't have that marker. Good news. We'll take it!

Chemo and radiation will start in a couple of weeks. Radiation is for six weeks, five days a week, with weekends off. First I need to be fitted with a special headpiece for the treatment, and they will give me a couple of weeks more to recover from surgery.

Chemo will start at the same time in the form of a pill I take at home. I will probably lose my hair at the radiation spot, but it will eventually grow back, maybe a little thinner. Chemo can make you nauseous, but they give you meds for that. Chemo will be for at least one year. Chemo and radiation may shrink the tumor as much as 20 percent, but the main goal is for no progression, no growth, and for me to be feeling good.

Dr. X and the oncologist were both optimistic about long-term survival. When I asked Dr. X about the effects of chemo on me, he said, "Are you planning on having any more children?" I thought that was so funny. Hey, Doc, have you looked at my chart? Besides the fact that I will be 43 next week, I have BRAIN CANCER. I think I'm done having kids. I thought that was a strangely optimistic question, though! It made me happy that he thought having more kids was even something to consider. I'm going to hold onto that.

There is some relief in that there are no more unknowns. The cat's out of the bag, and now we press on with full attack mode. I have to hold off on some of my supplements, like antioxidants and fish oils, because they actually make the radiation less effective, but other than that it's about maintaining the diet, exercise, and visualization to heal myself. Dr. X says attitude and support systems are everything, and I have the best of both I think.

Xo Katie

## 6/26/12

I had so much love and care yesterday. Lots of people were at my house, including my rehab guy and the psychologist from Dr. X's office. Unfortunately, I am not good at slowing down and resting because I want to hang out with my friends and chit chat, hang with my kids, and clean the house. All in all, it was too, too much because around 7:30 I had a mini seizure. I first started to feel my left hand tingle and then it went dead; it then crept up my arm and face, and even my tongue went numb. I was really scared and Micah was outside greeting my friend and nighttime caregiver, so no one heard me calling for help. Because it wasn't full-blown and I wasn't convulsing, I tried hard to calm myself, but it is next to impossible. The fear grips me and takes hold for a long time afterward.

Finally, I heard Micah and Krista come in and called them for help. I had already taken my seizure meds 30 minutes before, so the only thing to do was to take some anti-anxiety meds. We called my doctor and just let them know what was happening. Then it finally stopped. The hardest part for me is the fear that it will start again or become a full seizure. I was scared and shaking for a while after.

Xo Katie

## 6/27/12

I'm at Sherman Oaks Hospital for the night. I had a big seizure about 1:00 p.m. and called an ambulance. Very scary. I will fill you in more later.

Xo Katie

## 6/28/12

I've been outta touch. It has been a nightmarish 24 hours. OMG. Yesterday we had some visitors, and as they were leaving, Micah walked them out and I lay down to take a nap. I was in the house alone. Out of nowhere, my head jerked to the left, and because I was on my left side, my face went directly into my pillow. I couldn't move or call for help. I was paralyzed, yet my left side was convulsing. I could feel my throat, face, and tongue convulsing. I was desperately trying to get air through the pillow and I was hyperventilating. My thoughts went to, *What can I kick off this bed to make a loud noise?* and *My family is going to find me dead in my bed.* After about two minutes, I realized I could move my right arm, and I reached over and pushed the pillow down away from my mouth and nose. I was still having trouble breathing when I heard Micah in the kitchen. I made a guttural sound when I called his name, and he came running. I will never forget the look on his face when he saw me; it was sheer horror and panic. I could only imagine what he saw. By this time it seemed like it was starting to wind down and I mumbled, "Call 911."

After 911 was called, Micah called Dr. X's office. He got his assistant on the phone. Micah was simultaneously talking to the paramedics, who were now in my bedroom, and Dr. X's assistant. She was adamant that this was normal and that I did not need to go to the hospital, while the paramedics were saying, "She could have a blood clot; she could've had a stroke. You need to let us take her." When one paramedic said, "Man, if this was my wife, I'd take her to the hospital," that was all Micah needed to hear and off I went.

Of course they took me to the closest, crappiest hospital around, but my mom stayed with me. The worst part was saying goodbye to Lucky as the ambulance took me away. My mom stayed with me at the hospital. and I had another seizure at 3:00 a.m. that woke me from a dream. Luckily, I was able to kick the foot of my bed with my right foot and wake my mom up. There was nothing for anybody to do really except make sure I could breathe. My mom screamed at the nurses who were just standing there watching me, yelling, "Do something!" It was like a scene out of *Terms of Endearment*. The seizure lasted about three to five minutes, mostly on my left side, hand, arm, and face with the stiffness and out-of-control movements in my hand and arm, and lots of facial contortions and twitching. It's not pretty. Micah said later that he never wants to see me like that again. I looked terrified and stuff was coming out of my mouth. As I write this I realize that words fall short. There are no words to adequately describe how any of this felt for me.

We saw a seizure specialist today at Cedars via Dr. X. He says my brain is irritated, angry, healing, and got moved around and prodded with electrodes. There is probably swelling as well. It needs to heal and there is a chance these will stop, but I may continue to have seizures and have to remain on medication indefinitely. But for now, it's about getting the dosage of meds right and high enough without turning me into a zombie. I am already zombie-like because these drugs are new to me, so he hopes I will get used to the sleepiness. The seizures leave me tired, weak, and even affect my voice. My left hand is useless for hours afterward.

My anxiety level is through the roof, and I'm having small panic attacks for fear of having a seizure. They are incredibly scary; I can't possibly describe accurately how terrifying it is to be paralyzed, have trouble breathing, and not be able to speak, convulsing violently. Of everything I've been through, this is the worst by far. I'm in hell. This is worse than cancer.

In addition, the seizure meds and steroids for swelling can make me depressed, irritable, and angry, but really I only feel depressed, scared, and weepy. I can't control it. I just burst into tears. It's terrible.

When we returned home from the doctor, I went into the backyard to hang out with the kids. I sat down on the grass, and Haven came over and accidentally hit me on the head with a stick right on my incision. I had about one second to say, "I'm having a seizure." I instantly went into a full-blown seizure in front of both kids and Micah's parents, Jerry and RoseMarie. Grandma got the kids inside and Grandpa and Micah held me. This one was the longest yet, probably because it was caused by an injury, and my brain was saying, "What the hell are you doing to me?" It was awful. My incision was bleeding. I decided from now on I have to stay in bed out of harm's way and just take care of myself and heal. Now whenever Haven comes near me, I am hyper-conscious of where she is, and I protect my head at all times. Right now I can't be left alone, and I feel like the grandparents and Micah are exhausted. We need help. Maybe it just means coming over and watching TV with me or watching me sleep. We'll figure it out. Micah wants me to say he's sorry if he hasn't gotten back to you; it's been a crazy 24 hours. Thank you for all the messages, food, flowers, and love.

Xo Katie

## 6/29/12

I got to fulfill a dream today by taking Haven to her first parent/tot class at our Waldorf school. Yay!

I truly have the best husband in the world. I cannot believe how he has stepped up and how wonderful he is at taking care of me and the kids. It has been a complete role reversal to the extreme. He is organized, thinking three steps ahead all the time, loving, gentle, and nurturing, and he bathes me and has washed my hair. He holds my hand while I fall asleep. As hard as it is for me to ask for help, it's even harder to turn it away, so I'm sorry to have to do that. I know everyone wants to help in any way; we just need to keep it quiet around here for a few days. I cannot express enough what all of your support means to me.

Xo Katie

## 6/30/12

What day is it?

Oh yeah, Saturday. I tried to nap but couldn't really (I have a fear of falling asleep now because of the seizures, and I won't lie on my left side because I don't want to be smothered again). The cons of doing all my research are that there is so much conflicting advice and so many alternative treatments that there is the fear of making the wrong decision that will cost me my life. For example, since I am going to start radiation, which works by oxidizing tumor cells, I am not supposed to take antioxidant supplements anymore. No more green teas, berries, vitamins, or anything which could make the radiation less effective. Since you can only do radiation on a tumor once, it is essential that it works. So, since there is so much hype about antioxidants being amazing cancer fighters, I am scared and confused about whether or not to stop taking them.

Infrared saunas? Bovine colostrum? Grounding? Alkaline water? Rebounding? Should I travel to Peru or Brazil or Canada to seek out healers who have "cured" incurable cancers? Visualization? Guided imagery? Hypnosis?

I'm overwhelmed.

I just had to stop writing because I had another "mini" seizure, where the left side of my body and face go completely numb. It's scary but not a full seizure. I feel it's my brain healing from the biopsy because it seems to be getting better.

Just hoping and thinking that my brain is still healing and these will disappear soon too.

I had a complete freak-out meltdown last night. These drugs make me crazy and depressed, and I lost it because the kids came home in need of baths, hungry and tired, and I gave Haven a bath, and she was so grumpy, and I felt like I couldn't care for her or Lucky in the way that I want. I got very stressed and felt like I might do something crazy or like my head might just fly off or explode. It's the scariest feeling in the world to be so out of control of my mind. I couldn't even be in the same room with anyone or have anyone talk to me. I couldn't answer a simple question. I wanted to run out into the middle of the street or rip someone's head off. I desperately called for my neighbor Betsy, and she came and I clung to her and cried for an hour. Then we went and sat outside. I haven't been outside in days; it felt so good. By the end of the night, we were laughing. Thanks to Betsy and Klonopin, I had a good night's sleep.

From now until my birthday on Wednesday, I am placing a moratorium on research and just focusing on things that bring me joy in my life.

Xo Katie

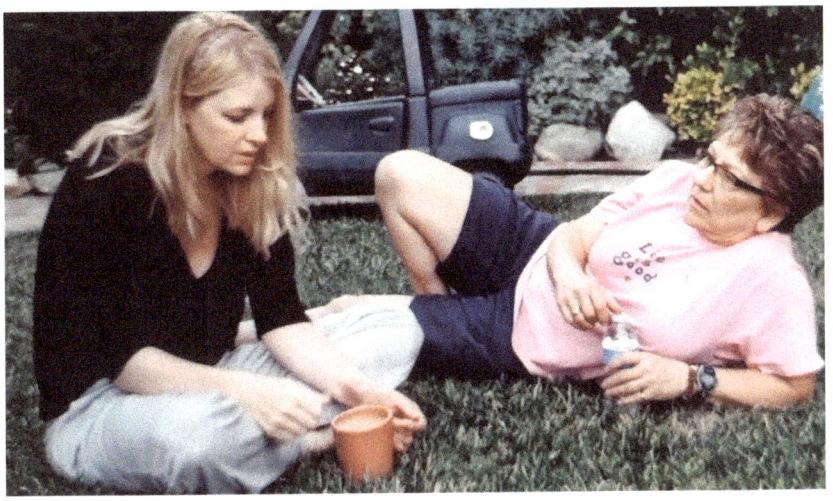

Betsy and I hanging out in my backyard

### 7/1/12

I had a nice day today. I got lots of rest, had a long nap, and even went through the mail and paid some bills. It actually felt great to do something "normal." I did a little gardening with Haven, being careful not to get whacked in the head, and she enjoyed hanging out with me and gave me a rare unsolicited kiss, pure heaven. These meds do mess with me, though. My taste buds are off, and I am still dizzy and unstable on my feet. My voice is better (it was messed up badly from the intubation, times two) but not completely. It's 10 p.m. and just now I had another mini episode. I wish these would stop!

Xo Katie

### 7/2/12

I'm doing pretty good today. I went for a short walk around the neighborhood with Micah, my mom, and Haven. It felt good. I got a full body massage last night from my mom with coconut oil (miracle stuff), and it felt amazing. I can't describe how much I need to be touched in a way that's not painful. That's not something people think about. Every time a cancer patient gets touched, it's to do something that causes pain. It's nice having my mom take care of me and it's nice bonding again together. I decided I'm going to break my diet for my birthday. I deserve it.

I did a little research on the meds I'm taking and their side effects. It's probably not a good sign when your seizure medication can cause suicidal thoughts. Oh, and itching. The itching alone will make you want to kill yourself!

Xo Katie

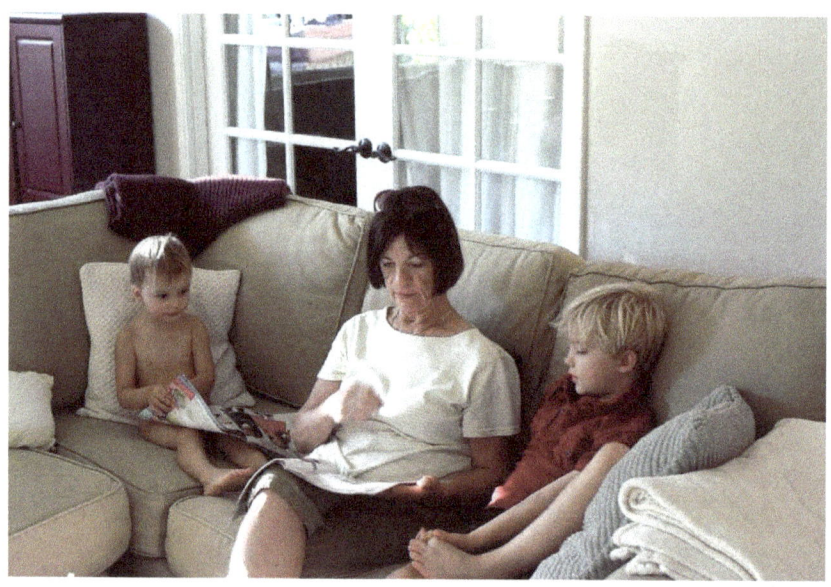

My mom reading to the kids while I sleep

## 7/3/12

I had a lovely day. I have to say I have been obsessed with food for the last two days! I suspect the steroids are increasing my appetite, plus just healing and feeling better.

It's funny, I thought that being diagnosed with cancer would make me feel like I was part of a "club." When I got married I became part of the "Married Persons Club," the same as having a child. Then I even became a member of the "Second Child Club." You just enter a different level. But truthfully I don't feel like a member of the cancer club, can't even really relate. There is definitely happiness that comes from hearing survivor stories because I relate more to the fighters, but I just don't feel sick. Apart from the effects of the surgery itself, I can't fathom that there is anything wrong with me.

There are only a handful of things I can think of that are worse or elicit more terror than inoperable brain cancer, but for some reason, I'm not freaking out. My perspective on life has changed. I don't worry about stupid stuff. I enjoy simple pleasures and am soaking up so much love. I am starting to actually enjoy being taken care of. My whole life has been spent caring for others, even as a child, so it's a relief to surrender to being held, loved, and cared for.

Don't get me wrong, there have been some REALLY bad moments; there has been a lot of fear and uncertainty; seeing worry, fear, and pain in my family's faces. I have a fear of not being around to see my children grow up, but I only let those feelings come in very briefly and then I push them away. Maybe I'm delusional, but I think I've got this :) My vision is me with Micah and the kids 10 years from now frolicking on the beach in Hawaii with all of us in perfect health.

Xo Katie

## 7/3/12

To top off my early birthday, I got my dream meal from The Smoke House and am still enjoying it, pacing myself so my stomach doesn't rebel!

Thanks to everyone for the cards, gifts, flowers, and food made with love.

P.S. Happy Birthday to all my July "Cancer" sign friends, a cancer group I'm proud to be a part of!

Xo Katie

## 7/4/12

Thank you to everyone for all of the wonderful birthday wishes. It's been a good day so far, lots of indulgence on my part! In honor of Independence Day, the theme song of the day is **"I'm Free" by the Soup Dragons,** an upbeat song about being free to do and be anything you want.

A nap is in my near future and then off to Pasadena to hang out with friends and see fireworks with Micah and Lucky while the grandparents stay with Haven.

Xo Katie

## 7/6/12

I realized that I used to say a prayer of gratitude every night that went "Dear God, thank you for keeping me and my family happy and healthy, safe and well." I haven't said it since I was diagnosed. I think I have lost faith. Clearly, it didn't work, so why bother?

It's been two weeks since surgery. This might be a long post because I'm overdue and I need to vent.

It's been a crazy two days, lots of activity and very little rest. I had a fun time watching fireworks and hanging out with friends. I was anxious to be out at first but was finally able to relax and enjoy myself.

I absolutely HAVE to get off this medication—it makes me crazy. I'm loopy, drugged, irritable, anxious, depressed, and tired. Today Micah and I went to Cedars to meet with my neuro-oncologist,

Dr. Hu. (My regular doctor is on paternity leave.) His name is pronounced "who," and his first name is Jethro. Jethro Hu is a big guy who looks like he is constantly stoned. He is always kind of smiling and has bloodshot eyes but doesn't say much. Because of the drugs, being out in public made me feel as if I was in a David Lynch movie or maybe dropping into the land of Oz. Everyone looks weird, and it feels like everyone is looking at me. Music sounds strange… It's like a bad acid trip in slow motion. Dr. Hu said when I am seizure-free for two weeks (the mini episodes count as seizures), we can try reducing my Keppra a bit, then watch and wait to see if I can remain seizure-free. The radiation I am going to start in a couple of weeks can cause swelling and irritation, which could possibly cause seizures, so we will have to take it slow on getting off the meds. I start the chemo the night before radiation, both for six weeks, and then I get about three or four weeks off from the chemo, do an MRI, then do chemo again.

I got a fairly definitive list of what he thinks is okay, what he wants me to avoid, and a couple of things he was unsure about. I asked him about juicing raw cannabis because I read it's good for tumors, and he said it was fine. He even did one better and said that in one lab study, medicinal marijuana was shown to SHRINK GLIOMAS! Of course, Micah asked him if this "study" was done in his dorm room!

So I got the green light to smoke up, plus he said it will help with nausea from chemo and works as an anti-anxiety medicine. I have been taking anti-anxiety meds every night. Why? Why didn't we hear about this before? Because they can't prove it shrinks tumors in people, only in a lab, but if it can't hurt and can even possibly help, then I should know about it. I also had read about things like melatonin being good for tumors and Viagra helping chemo work better. He said melatonin is fine, and Viagra has been shown to help chemo bypass the blood-brain barrier better and work more effectively. I said I want it! Again, why do I have to ask for these things? Thankfully I did my research, but what if I didn't? Should I ask if smoking rubber tires or eating gravel will help my tumor too? Jesus. I'm currently enjoying the last of my birthday sugar, a Napoleon pastry that Micah got me. It's so yummy, but I'm back on the wagon tomorrow.

I think Haven has a cold :( It's really the last thing we need. Hopefully, all of this clean, healthy eating will keep the rest of us healthy!

Xo Katie

## 7/7/12

It was a weird night. I decided to smoke a little before bed, courtesy of my neighbor, but I think I overdid it. It's not my first rodeo for sure, but it's been a long time. My brain went bonkers. I think it was 50 percent pot-induced crazy and 50 percent psychosomatic. I imagined I was having seizures and that I could feel the numbness and tingling in my hand and arm constantly. I felt like I was having an hour-long panic attack. As I lay in bed trying to calm myself down (practicing my visualization of breathing in white light and sunshine through the top of my head and breathing out any negative, useless energy), debating whether or not to wake up Micah, I decided that if I woke him and told him I was freaking out, then it would actually make it real when I knew I could make it stop if I really focused. I also hadn't taken my anti-anxiety med but decided to not take it on top of everything else. There were certain points where I had to remind myself to breathe. Basically, I just got really, really stoned. Not a feeling I like, but hopefully I can build up a tolerance and start slower. There is actually a lot of info on Google about marijuana and gliomas, so I want to make it work.

I think I have underestimated the power of fear and how strongly it can affect a person. I definitely feel it creep over me and wrap itself around me at times. It's weird because a lot of small things don't bother me anymore, but I am also feeling just how precarious life can be. Sometimes I get jealous of people who have only small problems; other times I think I would never want to go back to worrying about small

problems, and I feel relief from that. I'm in such a strange limbo right now. It's hard to imagine a time when I won't be afraid, when this thing won't consume my whole life, but I look forward to those days.
Xo Katie

## 7/8/12

Not a very productive day, although I hung out with Haven a lot. She was feeling better, so that's nice. I woke up this morning dreaming about the stupid tumor.

Yesterday too, so now I promised Betsy I wouldn't do any research after dinnertime to give myself a break and hopefully dream of happier things. I was planning on getting a mani/pedi today with my mother-in-law (RoseMarie aka Grandma Sippi), but I was having anxiety issues this morning so I took some meds and slept through my appointment.

I am still in awe of the massive amounts of continued support from family, friends, and my former clients (I was a child behavior specialist/consultant), who have become friends. You lift me up and warm my cockles! Oh, I plan on getting an MRI to find out exactly where my cockles are really soon!
Xo Katie

## 7/12/12

I had a good day considering most of it was spent at Cedars Sinai. Today was the first morning since my surgery that I got up with my kids and got Haven out of bed, and I made breakfast!

We left early to go to two doctor's appointments. The first one was for my radiologist to learn about my radiation treatment. I felt a little emotional and overwhelmed going into the "Cancer Center," which is all the way down in the basement. I got off the elevator and told Micah, "I don't belong here." It was so surreal. I just don't feel like I have cancer. I don't feel sick. What a nightmare.

The doctor was very nice, as are all the doctors at Cedars. Next Monday we go back for a simulation. They fit me with a special mesh mask and headpiece to keep my head stable. I will probably start radiation the following week. The side effects are that I will most likely lose a big chunk of hair in the area of the tumor. It will basically be burned off. He said it will "probably" grow back. Also, most people feel very tired, especially toward the end of the six weeks. The good news is they only irradiate the tumor and an area around it, not my whole brain, so I shouldn't suffer any lingering side effects like memory loss, etc.

The goal of radiation is to kill the tumor, which is different than having it disappear. It may shrink some, but really because the tumor is part of my brain, it doesn't just go away. What they hope for is to kill it and stop any cells from reproducing. This process can cause some swelling (which can look like growth on an MRI), but then they follow up a few weeks later, and he said they are pretty good at differentiating between swelling and growth. The combination of the radiation and the Temodar chemo pill is the gold standard of treatment for what I have.

He was optimistic about my prognosis and said if he had a grade-three glioma, he'd want the kind I have. Cool.

He also made me feel better because I have been lamenting the fact that they couldn't surgically remove the tumor, which was such a huge blow. The whole idea of it going from operable to inoperable changed everything. He said that it is actually more important with the grade-fours, and that's when surgery can have the biggest impact on survival. But for a grade-three, surgery wouldn't have changed the outcome that drastically. It would have only slightly improved the situation. So that made me feel a bit better.

He also said I could continue taking most of my supplements (yay!) and that it shouldn't counteract the radiation. Just no vitamin D or E supplements, but I can continue with my mushrooms, garlic, soy, turmeric, seaweed, and pot! He said, "Have fun."

Next we headed over to the oncologist, Jethro Hu, to talk about chemo. Just a light, lackadaisical day in the life of Katie and Micah. More discussion about side effects (nausea, constipation, low blood counts, and the ever so rare leukemia). I got all my prescriptions for Temodar (chemo), Zofran (nausea) and Viagra! He also decided to taper me off these steroids, thank God, so by next week I should be steroid free. Then he wants to wean me off the anti-anxiety meds I'm taking every day, and then we can talk about decreasing my anti-seizure meds.

It's a little scary because we are just starting to calm down and not be so nervous about seizures and leaving me unattended for short periods of time. Once we start changing the meds, we have to be careful again. The radiation could potentially cause seizures, and that scares me a lot.

Xo Katie

## 7/13/12

Today's theme song is **"Summer Rain" by Paul Kelly.** I just walked outside and hung out in my backyard, swung on a swing while being rained on during this beautiful weather. I was imagining being in Hawaii.

Today was a busy day, as usual, but I pushed myself too hard because I felt pretty good; then I felt bad tonight.

Last night was the first time that Micah and I had been alone in our house with the kids since pre-surgery. What a strange feeling. It feels good and scary at the same time. I wish I could live without fear. When I felt bad tonight and got scared, I had to send Lucky, my six-year-old, outside to the garage to get his dad to help me. I hate having to scare him like that.

I find myself getting so overwhelmed by my daily schedule, juggling the kids, their caregivers, my caregivers, doctor's appointments, and the day-to-day of paying bills, ordering supplies, talking to pharmacies, dealing with the disability office, etc. that I keep forgetting things. I had an appointment today, and I had it written down in three places and even discussed it with Micah, and I still forgot about it. Most of the time I'm not even sure what day it is.

Xo Katie

## 7/14/12

I had a more relaxing day today. I've gotta make a conscious effort to not do too much, even though I feel like I can, because when I rest I feel better. I've been sleeping well, smoking a little before bed, and taking the melatonin (20 milligrams), good for helping the chemo. I'm getting a huge calendar dry erase board tomorrow, so hopefully I can get my life organized. I found a part-time sitter a couple of days a week for Haven, which will be great; I feel like she needs some consistency. Her little world has been as nuts as mine.

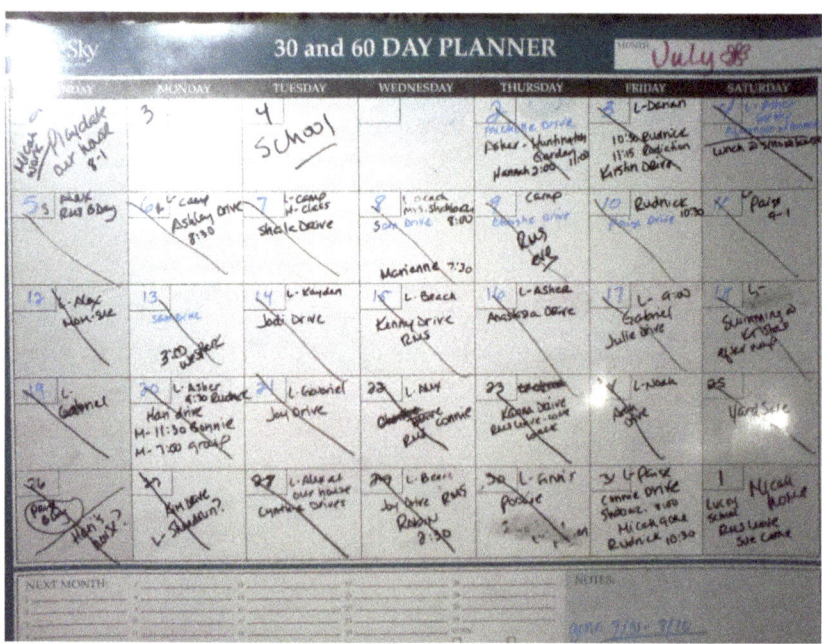

Our busy days

Haven has developed this amazing, hysterical laugh, and she sounds as crazy as I feel. It's this deep, guttural laugh, and it is delicious. It's very hard right now for me to not give in to my urge to completely spoil my kids. I just want them to be happy all the time.

Sometimes I wish I had known about the tumor years ago so that it would have been smaller and they could have removed it, but then I think that had I known I might have decided not to have Haven, knowing there was a chance I wouldn't be there to raise her. Ultimately I am glad I didn't know because we, as a family, are complete with her in our lives. Lucky said to me recently, "Mom, thank you for making Haven alive." How can you beat that? Perfection. Everything for a reason, right?

Xo Katie

## 7/15/12

I had a nice day, took a walk around the neighborhood with Micah and Haven; it's amazing how totally wiped out I get. I came home and took a long nap, then quickly got ready to take Haven to a friend's daughter's first birthday party. Even though we were very late, it was nice to get out and do normal things. I did have another *Terms of Endearment* moment, though. I knew a lot of people there would know my situation, and it reminded me of the scene in the movie when the best friend takes Debra Winger to a party, and everybody knows about (whisper) "the cancer." Also everybody tells me how great I look and how happy they are that I came and best wishes, making a point to touch me repeatedly—one last touch before I die.

I don't blame anyone. However, it's super important to me that people don't think of me or treat me as if I have one foot in the grave. Don't we all? As Betsy says, "Ain't none of us getting outta here alive." When people look at me like they're scared for me, then I get scared. Cut it out. I love ya, but cut it out.

I got my chemo drugs in the mail today, and all I can say is thank

God for insurance. Something like $8,000 for 45 days. Luckily I only had to pay my $500 deductible.

The hospital bill for my surgery came to $185,000. You just have to laugh. Especially after I hit the pipe :)

Xo Katie

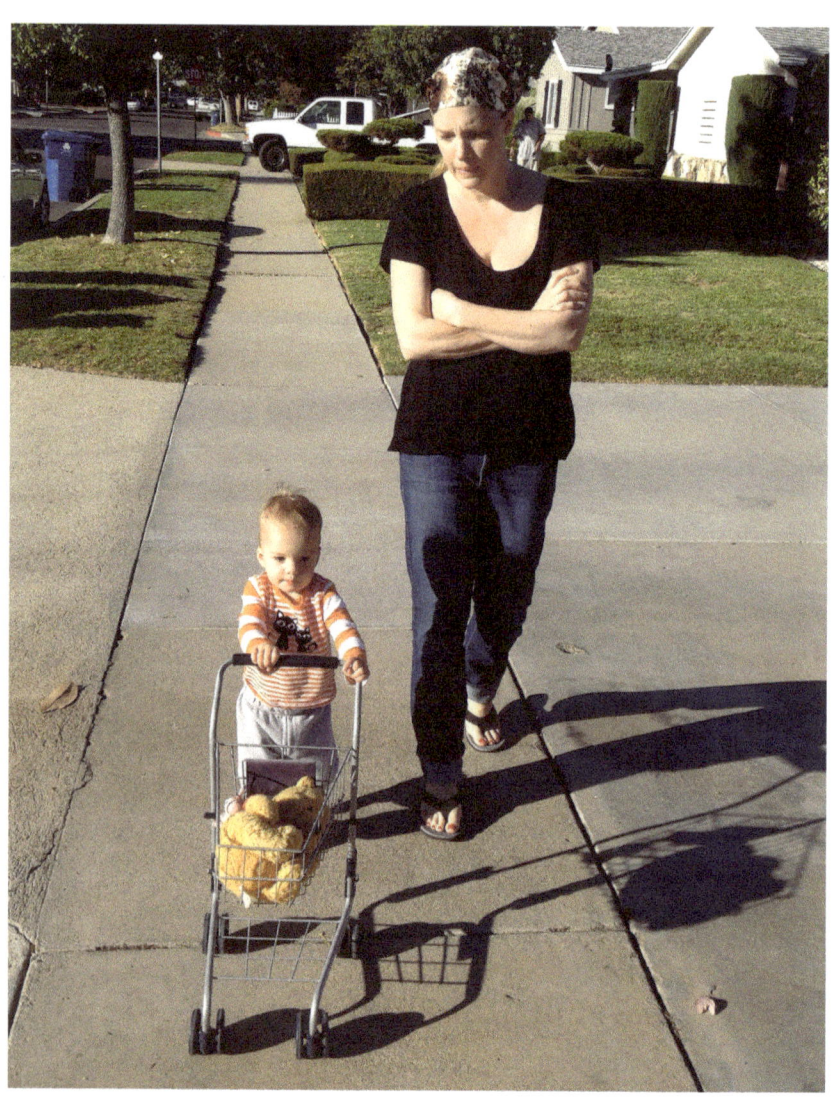

Walking with my girl

## 7/16/12

Feeling grateful today. I feel like I'm coming out of the fog a bit. I even felt inspired to take a brisk nighttime walk with my hubby around the neighborhood. It felt great. A friend gave me a book called *The Magic*. It's about gratitude, as well as a journal to write down things I am grateful for every day. I think I would rather write them here and share them with all of you and maybe inspire you to be grateful as well.

Today I am grateful for feeling good, for spending time with my kids, for being able to sing Haven to sleep, for friends bringing delicious food and helping organize my house and my life, for family helping me with the kids, and the joy on my kids' faces when they see their grandparents. I'm grateful that Micah is rubbing my back while I write this, that my housekeepers are coming tomorrow, that I get to go to the doctor tomorrow and start the process of my recovery, that I have choices and options, and that I have hope and joy in my life. I am grateful to friends and to strangers who are becoming friends. I am grateful for people's generosity and the human spirit.

I am thankful that I can still feel thankful.

Xo Katie

## 7/16/12

Radiation simulation today, whatever that means. I'll keep you posted.

Xo Katie

## 7/16/12

Something about being here at the Cancer Center is just so upsetting and surreal to me.
Xo Katie

## 7/16/12

I made it through my simulation. Basically they soak this rubbery mask that reminds me of those squishy rubber drawer liners or under rug mats that are full of holes. They heat it up in hot water and then while I lie on the CAT scan table, they come over and put it over my whole face, head and shoulders. It's squashed against my face with just the little holes to breathe and see through; you can't even open your eyes fully because your eyelashes touch the mask. They shape it to your face, tape it to your head, snap it to the table, and make marks on it. Then they took photos of me and I joked, "Are these for your Facebook page?" But I do get to keep the mask at the end and use it for wall art. My 30 treatments start Monday. It would be terrible if everyone there wasn't so freaking nice! You really are treated like royalty; it's surprisingly not depressing at all. They have bowls of fruit everywhere, all kinds of coffee, hot chocolate, tea, refrigerators full of snacks and sandwiches, and parking is even free valet! Plus everyone is so friendly, and I rarely have to wait more than five minutes. Today I am grateful for the healing to begin in such a nice environment. Grateful that I got to spend some quality time with my dad, who drove me, grateful for friends who visited, healthy chocolate pudding and sweet potatoes from Julia, a good nap, and amazing grandparents for my kids.
Xo Katie

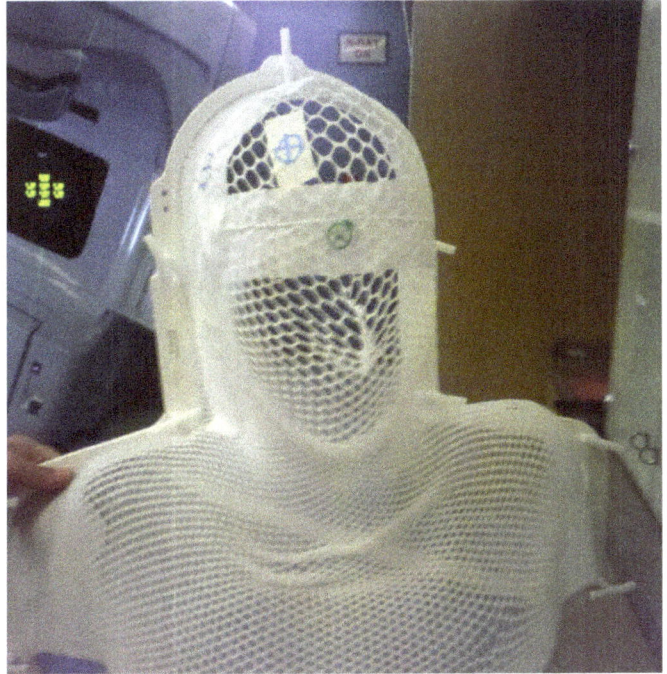

Radiation mask. X marks the spot.

## 7/17/12

Good evening. I got busy tonight and almost forgot to post! I have been reading my 100 page packet of info from a "cancer nutritionist" my oncologist referred me to. She specializes in brain tumors and has sent me a TON of info on diet and supplements meant to keep tumors from growing and what to take/eat to complement my chemo and radiation and what to avoid. It's pretty intense and detailed. She also recommends some blood tests because there are things that indicate whether or not I am at risk for tumor growth such as thyroid function. Ironically, low thyroid function is better for brain tumors than a thyroid that is functioning well. Who knew? I'll need to see what my levels are, and if they are not low enough, I'll need to make sure I avoid things that stimulate the thyroid, like iodine, which means no iodized salt, sea vegetables, seaweed, etc. That's just one example; there are tons more. My head is spinning.

The good news is today was my last day of steroids. Happy to be on one less medication, especially one that alters my mood and makes me crave carbs and sweets and makes my skin break out. UGH. My wonderful in-laws have offered to buy me the Cadillac of blenders—the Vitamix! Yay! We are taking a field trip to Costco tomorrow to see the roadshow demonstration in person! Now that my mom got me the Breville juicer and I will have a Vitamix, there will be no stopping me! I'm thankful. Just going into a store will be fun too, even if it is Costco!

Xo Katie

## 7/18/12

A day full of ups and downs, highs and low, lows. I'm going to choose to concentrate on the highs and focus on what I am thankful for. I spent the morning at Costco watching the amazing Vitamix at work! I'm so incredibly inspired and excited to start cooking. Up until now cooking has been the last thing I wanted to think about, but now I am getting excited. I made Lucky a spur-of-the-moment sorbet! I spent a portion of the day trying to get my Viagra prescription covered by my insurance, but it didn't work. They won't cover it for me because it's experimental in its use with chemo. Without insurance it's $700 a month. My chemo will be for at least 12-18 months. This is unacceptable, so I am turning to Canadian pharmacies. I can get it for $95 for a 40 day supply. Unbelievable.

I hope the radiation shrinks this tumor, because my hand seems to be getting a little worse which makes typing really frustrating. I keep hitting the caps lock with my left hand by accident, and then I have to erase everything I just wrote. I am still trying to use it, but I'm tending to use my right hand to type more. I am officially off the steroids, yay! Getting a little nervous about starting the chemo pill Sunday night and radiation on Monday. I've read that it's important to visualize chemo helping and curing as opposed to thinking of it as poison in your system, so that's what I'm going to try to focus on.

I'm hoping for an even better day tomorrow.

Xo Katie

## 7/19/12

I'm SO tired today! I think I have been staying up too late, and Haven has been teething and waking up at 5:15. Even with a nap I was exhausted. I had a headache too, so I am wondering if going off the steroid is causing me some withdrawals. My left hand seems to be getting worse also. I'm struggling with it today. I get very frustrated when I can't do something simple. I'm excited to see what wonderful changes come on Sunday with the chemo. Do I sound bitter? It's hard when you already feel bad, knowing that it will probably only be getting worse. It's been a long, tiring week for Micah and me.

Okay, enough of the pity party.

I've gotten a few things accomplished today. I had some blood work done that my nutritionist requested; hopefully, this will give her an even clearer picture of what is happening with me and what I need to do to fight this SOB. I've got one week's worth of levitra(generic for Viagra)for over $100, but even better, I got a prescription to fax to the Canadian pharmacy; done.

I made some homemade almond milk in my Vitamix! Yum.

I am reading more and more about how cancer is becoming more of a chronic illness like diabetes that has to be managed, not "cured." Realistically, many types of cancer come back. That's why changing your lifestyle and diet and doing alternative treatments are so important. It's becoming less and less important to remove tumors and more important to keep them dormant, stable, and unchanged. The whole idea of a five-year "remission" is a false sense of security. Again, it's hard to imagine living with this long term, not ever feeling "cured" and free from worry, but I also think the fear of recurrence or progression will help to keep me on the straight and very narrow path of ultimate health.

Xo Katie

## 7/20/12

I'm having a hard day. So tired, and Micah and I trying to manage the kids by ourselves in my present state is proving to be very difficult. Even though I haven't had a seizure in a while, I am afraid to be left alone with the children. I'm afraid to be left alone, period, but especially with the kids. In the last couple of days, it's been necessary and it was okay, but once I start radiation, they said it could trigger a seizure, so we will have to be on guard again. Still my biggest complaint is how tired and drugged I feel all the time. Most days just don't allow for me to sleep as much as I feel like I could. BTW, to take the chemo pill I'm supposed to wash my hands, put on rubber gloves, take the pill out of the bottle, wash my hands again, then eat it! Nothing to worry about there! Yikes! I will take Viagra an hour before the chemo.

Xo Katie

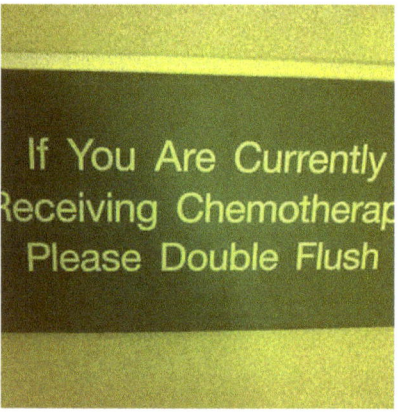

Cancer and cooties?

## 7/21/12

So, of course I had to do some research on my symptoms of late, and it is definitely related to going off the steroid. Extreme exhaustion (some people said they slept 20 hours a day), mood swings, rage, dizziness, headaches, swelling, numbness, joint pain, weakness in arms and legs, and psychosis. Just to name a few. Once again I feel I was not prepared appropriately by my doctors. The only thing they warned me about was a possible headache. I have been crying all day wondering what the hell is wrong with me? Why can't I keep my eyes open, why does my hand seem worse, why am I so moody? Jeez, the brain tumor I barely noticed; it's the treatment and "care" that make me feel like I'm dying.

I am at least relieved to know that this will hopefully pass, probably just in time for the nausea to kick in :)

Thanks for all the support. On the brighter side, I had a date with my husband for dinner while my friend Paige babysat. I was so tired and grumpy that I canceled once, then decided to try to rally, and I did. It felt good to get out.

Xo Katie

## 7/22/12

Started out like it might be a bad day, but ended up being pretty good. Had lunch with a friend I haven't seen in a very long time, and it was so good to reconnect again. I'm so happy that my situation helps people realize what is really important in their lives. That's what she shared with me. Then I was escorted to Whole Foods by my personal chauffeur, Betsy, and it was great to get out and shop for myself. We had a lot of fun. I haven't been to a grocery store for over a month! I found maple syrup made with xylitol! That made me so happy. It's the little things. I'm going to make pancakes with spelt flour and use my xylitol syrup.

Drinking my disgusting fermented wheat germ and watching a funny movie. So tired again, but feeling better today; maybe I'm on the upswing.

Xo Katie

## Later…

Starting chemo tonight and radiation tomorrow. Freaking out a bit. Still having headaches, weakness, and tiredness from steroid withdrawal. How will I feel tomorrow?

Xo Katie

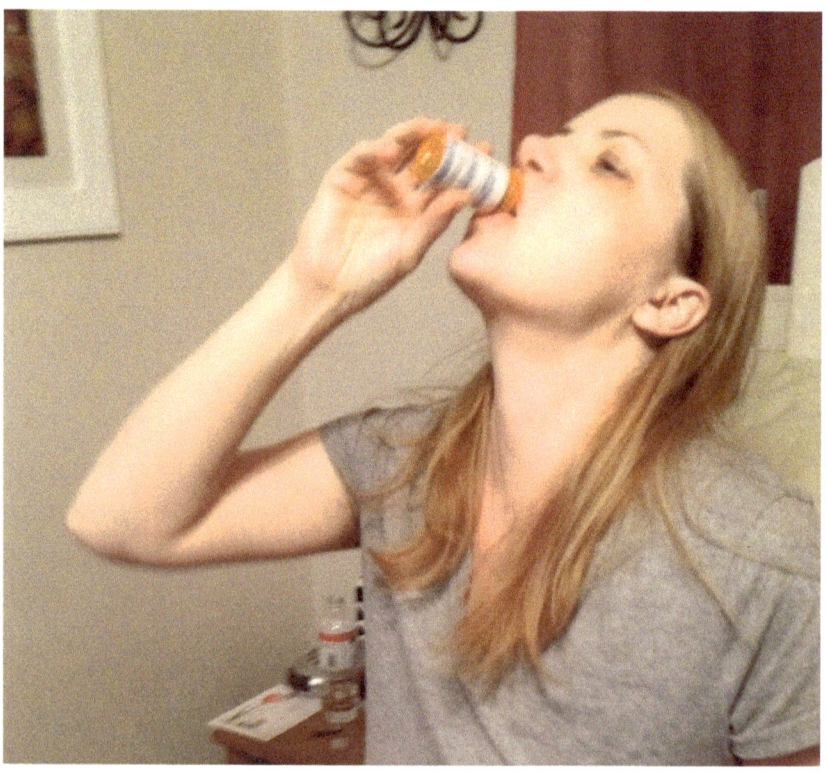

Taking the chemo straight from the bottle so it doesn't touch my skin

### 7/23/12

Woke up this morning feeling okay except for a throbbing headache, most likely still due to the steroid. Glad I didn't wake up nauseous. Had a fun time last night seeing *Magic Mike* with good friends! Nice escape from reality. Will check in later.
Xo Katie

### 7/24/12

Hi. So chemo went okay last night, no side effects or nausea so far. Had my first radiation today, very easy and quick.
Xo Katie

### 7/25/12

Fourth day of chemo/radiation. Things seem to be okay so far. The Viagra seems to be giving me some nasty, throbbing headaches that are waking me in the night, though. I am not going to take it tonight and see if I get a headache. So far I haven't had any nausea, so I am grateful for that. The radiation is pretty easy so far; they say my hair will start falling out around week three, and the fatigue will be cumulative and get worse as the weeks go on. It takes about two weeks after radiation ends to start feeling better. So far it's fast and relatively easy. Starting the serious search for a nanny now. It's inevitable that family and friends get burned out, and I really am going to need the help as the fatigue gets unbearable.

I'm grateful to reconnect with friends I've been out of touch with and enjoying spending time with them and all my friends. Thinking about my friend Dana today who I think is having a baby! Hoping I can visit her and baby tomorrow at Cedars!

I have an appointment with my oncologist tomorrow before

radiation. I haven't seen this one since surgery and I really liked him, but it's so confusing because he has yet another opinion about what supplements I should take or avoid. I will get my blood test results that the nutritionist recommended tomorrow. Hopefully I can get her advice soon and be done with it. So tired of the mixed messages. Have to post this ASAP cuz I'm getting texted by (you know who you are, Shadi) that I haven't updated everyone today in a timely manner! Cut me some slack! You know I love you!

Xo Katie

## 7/26/12

Today I woke up with no headache, thanks to the fact that I didn't take Viagra. This creates a dilemma because I want to take it. I met with my oncologist today, the one who was on paternity leave, Doctor Rudnick, before my radiation. I really like him. He wants to keep me on the seizure meds until radiation is over but wants me off the heavy-duty anti-anxiety med. That's been a hard one for me because I have a ton of anxiety, especially regarding the seizures.

He asked me to explain to him what happened, and just telling him the story of my first seizure and how I was alone, with my face smashed into my pillow, unable to breathe or make any sound had me crying in his office. I said I felt like I had post-traumatic stress disorder, and he said I do. He said, "It's as if you're walking around the house expecting that someone will come up behind you and start choking you at any minute." I said, "Exactly." My mind plays tricks on me, making me think that I am about to have a seizure when I'm not. I have panic attacks that come out of nowhere. Usually I can talk myself out of them but they are scary. I never knew that people could have seizures while being fully conscious. Lucky me.

In order to get me off the anti-anxiety pill, he wants to put me on an antidepressant, which would take care of my PTSD, panic attacks, and weepiness, without the highs and lows of the anti-anxiety med.

He thinks once radiation is over and I am feeling better, I can get off all of it. We won't be so nervous about the radiation causing a seizure, and hopefully I can start to relax.

I'm still having withdrawal issues from the steroid Decadron. Now I have bad pain in my legs and a rash on my arm. My left hand continues to not function well at all. Typing this is torture. So many mistakes, and I'm dropping things like crazy. It's really frustrating and scary; it's like I had a stroke or something. Hopefully it's just rebound swelling that will pass. Dr. Rudnick basically left the decision about taking Viagra up to me. I am going to hold off for another day and then try half a dose and see if I get a headache. I have to weigh the pros and cons.

I seem to be tolerating the chemo pretty well so far. I'm grateful for my doctors and my friends.

Xo Katie

## 7/27/12

Having radiation every weekday gives new meaning to the phrase TGIF! I can't believe this is my life for the next five weeks. But one down! My head is starting to itch a lot and it's sore.

I have a decision to make about my hair. Confession time: I'm not a natural blonde. I used to be, a long time ago. Now I have my roots coming in as well as a seven-inch strip of hair that is dark and standing straight up. Do I just leave it all and say to hell with it since I have to wear hats anyway to protect my head from the sun? Or should I dye all my hair darker? It's expected that I may have multiple bald spots from the radiation from where the beams go in and then exit. So factor that in too. Good times.

I'm not too happy with the new antidepressant. I felt worse yesterday on it then I have felt not being on it. I am now having heart

palpitations, trouble sleeping, nausea, and MORE anxiety. WTF? I called the doctor this morning and started crying when I was talking to the nurse. I said, "I cannot handle anything that's going to make me feel worse than I already feel, even if in two weeks it will make me feel better! I just can't do it." I will probably stop it for now. I will see him next Friday and discuss it. A person can only take so much, seriously. On my list of things I'm grateful for: Good friends driving me to treatment, having lunch out, a weekend to spend with the kids, yummy (really) green juice every morning, and good health!
Xo Katie

## 7/29/12

I had some ambitious plans for today but only got about 30 percent done. I took a bath, washed my hair, took a walk, napped, took Lucky out for lunch, then had a home visit from Lucky's new first grade teacher, Kathy. That was nice. I like her very much. That's about it. Going through emails, mail, and returning calls takes up a lot of time. I feel pretty good today. I have a stiff neck, which is giving me a headache, but otherwise okay. I'm so frustrated with my hand. I'm not using it to type anymore; it's not worth having to go back and correct all the mistakes. I really hope that this is caused by swelling and irritation from the radiation. I want to get my function back. You don't realize how much you need both hands to do almost everything. Try opening a jar or even a tube of toothpaste, or putting your hair in a ponytail, with one hand tied behind your back. My head is getting pretty itchy and sore too.

P.S. Many of you are suggesting that I shave my head, but I am not supposed to lose all of my hair, just a patch or two where the radiation beam enters and exits. They say some people don't lose their hair at all. The chemo I'm on is not the kind that makes your hair fall out. I am leaning toward dyeing my hair brown for a while. Can't do the blonde with brown roots. Yuck.

I'm thankful today for being able to go out to lunch with Lucky. I'm thankful he has a lovely new teacher, thankful that Haven has only one more tooth to break through until her two-year molars!

Xo Katie

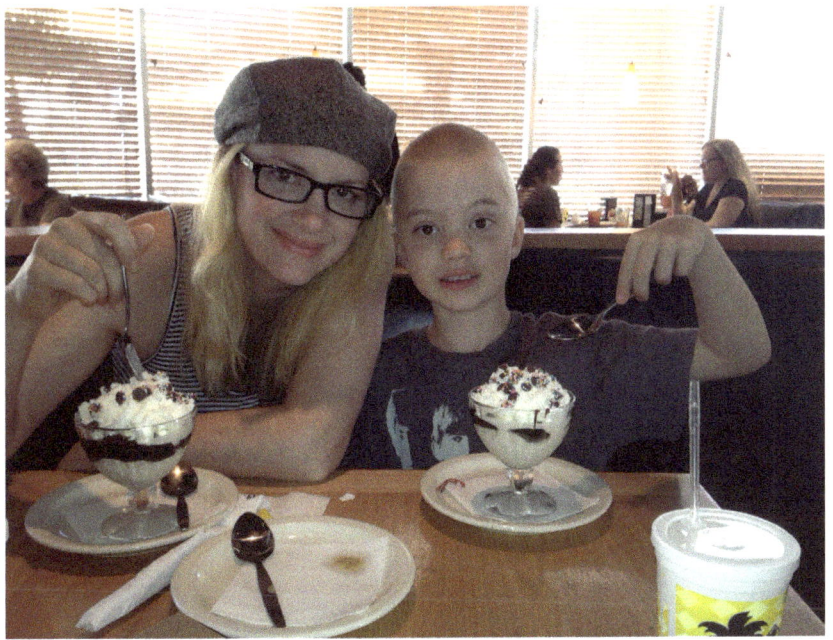

Lunch and sundaes with my boy.

## 7/30/12

I had a nice day, very busy. Up at 5:30 with Haven, damn that tooth! I let Micah sleep in out of the kindness of my heart. I interviewed a nice nanny who got the full Haven experience. I took a long nap, and then my mom took me shopping. This weekend was sort of like a mini vacation. A mini vacation where you still work all day :) I do look forward to spending time with friends I never get to see.

Big news, I didn't take any anti-anxiety medication today! I figure if I'm not going to take the antidepressant, I'll just have to get off the anxiety meds myself. I managed to stay calm today; I actually started feeling anxious around 7:00 tonight so I just took a lightweight anxiety pill, and only half, not the big guns I've been taking every day. I'm proud of myself. Maybe I can beat this anxiety with sheer willpower. I dumped the therapist from Dr. X's office; she wasn't helping at all and she was very expensive. I'm going to see my longtime therapist, who I love, this week.

Between her and my neighbor Betsy, I should be good. Too bad I had to explain to the nanny, Hannah, that I can break out crying at a moment's notice, as I started crying. Oh well.

Xo Katie

## 7/31/12

This morning started off rough, tensions were high, but the day went well after that. Cancer is hard on marriages. It's like navigating a whole new relationship. Sadly, I am no longer the person Micah married. I am depressed, anxious, moody, and handicapped. I got my hair colored brown. I always think of myself as a blonde, but I think this is for the best for now, low maintenance.

I talked with a 12-year survivor of the same kind of tumor as mine. It's so inspiring to talk to long-term survivors. Every situation is unique, but it helps to talk with someone who knows exactly how I'm feeling. I thought of joining a support group, but there are too many depressing stories out there. I know because I've talked to a bunch of brain tumor people, and they aren't all fighters; some people choose to do very little to save themselves. I also didn't want to join a group where there was the chance that someone might not show up one week because they had died. I need to surround myself with positivity and like-minded people.

I had a 1.5-hour phone consultation with my brain tumor

nutritionist. It was very helpful. I'm going over my list of supplements and additional supplements she suggested that would complement my treatments and what to avoid. I feel like I have a clearer picture of what I need to do.

Xo Katie

## 8/1/12

I waited way too long to post, and now I'm too tired and stoned to write much. I was able to go to Haven's class today. I had a great day. Feeling pretty good, weaning off the Klonopin (the anti-anxiety med), chemo is treating me well, but radiation makes my head sore and itchy.

Xo Katie

## 8/2/12

I had a good day, radiation, then a nice lunch—BLT with tempeh bacon. Who knew? But it was delicious! I traded in my nap today for therapy so it was hard getting through the afternoon. My head is getting really sore; it's hard to imagine how it will feel a few weeks from now. You know how when you get a bad sunburn and it itches, and then you scratch but you forget it's a burn and there is that immediate "oh shit" moment right before the excruciating pain? It's like that. The more I touch it, the more it itches too.

I Just spent two hours going over my new supplement list from the nutritionist. Still not sure if I will take all 20 of them. I'm so nervous about them affecting my radiation and chemo. Tough decisions. I wish all my practitioners could agree on something.

30 more minutes and I can take my chemo and go to bed. Sweet dreams.

Xo Katie

## 8/3/12

Not a good morning, that's all I'll say. One of those days that makes me want to run away from home. I am using something for my head. The doctor recommended argan oil; it helps some.
Xo Katie

## 8/3/12

Yes, I am posting twice today, you lucky people! My day did turn around, as soon as I got picked up by a friend and left my house! She made the comment that at least radiation gets me out of the house! Quite a silver lining :) I think I have made the decision, after even more research on my part, to take the antioxidant supplements. There is just not enough evidence that it affects radiation in a negative way, and there is more evidence that it can actually help it work better and definitely helps with side effects. I have to trust my judgment at some point and believe that God led me to the nutritionist for a reason.
Xo Katie

## 8/4/12

Good morning. I had a major meltdown last night. There are days when I just can't take it anymore, and by "it" I mean all my worst fears, anxiety, and stressors. Life goes on and in some ways that's not always a good thing. Bills still have to be paid, taxes still have to be done, the house still needs to be cleaned, and kids still need you all day long. There are times when I just want to scream, "I can't deal with this right now! Don't you know I have brain cancer? Do you have any idea what I'm going through? No, you don't, and you can't possibly." If one more person tells me that we could all walk out the door and get hit by a car, I'll punch them. It's not the same thing! What if someone told you that you would **definitely** get hit by a car and die—you just don't know when. Then you might have an idea what I'm feeling. It's all just too much.

UGH.

I'm struggling a lot with the fact that I can barely use my left hand. It's VERY frustrating. Trying to teach Micah how to clip a tiny piece of cuticle off my right hand (which he couldn't do, but he tried) and I almost burst into tears because I am angry and frustrated! I saw my oncologist yesterday, and he told me that he thought I could get the full function of my hand back, and I did burst into tears. That was such a relief. He thought that in a few weeks when the radiation has shrunk my tumor (which he said can actually take up to six months to see the full effects), then I can work with a physical therapist. He said I shouldn't avoid using it, that the brain can make new pathways, and I should practice the tasks that are difficult for me. So I am trying to type now using both hands.

He also told me that the genetic marker I have (IDH1), which makes my tumor less aggressive, is more of a predictor of prognosis than getting the whole tumor out with surgery.

Xo Katie

## 8/6/12

It's official, my hair is falling out. It's very depressing. It is, don't tell me it's not.

No matter how prepared you are, you are never really prepared. On the brighter side my hand feels minutely better, I think; it could be wishful thinking. We'll see. I'm bummed about my hair. I already have a sideways mohawk. I'm going to be a freak.

Xo Katie

## 8/7/12

This whole hair thing has been harder on me than I thought it would be. I knew it was going to happen, but I just thought, *So what? It's not important in the big scheme of things. I just want to live.* But it's still shocking. When Haven touches my hair so gently and comes away with ten strands in her tiny little hand, it's disconcerting to say the least.

My hand is definitely a bit better, though. Last week I couldn't cup my hands together under the faucet to splash water on my face; now I can, and I am typing using both hands. I'm trading my hair for my hand. A pretty good deal, I think.

Something I realized I've been missing is driving in my car and listening to music. I love to drive by myself, turn music up loud, and sing in my horrible voice. Tonight I decided to go outside after dark, lie on my hammock, look at the stars, and listen to my iPod. First I listened to sad music, which I actually enjoy doing, and cried. Then I listened to uplifting music and sang; then I got up and danced around my yard. It felt so good. I'm going to try to do it on a regular basis. It's good for the soul. It's good for my soul.

Xo Katie

## 8/9/12

Now I have a bald spot on the top of my head about the size of a 50 cent piece, and the hair next to my right temple is very sparse. Hair is still falling out nonstop. I had to shower this morning, and I dreaded it as I knew how much hair would fall out in the process. As I was combing it out afterward, my sink filled up with hair.

On the bright side—thank God there's usually a bright side—I found this amazing cancer support center called WeSpark! It is this amazing non-profit place with support groups for cancer patients, family members, caregivers, and friends. They have free classes in tai chi, qigong, meditation, Reiki, the list goes on. They also do comedy nights with stand-up comedians, nutrition experts, and guest speakers. I'm excited because their support group will be just for cancer patients, but not specifically brain tumors, which would be too hard for me. But being with other cancer people where we could just vent about treatment, etc. would be helpful I think. Maybe.

Xo Katie

## 8/10/12

One of the sadder aspects of the last few months for me has been the fact that I was forced to stop nursing Haven before either one of us was ready. I know that I was fortunate to have been able to nurse her as long as I did, 16 months, but because I knew she was going to be my last baby, I thought we would just go until it felt natural to stop. I stopped nursing Lucky at 15 months because I wanted to start trying for another baby, and he couldn't have cared less, but Haven continues to talk about it every day. Now that she has so many words, she will say, "Boobies, milk, sip," looking up at me. I tell her it's all gone, and she can have a milk bottle. But her latest thing is to offer up my breasts to all her stuffed animals, babies, even a wind-up toy, and pretend they are drinking. She sees the other children in her baby class nursing and is very curious. I decided to offer it to her and see what she would do, knowing my milk was gone so there was no danger of her getting any of the meds in her system. She couldn't remember what to do. She knew she should sit in my lap, but then just rested her head on me. She seemed satisfied with that. It broke my heart. She is a funny little girl; she melts my heart. We were robbed, and my sadness about this runs very deep.

I saw my radiologist on Tuesday, and I told him I was getting some of the function back in my hand, and he said that was a really good sign because most people don't see any improvement until the end of radiation because it causes so much swelling. The fact that my hand is improving means that the amount that my tumor is shrinking is more than my brain is swelling. A very good thing :) I attribute it to all the alternative things I'm doing, including visualization.

One of the most anxious times for me is when I am bolted to the table during radiation, mask on, hands and legs strapped to the table. I worry that if there was an earthquake, I would be left there bolted to the table, so I try to use that time to practice my visualization. I imagine that God's hand is reaching into my head, and His fingers are the beams of the radiation. And as he touches the tumor, it shrivels up and dies. It gets me through.

Xo Katie

## 8/11/12

I'm halfway through radiation, but it feels a lot longer. My bald spot is now the size of a baseball, at least. I saw my oncologist today and was complaining about it. He said, "Let me see it," so I took off my hat, and he laughed and said, "Yeah, it's gonna get a lot worse." You gotta love him. I look like a rabid animal with mange. Even worse is how bad it hurts and itches. Some spots feel like bad sunburn, and other spots feel like I was hit on the head with a hammer. I can barely touch them to put on my calendula/aloe mixture. The baldness is all on the right side, but the left side is thinning out too. I won't go bald on that side, though. No, I'm not going to shave my head. When it's all done I will eventually get extensions. I need to feel good about myself, and shaving my head will not accomplish that. I need a full head of hair. For now, I can still pull off wearing a hat, and you couldn't tell that I lost any hair. I will do that as long as possible.

I'm going to enjoy a date with Lucky tomorrow. I'm going to take him bowling and to lunch. I'm looking forward to it. Twice this week

he told me, "I miss spending time with you." It breaks my heart. I miss him too. I can't wait for radiation to be over. I think I'll go outside now and enjoy the cooler night air and listen to some music.
Xo Katie

## 8/12/12

I can't post tonight. Too many panic attacks, too much anxiety. Hopefully I will feel better tomorrow.
Xo Katie

## 8/13/12

I had a rough couple of days in terms of anxiety. Not quite sure where it's coming from, besides the obvious. It's probably the hair loss. I took a shower yesterday afternoon and probably lost 20 percent of my hair in that one shower alone. The top of my head and right side are completely bald except for the sideways mohawk of new hair that was growing after my surgery. But even that is falling out slowly. The left side and back have lost at least 50 percent of the total volume, maybe more. I think the anxiety started after that shower. Plus I've been feeling nauseous the last two days. I wasn't sure if it was the chemo finally making me sick or if it's the 40 supplements I was taking a day. So I stopped all supplements and am feeling better today. I think I'm going to have to build up to those more slowly. 40 pills is a lot.

Back on the Klonopin for tonight, and I feel better already. Can't deal with constant anxiety along with everything else.
Xo Katie

## 8/14/12

I am perfecting the art of the comb-over. I'm holding on to what hair I have left, for as long as I have it. Sorry I'm obsessing over my hair; it's just that I'm obsessing over it. I told Lucky I was going to my treatment today, and he said, "I bet more of your hair is going to fall out!" I said, "I bet you're right!" He thinks it's funny.

I went to the cancer support center today—WeSpark. It was great. I'll start using the facilities probably after I'm done with radiation. I'm still having anxiety. I'm wondering if the radiation is actually causing it and it's not all "in my head" literally. I'm going to ask the doc tomorrow. More good news, I'm becoming allergic to the chemo pill. I have been breaking out in a rash and itchy hives all over my legs. My doctor said to take Benadryl so we can hopefully get through the end of the six weeks.

Xo Katie

## 8/15/12

I went to radiation today and met with my radiologist beforehand. I had a bone to pick with him. I was very upset about my hair. (OMG she's talking about her hair again!) I was crying and telling him that I was completely unprepared for the amount of hair loss. First I was told I would have a bald spot the size of a small lemon; then they said it would be the size of an orange; then they said I would also probably get a bald spot on the lower left side where the beam exits my head. I was prepared for all of that. I was not prepared to have the entire top of my head be bald and all the rest of my hair thinned out by more than half.

When I took off my hat and showed him, he was genuinely shocked. He said it was one of the worst he had ever seen. He said very rarely has he ever seen anyone lose as much hair as I have. I actually felt validated. I had felt angry and deceived, but he was so surprised and felt so bad about it. At least I know now that what I am feeling is appropriate. He said, "What can I do to make it up to you?" I said, "Kill my tumor."

He said obviously my hair follicles are very sensitive to the radiation. Sometimes that can be an indication that the tumor, especially one like mine that is on the surface, is also more sensitive to the radiation. We hope so. He said it can take anywhere from two to six months to start growing back, and I may end up with a permanent bald spot where the strongest beam is directed. My hair could also be thinner in those areas. Who knows what I will end up with?

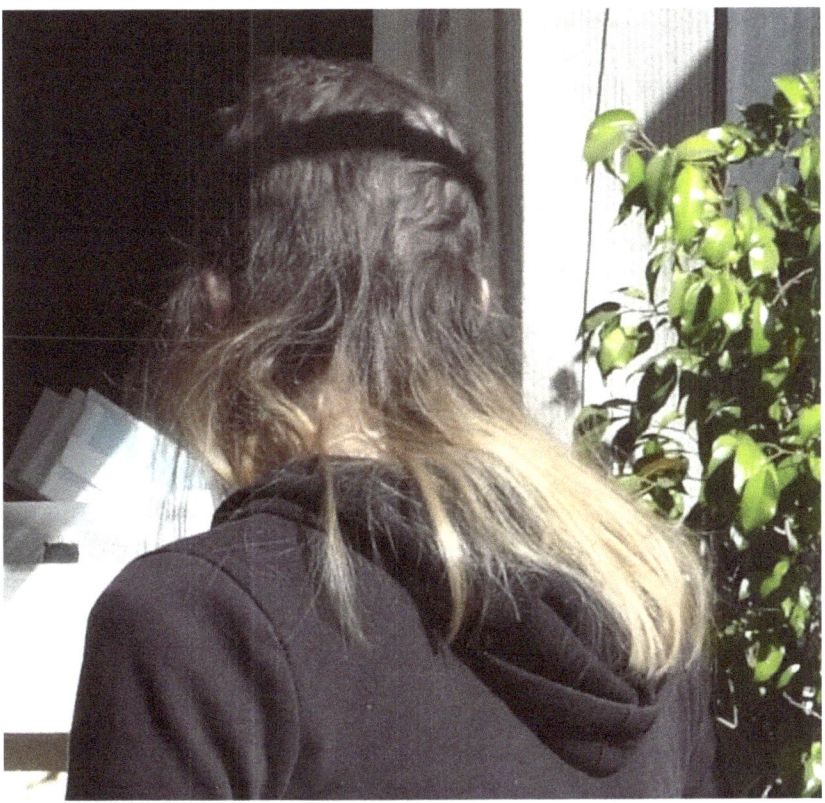

The only picture I have of the back of my head about a month after it started growing back. The black line is a shadow.

I tried taking Benadryl with the chemo, but it's not working; the rash and hives are getting worse and now climbing up my torso. I can't take it anymore. I'm going to have to stop the chemo. It's scary since Temodar is the gold standard of treatments for anaplastic astrocytoma. Maybe we'll try a different chemo later. I just can't take the hives anymore. It's unbearable.

Xo Katie

P.S. The radiologist said that my anxiety could be caused by the fact that now I actually look like a cancer patient, whereas before nobody could really tell. Hmmm....

## 8/16/12

Haven is 18 months old.

Not much going on. I'm almost done with my fourth week. I'm crossing off the days like a prisoner waiting for parole.

Xo Katie

## 8/17/12

I apologized to Micah the other day because I felt like this is way more than he signed up for. We've had nonstop medical issues for the past seven years, and just when we thought we were done with it— blamo! Brain cancer. I feel so unattractive on top of everything else. I've been listening to a song by the Verve Pipe called "Colorful" and there's a line that basically says you bought a ticket to a fun rom/com and you ended up in a horror film, but you love me anyway. That's how it feels to me. Of course he was wonderful and said he loves me and is still attracted to me, but it would be a lot for anyone. In sickness and in health—you never think it's going to happen to you, at least not until you're much older.

I have to say that it's almost offensive to me to see people not take care of themselves. I rarely drink, never smoked, or took drugs (excluding some experimenting in my youth), and it's not my place to tell people how to live, but in my down moments I can't help but think, *Why are they fine and I'm not?* It's not a blessing, or a gift. It's like when I was trying to have a baby, and you see drug addicts popping out babies, no problem. I guess no one said life is fair, and it definitely isn't. With all that said, I do believe there is perfection in everything and a reason for everything. It's not clear now, but someday it will reveal itself, and I'll be here to see it.

Xo Katie

## 8/17/12

I had a rough night, didn't sleep well. I'm pretty sure that if I didn't have children, I wouldn't even get out of bed. Ever. It's amazing that I've had this tumor since before I even had children or a husband, and now they are my reason for living. I can't imagine having to battle something like this without such strong motivation. The depression and exhaustion would become too much and I'd want to give up. I'm grateful for my family.

Xo Katie

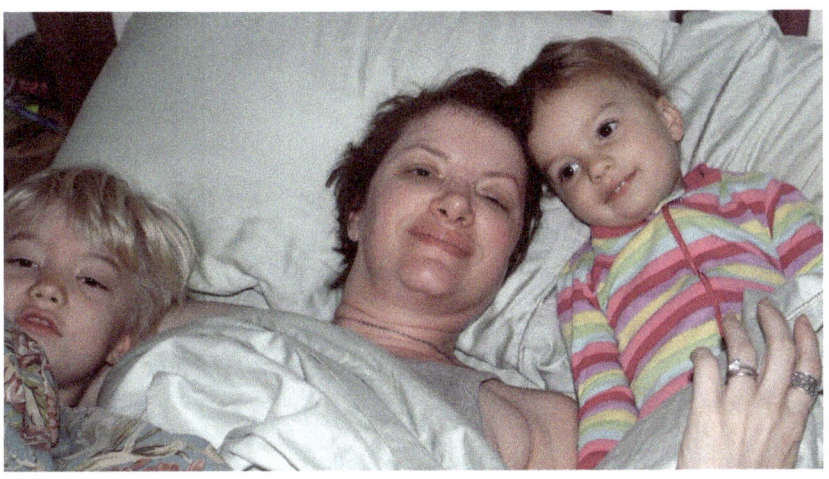

My reasons for living (looking really rough in 2013)

## 8/17/12

The countdown begins…

The other night after one of my many meltdowns, Micah and I were talking and I said, "At least we'll always have something to talk about. One day we'll be old and I'll say, 'Remember when I had fucking brain cancer!'" and he said, "And I'll say, 'You had brain cancer? Where was I?'" We laughed hard at that one, because it's true! Typical Micah.

We're taking Lucky bowling again tomorrow. I'm grateful that I'm right-handed. I plan on kicking some ass!

Xo Katie

## 8/19/12

I'm posting a photo of me in radiation. Thinking of running over my mask with the car when I'm all done, or maybe crushing it with a sledgehammer. I can't wait for this to be done. My hair is still falling out. I talked to a friend yesterday who said losing her hair was harder than losing her breasts. I would have to agree. It's been one of the hardest things so far.

I did some research on people who lose their hair to radiation, which is very different from losing it to chemo, because radiation is more like a burn. Sometimes it doesn't come back, sometimes only parts of it come back, and it usually comes back different. If it does come back, it can take months before you see any growth at all. I think I'll call my nutritionist and my dermatologist to see if there's anything I can take to help or what they recommend. My radiologist says to only use calendula right now for the itching and pain because anything else will damage the hair follicles. Who knew?

Xo Katie

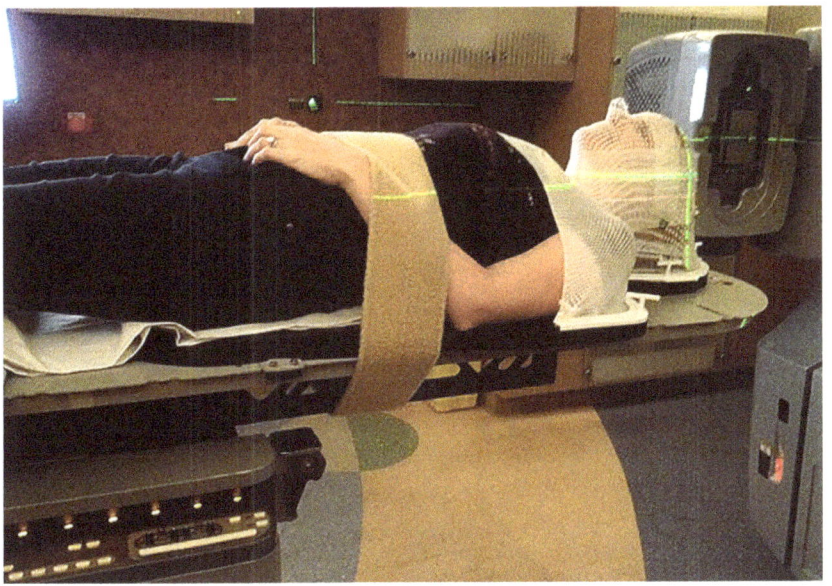

Being radiated

## 8/20/12

    I had a good appointment with my oncologist today, and Micah got to come with me. I asked him about the clinical trial, and he said I'm in a "clinical trial wasteland." The doctors/pharmaceutical companies running the studies wouldn't want to invest in me because I would live too long and it would cost too much to follow my progress. Since my tumor is not an aggressive tumor, they wouldn't qualify me. It's good news. He said, "I would rather be in your shoes than qualify for the study." He also said that in a year or two, if the vaccine shows promise, then the FDA would approve it and it would become "off the shelf," meaning he could just prescribe it for me. I wouldn't have to be part of a trial. Good news.

    We asked him if we would be seeing Dr. X again and he said, "Probably not." We were surprised and he explained that you only need Dr. X if things aren't going well. He was happy about the progress in my hand, which gets better every day; I barely notice it anymore and haven't dropped anything in two weeks. Awesome. He also concurred that it's possible my tumor is more sensitive to the radiation because of the way my hair and hand have responded to it. More good news.

I felt really good about the visit. He said everything is going great, my blood work is great, and I feel good except for the obvious itching, irritation, and fatigue, and he isn't worried about me. And I got to wear my new shirt that says, "My Oncologist Is My Homeboy." Micah took my photo with him. He said it was the best shirt he'd ever seen and wants a copy of the photo. All in all a good, uplifting day. It's funny how I hang on every word he says and look for any nuances that indicate anything positive, and then hang on to those for dear life. I wonder if he knows how a simple sentence from his mouth can alter someone's perception of their future. No pressure.

Xo Katie

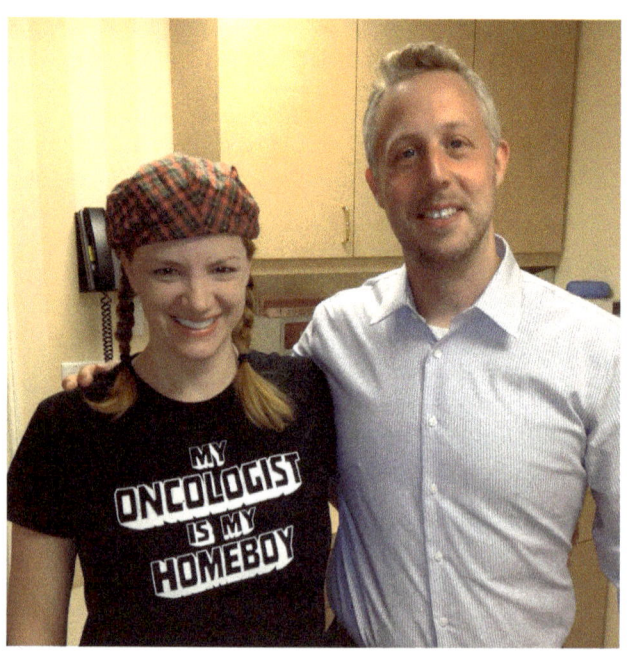

## 8/21/12

My theme song of the week is **"One Way or Another" by Blondie**. I heard it the other day on the way to my doctor's appointment, and it seemed very appropriate cuz I'm going to getcha, you fucking tumor, one way or another.

Some tumor humor: My radiation techs (who are all younger than I am; when did that happen?) always ask me how I'm doing, and I always say, "I'm having a bad hair day." Funny things people say: "You look radiant!" Me: "Must be all the radiation! I'm glowing (in the dark)!"

Eight more days…
Xo Katie

## 8/23/12

Bad day. Song of the day:
**"Trouble" by Cat Stevens:**
Basically a song about someone who is begging trouble to leave them alone, that they have had more than their share and want to be free to just suffer now.
Xo Katie

## 8/24/12

Clearly I had a rough night last night. Something set me off, and it was a downward spiral from there. I'm better today. Cancer is a full-time job, I have to say. Not for just the obvious reasons like treatments, appointments, research, bills, etc. But sometimes it feels like it's my job to make people feel better about ME. I'm not talking about anyone in particular but everyone in general. Obviously everyone feels better as long as I'm perky and funny and cute and positive.

But the minute I have any negative feelings, it's just not tolerated. Turn that frown upside down! Think of all the things you should be grateful for! (Like I don't realize there are things to be grateful for.) It'll grow back! You're almost done! (I'll never be done.) Cancer isn't pretty, people, even with whimsical braids and a kicky hat.

Last night what I was missing was someone who would throw their arms around me and cry WITH me, not FOR me or for themselves. Someone who wouldn't try to talk me out of feeling bad. I guess that's what support groups are for. Okay, venting over.

Obviously I am eternally grateful for my friends and family. My support system is amazing, and it's impossible to know what I will need or want at any given time. I have had 25 radiation treatments and at least 20 different drivers and more next week. That's amazing. I LOVE my support. I even pulled off a joke today with my radiation tech. When my treatment is over, he takes my mask off, then puts his arm out and says, "Take my hand." This time I said, "But that would leave you with one!" He laughed out loud. Extra bonus points if you can name the movie that's from.

Xo Katie

## 8/26/12

I had a decent weekend with the usual ups and downs. Started off my morning with my son punching me and losing his playdate privilege, which is more of a punishment for me and Micah as he is then here all day. His real punishment was having to go grocery shopping with us.

Five more days and counting… As of last Tuesday I am getting one-fifth the amount of radiation as I was before. This is called "the boost" because they are targeting more of the actual tumor and less of the surrounding brain. My hair is still falling out in handfuls.

I can't wait to start healing from this ordeal. My head itches like poison oak 24/7, and my incision had barely healed when they started radiating it. It is as red and sore as the first day. Today I broke out in an itchy red rash all over my arms and legs, some kind of allergic reaction. Ah, good times.

Micah's high school friends in Biloxi, MS, threw a huge party/fundraiser for us last night. We heard it was a big success. A huge thanks to everyone who participated. You are great friends.

Xo Katie

## 8/27/12

I woke up this morning covered from feet to neck in an angry, itchy red rash that turned into welts. So much for this being the downhill part of my treatment. I swear I can't catch a fucking break. After radiation I went to the oncologist, who determined it is a cumulative, delayed reaction (sensitivity) to my chemo pill. So now I am on a heavy dose of steroids and Benadryl and Claritin to get me through this last week. UGH. Other than that things are good, I guess. I really like our new babysitter; Haven loves her and I think Lucky has a crush on her. I just filled out 30 pages of paperwork for the disability office trying to convince them that I deserve the disability money I've been paying into my whole life. This has been going on since May.

Four days and counting…

Xo Katie

## 8/28/12

In the emergency room…

## 8/28/12

Hey guys, it's Micah, the hubby... Didn't want to keep you guys guessing here.

Katie had an allergic reaction yesterday that went loco last night, and she woke up with red welts all over her body, itching like crazy. Yet another thorn that she has to deal with...anyway they shot some meds into her veins, and she's feeling better now. Poor dear needs a break from this soooooo bad.

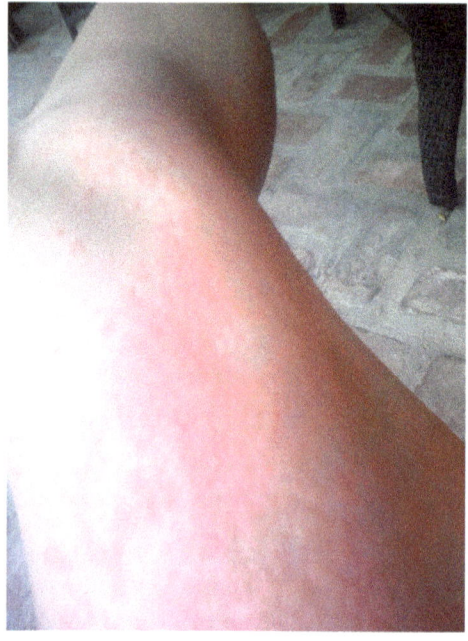

The rash on my leg

## 8/29/12

Sorry to leave everyone hanging. I do like to keep you on your toes, though. I had to go to the emergency room first thing this morning. In the middle of the night, I could feel the rash spreading all over my body, especially up my back, my arms and legs, and the back of my head. When I got out of bed, I could see how bad it was; there were no individual bumps anymore but huge patches of redness that blended together to cover my whole body. When I noticed that it was going up my neck and head, I worried about it getting into my throat. We had been calling and paging my doctor for an hour with no response, and I had already taken more Benadryl and steroids to no avail, so I asked Micah to take me to the ER. Once there my doctor called and we talked for a minute. He told me not to take any more chemo pills, that I was having a severe allergic reaction that was getting worse rapidly.

I talked to my oncologist again this afternoon, and he said I am off the chemo, potentially forever. That usually these reactions get worse and he said it could kill me. I'm actually upset about it because I want to do everything possible to kill the tumor and I want to do the gold standard of treatments.

He said that what was really important to him was that we got at least four weeks of chemo concurrent with the radiation. We actually got 5.3 weeks, so that's even better. He said to pat myself on the back. I made it. So I won't do the last four days of chemo, but I will continue with the radiation till Friday.

Both my oncologist and radiologist said that the radiation is the more important one anyway.

My doc said that there are other chemos, but they have more side effects.

He suggested doing allergy testing to make sure it's the Temodar, and maybe after a month break we can try a small dose and see what happens, or load me up on heavy doses of steroids (yippee) before trying the chemo again. Or maybe I will never take it again because my tumor looks fine and isn't changing. We just watch it with the MRIs, and if a problem arises, we deal with it then.

For now he says just take a break and enjoy this month of no more treatment and try not to think about it. Is that possible? I'm sure gonna try. I am so excited to start my life again. What a nightmare three months. My friend Betsy said, "Maybe your body is telling you that it doesn't need that anymore." I'd like to believe the tumor is dead and doesn't need the 12-18 months of chemo.

I just took my steroid and Benadryl and Pepcid and Claritin. Gonna pass out soon... No more Viagra, Zofran, or Temodar!

I suppose if I didn't have all of this drama, there would be nothing to write about :)

Woke at 3:00 a.m. with the rash back. I have to take Benadryl around the clock because after exactly six hours the rash starts coming back and I start itching badly. I don't know how long it's going to take to get this chemo out of my system. Called the doc this morning when I woke with the rash, and he put me back on the hard-core steroid Decadron, which is what I was on after my surgery that made me nuts. Should bode well with my pms. Everyone has been forewarned. Doc wants me to come in on Friday; I guess we will discuss my options. He told me on Monday that if I stay on my seizure meds, I can start driving in October, but if I want to taper off them, I won't be able to drive until December or January. Tough choice. I think I am leaning toward staying on them, not just so I can drive sooner but because I will feel safer as a driver if I am assured I won't have a seizure. I don't really think I'll ever have another one, but I would still be anxious driving my kids around if I wasn't "protected" by the medicine. I'm sure that as time goes by and I get farther and farther away from my last seizure in July, I will be able to relax more. Two more days!

Xo Katie

## 8/30/12

Big day tomorrow. I think it's ironic that my surgery was the day after summer started, and my last day of radiation is our last day of summer vacation. So, how was your summer? It's always been my least favorite time of year. I hate heat. I am looking forward to fall and to getting my life back somewhat. The strange thing will be that there are no more sign-up sheets for driving or playdates, everybody gets back to business and life, but in one month I have my first MRI, which will tell us how my tumor has responded to the treatment. Then it's MRIs every two months. I get anxious just thinking about it. A few weeks of peace before my anxiety builds again. And again.

It's hard for me to not get into thinking *What next?* I have learned to expect the rug to get pulled out from underneath me just when I think things have settled down and I am feeling confident. At this point I would love to just be bored. Enough excitement already. I want a mundane, ordinary, happy life. I'd like to enjoy my kids and my hubby, go on vacations, and make memories. Micah keeps joking, "What did you do in your past life to deserve this?" I wonder... And I wish this was the only time I wondered this, but it seems to be the story of my life. My cross to bear. I'll take the suffering as long as it always has a happy ending.

Xo Katie

## 8/31/12

Happy last "Fryday" to me. What a strange, surreal day. I feel a bit like a baby bird that's been kicked out of the nest. *What? That's it? You're done with me? That's all you've got? What am I supposed to do now?* Then I got a book in the mail from my friend Jodi about a woman who got cancer, had a near-death experience, and discovered why she got sick in the first place.

I realized in reading just the foreword and first few pages that my journey from here is mental and emotional. I've done all of the physical work and will continue to do so, but now it's about figuring out why this happened to me. Micah is not here so I will wait to celebrate with him tomorrow; besides myself, he has been the most affected by this, and I can't celebrate without him. For now I am eating his bag of M&M's that were stashed in the freezer. Sorry, Babe, I deserve it.

My original thought was to destroy my mask, this ugly thing that would only serve to remind me of this terrible time in my life, but after thinking about it, I might save it and view it as the thing that saved my life. I had an appointment with my oncologist today before my final radiation and I asked him, "How bad is it that I can't finish the chemo?" He said, "We don't know." He said that right now he's conducting a clinical trial in which patients only do chemo for the six weeks of radiation and no more because they (the doctors) don't know if more is better. They do know that the most important part was doing them concurrently for a minimum of four weeks, and I did that. He said I could have easily been one of the patients in his clinical trial and I wouldn't have been scheduled to do any more chemo.

In the next nine days, I will taper off these horrible steroids and then the only medication I will be on is the seizure medicine. Hard to believe. I had geared myself up for 18 months of chemo. I'm a little lost. MRI in one month. I asked him if I would ever be able to say "I don't have cancer" and he said, "We all have cancer." Gotta love him.

He said he expects about 30 percent shrinkage, and if the rest doesn't change, they consider me in remission. I don't think I'll be satisfied with that. I have higher expectations.

Even though this chapter is closed, I will continue to write to keep everyone updated and also to explore all of these thoughts and ideas I have. Hopefully I can prevent someone else from having to go through this "learning experience." I hope so. Thank you all for your continued support. My "journey" continues... I hate that word. I'm not on a cruise! I'll call it an ordeal.

Xo Katie

## 9/2/12

I took a break from posting last night. Still reading and processing my emotions. Plus these steroids make me feel jittery and crappy. Seven days left of that nonsense. School starts on Tuesday! Once again Micah and I are blown away by the generosity of people. Often it's people who don't even know us personally but are moved by our situation. We are eternally grateful. I washed my hair tonight, which I hardly ever do because it's so depressing. Losing a little every day is hard enough, but when I wash it, I lose a ton, and it's so hard. I'm hoping that after a week of no radiation, it will stop falling out finally. I can't use extensions if there's nothing to attach them to. Looking forward to a week of catching up on things at home: organizing, cleaning, paperwork…Things that have been put aside for far too long. I also hope to start cooking again, going to the support group, exercising, going to movies, etc. In other words, normal life.

Xo Katie

## 9/3/12

So I had an adventure today. My friend Birdie drove up from San Diego (two hours away) to pick me up and drive me to Palmdale (another hour away) to see a famous, visiting Thai healer, psychic, and herbalist. He has been in California for a couple of weeks doing television shows and private appearances where people wait for hours to have a reading with him. She had made an appointment for me to see him at this private appearance, so when we arrived I was able to bypass the line and get a reading right away. There were also many Buddhist monks doing prayers and chants, and lots of Thai food. People were eating and socializing while waiting in line.

"The Master" didn't speak English, so my friend translated for us. He said that he has been working with people who have cancer for 50 years, and he can smell it in people. He said I do not have cancer. He said I have a tumor because I have toxicity from something called formalin from formaldehyde and melamine, a common ingredient in plastics and tableware among other things. He asked if I put plastics in the microwave, and I said I used to a lot. He also said I have a parasite which contaminates the blood. It comes from red meat or fish.

He prescribed 400 pumpkin seeds a day mixed with any kind of milk (cow, almond, soy) for 30 days to kill the parasite and half a pound of red chard every day for 30 days to cleanse my system of the toxins. He also wants me to have milk with yogurt and honey and lime for protein, vitamin B complex and vitamin c.

Birdie asked me to list my supplements, and she read the list to him. He said something to the effect of, "Oh yes, those are for cancer; you don't have cancer."

He also did a reading for each of my children and Micah. The last thing he said to me, translated by Birdie, was "Congratulations. You are going to live for a very long time." I turned and burst into tears.

As you all know I am very open-minded, so I will try what he says and see what happens. The things he said about Micah and the kids were interesting; for example he said Lucky's back is out of alignment, and it prevents him from sleeping well and causes a temper. Hmmm... He said Lucky would become a doctor and Haven will be very athletic. He recommended certain foods for them.

Obviously anyone would be happy to hear they do not have cancer, and that could very well be true, especially after my radiation and chemo. Plus the fact that they only found one cancerous cell in my biopsy. His take on the causes of the tumor are interesting. Like I said, I think the doctors have done what they can for me, and now the rest is up to me. Exploring all avenues, and all potential causes, environmental and emotional. No matter what, I believe that people do not get cancer for only one reason; like my doctor said, we all have cancer.

Why it grows out of control in some people is the real question. This is a fascinating journey that will definitely change me forever.

Xo Katie

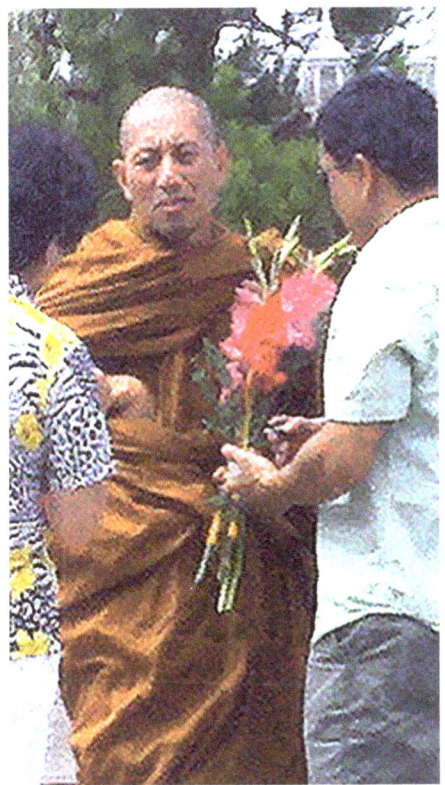

The Thai Healer

## 9/4/12

Okay, so yes, I ate my 400 (approximately) pepitas today and my red chard, though I don't think I ate a half a pound. I ate a lot, though. I put the pepitas in my Vitamix (yay!) with plain, whole fat yogurt, almond milk (unsweetened), and some honey and blended it into a smoothie. I didn't have any lime but I will get some. It was good. After no dairy or sugar for months, it felt decadent to eat yogurt and honey. Micah had a glass, and Haven liked it too. We literally bought a bucketful of pepitas (pumpkin seeds), raw, from Whole Foods. When blended with all the stuff, it's just a nutty smoothie. I guesstimated the amount. I sauteed the chard with olive oil, garlic, and salt. It was pretty good, like spinach.

Today was Lucky's first day of first grade! There was a lovely rose ceremony, and he got two 12th grade buddies who are very sweet. An exciting day that I was thrilled to see. The program listed the names of the first graders and said "Class of 2024," at which point I started crying. So hard to believe. It seems so far away yet I know it will go by so fast. I look forward to seeing him as a senior and getting a little six-year-old buddy.

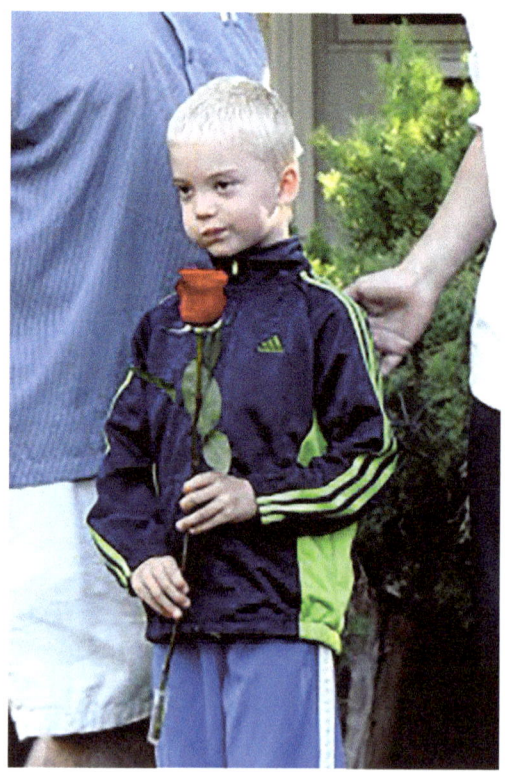

Lucky at his rose ceremony

I was so looking forward to having a normal week where I could get a bunch done but ended up with a baby with a fever and runny nose all day. At least she waited until radiation was over so I am able to really be here for her.

Four more days of steroids. UGH! I HATE the way they make me feel.

Still debating whether to go to the cancer support group at WeSpark. I don't think of myself as someone with cancer, and I'm not sure I want to surround myself with people who have cancer. We'll see, maybe I'll go to one. I would like to utilize their other services like yoga, Reiki, qigong, etc.

Xo Katie

## 9/5/12

Had a good day of cleaning, organizing, and being with my kids. Lucky had a good second day of school (his favorite class was German!) and Haven is feeling much better!

In my exploration into why this has happened to me, I am discovering that since childhood I have been a "people pleaser." I grew up feeling totally responsible for other people's happiness, but not my own. Because my sister was "the bad one," I made an unconscious decision at a very young age to compensate by being extra good. I had to be perfect, had to make my parents happy and proud.

I couldn't possibly compete for attention with my sister because we all know that bad behavior gets more attention than good, so I never expressed any anger, or frustration. I was never rude, selfish, or unpleasant in any way. I've never yelled or screamed in my whole life. I don't even know if I can. I was virtually invisible. My parents divorced when I was six and have been single the majority of my life, and my sister is not in the picture, which makes me feel even more responsible for their happiness and fulfillment. This is not to say that they are responsible for this, but they didn't notice what was going on and unknowingly encouraged it. It is something that carried over from my childhood and never left me. To this day, even though it's denied, I am still expected to be perfect, to say and do all the right things, and to look a certain way. I also felt I had to be the perfect girlfriend, wife, and mother. There are obviously many details I am leaving out, but you get the idea.

As far as I can tell I am the only person in my whole family who feels the need to be perfect, happy, pleasant, polite, pretty, selfless, and thoughtful ALL THE TIME. I am also the only one with cancer. Most of my grandparents and family members also drink or smoke or both, but I don't do anything, yet they live into their eighties and nineties. Are you getting the picture?

Someone recently wrote to me and said that meningitis (which I had at 13) is caused by extreme anger and that cancer is caused by resentment and hurt held over from childhood. Hmmmm...

I've been to the emergency room nine times in my life. That's a lot for someone who doesn't participate in any sports! Two visits were for seizures, once at 13 when I had meningitis and encephalitis from chickenpox which is very rare, and once from the brain surgery. Why did a simple case of chickenpox turn into a life-threatening illness? Because I was harboring extreme anger? Maybe.

Twice I have been to the emergency room for extreme allergic reactions. Once at 15 (we never found out what it was from—interesting) and once from the chemo, again, rare.

Also very interesting is the fact that all of my illnesses and emergency room visits happened in my first 15 years of life and the last 12. None in the 15 years when I was living on my own and only taking care of myself.

I'm not trying to blame anyone or throw anyone under the bus. I have talked to both my parents and Micah about all of this. I'm writing this in the hopes that it will help me figure out why I do this and also so that someone else may recognize themselves in my story and stop the madness!

My new life is going to consist of always finding the joy, taking care of myself, spending time with my husband and children as much as possible, allowing myself to express any emotions I'm having, including anger, and not feeling responsible for making everyone happy all of the time.

Xo Katie

## 9/6/12

I realize that because I always had strange and difficult things happen to me, especially medically, I assumed that that was my "lot in life" and somehow I had earned or deserved it in some way. My job would be to suffer, and I would suffer over and over again. I would also persevere and overcome, but first I would have to suffer. I was a walking Murphy's Law. If there was something that could go terribly wrong, it would. Even something simple like a crown on my tooth would have to be redone at least twice. This was typical, expected.

So was I surprised they couldn't get my tumor out? That I had cancer? That I would lose more hair than most people? That I would have a severe allergic reaction to the chemo? What do you think?

Having children was something I wanted since I was a little child. I was obsessed with babies. My friends would get mad at me because I always wanted to play with their little brother or sister. As I grew, my passion for babies only got stronger. I wanted children desperately. Because of my past history, I always had the fear that somehow, because it was so important to me, I would be denied this one thing I wanted more than anything. When I had my first miscarriage, I can't say I was all that surprised—devastated, but not surprised. Of course, this was the pattern. Why should it come easy? And of course the doctor would screw up the D&C, and of course they would diagnose me with some very rare uterine birth defect, and of course I would be a carrier for a rare fatal disease. Of course I would lose more babies. I would suffer over and over but persevere. This was my destiny. Botched surgeries, drug reactions, four miscarriages, misdiagnosis, pain and heartache.

I no longer believe I deserve to suffer, or that it is necessary in order to achieve what I want. There are things I couldn't control, but I also think my fear was so deeply rooted that it manifested as panic, which led to some bad decision-making and me responding by making choices based on more fear. One of my favorite books, *Conversations with God* by Neale Donald Walsch, states that every decision we make is based on either fear or love. Most of my decisions in the past were based on fear.

Now I see that I can change my future so that the next 50 years of my life don't have to be full of suffering, that things can go smoothly, that everything is perfect. I don't want to live with fear or the feeling that I never have enough, or that there is something right around the corner that will ruin everything.

Not to toot my own horn but I am truly amazed at my ability to remain optimistic at all, even with everything I have gone through. It's a true testament to the human spirit. The fact that I always knew in my heart that everything would turn out all right, despite the pain I would have to endure, made it bearable. I have everything I always wanted. I did it.

This is going to be a work in progress for me. I still feel the fear creep in at times. Changing your thoughts is easy; really believing it, deep down, is harder. But I can do it.

Xo Katie

## 9/7/12

An interesting piece of information. Most people don't know that a brain tumor can't spread to other parts of the body. Other cancers can spread or metastasize to the brain, but it doesn't happen the other way around. My tumor is called a primary tumor; it started in the brain. It can infiltrate to other parts of the brain depending on how aggressive it is, but as opposed to other kinds of cancer, I don't have to worry about it showing up somewhere else. So I've got that going for me.

Nothing profound tonight, just feeling good.

Xo Katie

## 9/8/12

There have been three times in my life, all in the last 12 years, when I feel that God or some higher power has spoken to me. Not in words but in a "knowing" that comes over me from out of nowhere.

The first time was 12 years ago. Micah and I had been dating again after a 10 year break, and things weren't going too well. He wasn't thrilled about the idea of being in a serious relationship with someone, so I had decided to call it quits. I was fairly devastated as I very much wanted to be with him and missed him terribly. One morning as I was putting my makeup on, getting ready for work, an overwhelming feeling came over me that Micah and I were going to get married. Now we were broken up at this time, so I had no real basis for thinking that, but a calm came over me and I just "knew" that he would one day propose.

The second time this happened was when I was struggling to have another baby after Lucky. As I've mentioned, I had loads of trouble in this area. Not only did I want another baby but I desperately wanted a baby girl. Having a girl was so important to me that if I had had another boy, I probably would have tried again for a girl, which would have been nuts and even dangerous. After two years of struggle, I was pregnant for the sixth time and was so anxious about the baby surviving and whether or not it was a girl. Again the feeling came over me that I would have this baby and it would be a girl. Complete certainty and a sense of calm and peace I hadn't felt in two years.

The last time it happened was a few nights ago. I was lying in bed, about to fall asleep, and I guess I was thinking about Haven. Obviously my biggest fear since my diagnosis was that I wouldn't live to see my children grow up. My anxiety about Haven was worse than Lucky because I knew that he was old enough to remember me a little, but if I died in the next few years, she probably would not.

Suddenly I felt such incredible happiness, and a knowing surrounded me like a warm blanket. I became sure that I would be around to watch her grow up and become a woman. I felt so much happiness and calm. If I hadn't had the other two experiences, I probably would have written it off, but I was familiar with this feeling.

Ever since then I haven't been afraid of dying.

Xo Katie

## 9/10/12

I really need to go to bed earlier. I was so tired today that I barely accomplished anything. Yet here I am again posting at 11:00 p.m. I have some really important things to say, but I'm just too tired to tell you. Just kidding.

Xo Katie.

## 9/11/12

I just wanted to let you know, because some people are hearing it already, that I had another seizure today. It was a very bad one. It was the scariest moment of my life. It lasted at least ten minutes. I was at Hugo's restaurant with my friend Nicole, and we were waiting for a table. Within a minute of talking to each other in the waiting area, I felt a familiar tightening in my left hand, and I was able to get out the words "I'm having a seizure" before I lost all ability to communicate and started to collapse. Nicole grabbed me and held me. The restaurant was packed, and we were standing right in the entranceway when it happened. Nicole held me for a minute, but I was having trouble breathing, and because my chin was resting on her shoulder, her hair was in my face, which amplified the feeling of not being able to breathe. I was dead weight and she was holding me up. At some point we collapsed down to the floor. My legs were bent under me, and it was hurting me, but I couldn't say anything. I was gasping for air the whole time, and Nicole said later that my tongue was kind of hanging out. Nikki started yelling for someone to call 911. My whole body was convulsing, and I was making moaning sounds and trying to get some air. A group of people were standing around watching, and some were discussing whether I had epilepsy or not. I remember a guy saying, "Oh, she won't remember this; she won't even know who you are." Oh shut up. Nicole was great, talking to me the whole time and telling me everything was okay as she would shout out again for 911 and say, "She has a brain tumor!" I was finally able to gesture to my left leg because it was hurting me due to the awkward position and how I was lying on it. Finally Nicole understood me and had a guy help her lift me enough to get my leg out. It had bad, bloody rug burns on it. I was still in full seizure at this time. I couldn't move anything on my left side; it was dead and I could barely hold my head up and I was still feeling like I couldn't breathe. Someone got behind me and lifted my shoulders off the ground.

 I heard the sirens and was so relieved but also scared because I knew they wouldn't be able to do much for me. I carry Ativan in my purse because you can squash a seizure if you can get it down in time. Unfortunately I only got a couple of seconds of warning, so there was no time. Right before the ambulance came, I managed to tell Nikki to get the Ativan and she did. They put it under my tongue. I was starting to come around when the paramedics came, but I could barely talk. Nikki did her best to answer their questions. She also tried to call Micah for me. They took me away in an ambulance, and I was still in full panic mode. This was the longest, worst seizure I had ever had. I was trying to answer their questions but so out of my mind I couldn't catch my breath.

I arrived at Sherman Oaks Hospital—UGH. I hate that hospital, but it was the closest. Micah and Nikki met me there. I felt so bad for Nikki that she had to witness something so scary. I could tell she was really shaken up. I told her she did all the right things. They started an IV and finally after much begging I got some more anxiety meds. Before Micah and Nikki arrived, the nurse kept leaving me alone with the curtains closed on a small gurney, not even a bed, no rails. I was having panic attacks and started screaming at her that she couldn't leave me alone. It seemed as if she couldn't care less. I was terrified. I thought I might fall to the floor if I had another seizure, and no one would notice. The place seemed dark and deserted.

Finally a doctor came in and we told him what happened. Here's what we think: I just stopped the steroids two days ago, which can cause some rebound swelling and withdrawals. I'm still healing from radiation, which causes irritation and swelling. I took my seizure medication two hours late this morning. I exercised for the first time in months. I was really tired and needed a nap and hadn't eaten yet. A perfect storm. My doctor at Cedars has increased my seizure meds, plus we're switching to a brand that lasts longer and doesn't wear off so fast, plus he's having me take one milligram of the steroid again. We will talk to the doctor tomorrow and probably see him soon.

I'm devastated that this has happened again. I've been crying ever since. I thought I had passed all this bullshit. I had quite literally just gotten to the point where I felt comfortable alone, not worried that I would have a seizure. Now that starts all over again. I was hoping to drive next month, but now that's out of the question. I'm devastated. There are no words.

**Song of the day:**
**"Mockingbirds" by Grant Lee Buffalo**
A song about devastation
Xo Katie

## 9/12/12

I want to say thank you to my friend Nikki. Thank you for not letting me fall; thank you for your calm and comforting presence. And in true friend spirit, Nikki went BACK to Hugo's and brought us lunch to the hospital. Now that's a friend. Small joke for some levity: What's an epileptic's favorite food? Seizure salad. I said it was small.

I woke up feeling like I had been hit by a truck. I am so sore and bruised and still very weak, especially my left hand. I have been dropping things all morning.

I am completely traumatized. I'm in constant fear right now, right back to where I was two months ago. Every five minutes I feel as if I am having another seizure, and my mind plays constant tricks on me. I can't sleep without someone lying next to me, and I panic if I am left alone in a room. I HATE THIS. I had only just gotten rid of this constant fear a couple of weeks ago. I was feeling so free and good. I was at the top of the mountain, and now I am at the bottom again.

How can I keep picking myself up again?

I'm so sad. Help me, God.

Xo Katie

## 9/13/12

Today was a challenge. Micah was working in Palm Springs, so I needed to take Lucky to school, and today was Haven's first day of toddler class. Micah's mom, Haven, Lucky, and our sitter Hannah all piled in the car, and Hannah drove us to school. I had an Ativan hangover, so I could barely keep my eyes open. Everyone I saw gave me a big hug, and I pretty much burst into tears every time. My emotions are right on the surface. Many times today I started crying out of nowhere. Mainly I just keep reliving the nightmare over and over again.

My mother-in-law, RoseMarie, joked that this last seizure was the "grand finale"; that's why it was so big and needed to be in front of a large audience. I pray that's true. BTW, she told me to post that she loves me. I love her too. She's held me while I've cried all day and she braids my hair. Among many other things.

I spoke with my doctor today. He said that it was probably due to the radiation as it causes a lot of irritation and swelling, and often it's worse after radiation is over; that's why they don't do the first MRI for a month, to give the swelling time to go down. He did say he was surprised just because of the fact that I had been doing so well. So even though it's common, it was not necessarily expected.

I asked him what he thought the chances were that it would happen again, and he said low. Mainly because we have upped the dosage of my meds and switched to an extended release form so it won't wear off, and I'm also back on steroids. I told him how difficult it was for me to breathe during the seizure and I asked him if it was physical, as in my lungs are seizing as well, or just from the panic, and he said there can be some constriction from the seizure, but the panic component is huge. He told me no one has ever died from not being able to breathe during a seizure(unless they are choking on something), and I made him promise me that it was true. I think it was so bad because I was in a strange place surrounded by strangers and I panicked big time. I don't even remember convulsing or the usual twitching or arms and fingers flailing. I literally felt like I turned to stone.

I feel connected to Nikki now as if we have been through war together. She is in the unique position of being the only person outside of my family (and 100 strangers) to see me have a seizure. She knows what it looks like, the look of fear on my face, the gasping for air. It's incredibly intimate in a way I can't describe. I can still picture her face looking at me with such concern.

I have talked to my therapist about helping me with my post-traumatic stress disorder. I said I feel like those people who come back from war and duck when they hear a helicopter overhead because they feel as if they are being shot at. She said, "You don't have POST-traumatic stress disorder because the threat is still real. The helicopters ARE shooting at you." It's so true. How do I deal with that?

I am trying to access that place I was in a week ago, living fearlessly. The book I'm still reading, *Dying to Be Me* by Anita Moorjani, is an inspiration. One foot in front of the other. Living in fear isn't living, so I have to get through it. This is really, really hard.

Thank you for all of the words of support. I need them really badly right now.

Xo Katie

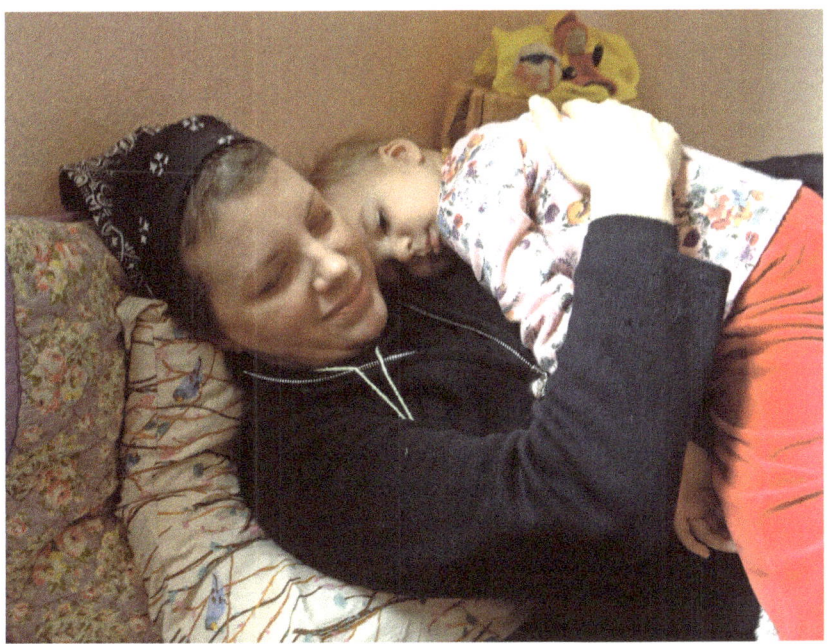

Lying on the ground at Haven's class trying to at least be there for her

## 9/14/12

So much for the grand finale. I had another seizure at my son's school this morning; luckily he had just gone into class and shut the door. I was literally on the ground outside of his classroom. Fortunately I was surrounded by familiar faces of people who care about me, so I was able to keep myself relatively calm and it only lasted a few minutes. Thank you to all of you who held me and comforted me. Amy, thank you for just smiling so big and telling me everything's okay.

Unfortunately, I just had a seizure a few minutes ago. It lasted longer because I was alone for the beginning. Two in one day :( This is horrible.

My doctor is sure that this is a result of the radiation, and it is peaking right now at the two-week post-radiation mark. He may move up my MRI to next week instead of two weeks from now.

I need people who can come and be with me during the day. I cannot be alone for even two minutes. I'm terrified. I keep my Ativan within arm's reach at all times or walking with it in my hand everywhere I go. My mom or MIL will also be here as well as Hannah and Micah. It takes a village to take care of Katie.

My seizures are not like in the movies. I do not lose consciousness. I wish I did because then I would have no memory of them. Since I am awake, I need certain things to happen, and it was suggested that it would be very helpful to make a list because most people don't know what to do. You will get a written reminder when you arrive, but for anyone else who may be around me:

Here it goes.

If I have a seizure:

1. Make sure I do not fall.
2. Make sure my face is not obstructed by anything, even your hair or face; do not hug me.

3. I prefer to be sitting up, legs crossed or in front of me, not under me, sit across from me so I can see your face.
4. If not possible then lay me on my left side so I am able to use my right hand.
5. I have Ativan (lorazepam) in my purse (middle compartment). Put one under my tongue ASAP.
6. Call 911 or have someone else call if the seizure is lasting more than five minutes or if I have been injured.
7. Talk to me, smile, tell me everything's okay, and remind me to breathe and calm down.
8. Don't attempt to hold my left arm or hand. They will be rigid. You can hold my right hand.
9. Call for Micah if he is home or call his phone.
10. Other than Ativan do not put anything else in my mouth, especially your fingers!

If you think you are up for the task, please sign up. Hopefully I will not have any more. I won't be great company because of all the drugs, but I would love to eat, watch TV, or nap with you.

I certainly didn't think I would be back in this position of needing round-the-clock care again this soon, but so it is.

Xo Katie

## 9/15/12

No seizures today but I am an absolute zombie. I guess if you tranquilize someone enough, their brain just shuts down. I want my life back. I got just enough of a taste of it before the shit hit the fan again. Now I'm back to not even being able to leave the house, shower by myself, put Haven to bed by myself, forget about exercising or the parties I'm missing out on. I can forget about driving again until December. What kind of life is this?

My in-laws stayed an extra day because we needed someone here for me, someone for Haven and someone for Lucky. Having just one extra person here isn't enough. I'm so nervous when Lucky is around because so far he has never seen me seize, and I don't want him to. I think it would be traumatizing. I did explain to him what's going on, but if he can avoid seeing it, then so much the better.

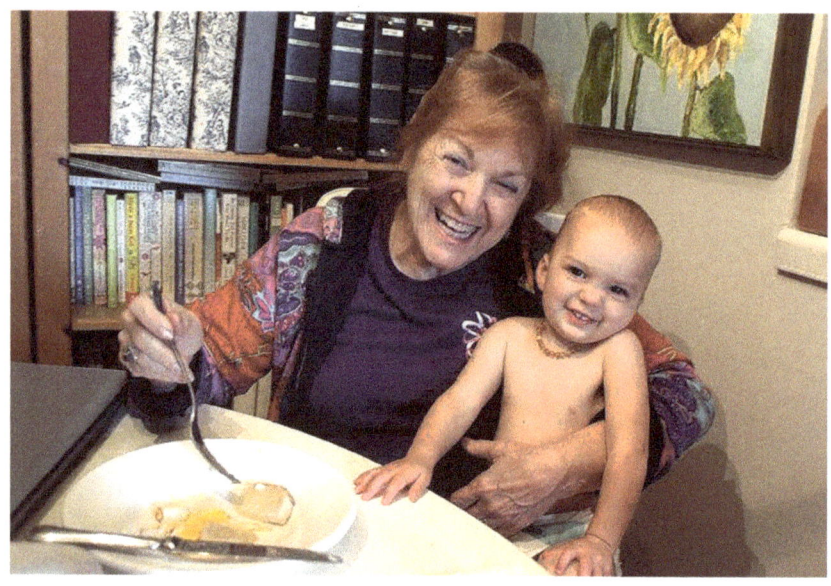

Haven and Micah's mom, "Grandma Sippi"

## Later...

I'm still trying really, really hard to not live in fear. The panic rises in me and I usually reach out to touch someone close by because it calms me down. I just don't want it to take two months again for that fear to go away. Please help me, God.

Xo Katie

## 9/16/12

I woke up at 5:00 a.m. to a seizure out of a dead sleep. Then another one two hours later. I'm so scared. The doctor upped my steroid and is adding another seizure drug. He also wants me to move my MRI up to this week so they can see what's happening. It could be possible bleeding from the tumor. I don't want to die. I'm so scared. I'm so drugged I can't even think straight. I need help. Please, God.

### Later...

Thank you for all of the kind words and support; it really does help. I am a wreck today. Afraid to sleep, afraid to eat in case I might choke, afraid to be around my kids, afraid my brain is bleeding. Back on all the hard-core meds I was on right after surgery, the ones that make me crazy, plus some new ones. All of them have side effects like irritability, rage, suicidal thoughts. I'm trying really hard to move through the fear.

Please pray for the swelling to go down and for my brain to be peaceful. I'm hoping that the dead tumor cells are shedding and causing swelling and irritation. I will focus on that.

I'm feeling really low,
Xo Katie

## 9/17/12

I spoke to my doctor again this morning. He doubled my steroid and second seizure med, but he is happy that the seizures seem to be isolated to just my left hand for the most part. He says my brain is still firing the signals for seizures, but the medication is working to keep them from spreading. Now we wait for the inflammation to go down and my brain to heal.

He will try to schedule an MRI for this week just to make sure everything is okay, but he basically said that even if the tumor is bleeding, they can't do anything about it, just wait for it to heal. I did ask him if this means my tumor is getting worse and he said, "No way." This is supposedly very common. Yay!

Xo Katie

## 9/18/12

Heading to Cedars ER this morning. Four seizures since 1:30 a.m. I will probably stay overnight. I'm scared. I'll try to post if I can.

Xo Katie

### Later...

Seven seizures so far today. It's unreal. I had my MRI and I am now hooked up to an EEG all night long to capture any seizure activity that we may not be able to recognize as an obvious seizure. I spoke to my oncologist tonight. He will come by in the morning to give us the results of my MRI. I could be hooked up to this EEG all day, I don't know yet. Hopefully I will get to go home tomorrow at some point. I miss my kids and my husband. But I'm lucky to have my mom and my best friend, Krista, with me in a nice room with a nice view.

I'm very sleepy now, going to bed soon. I'll post more in the morning.

Xo Katie

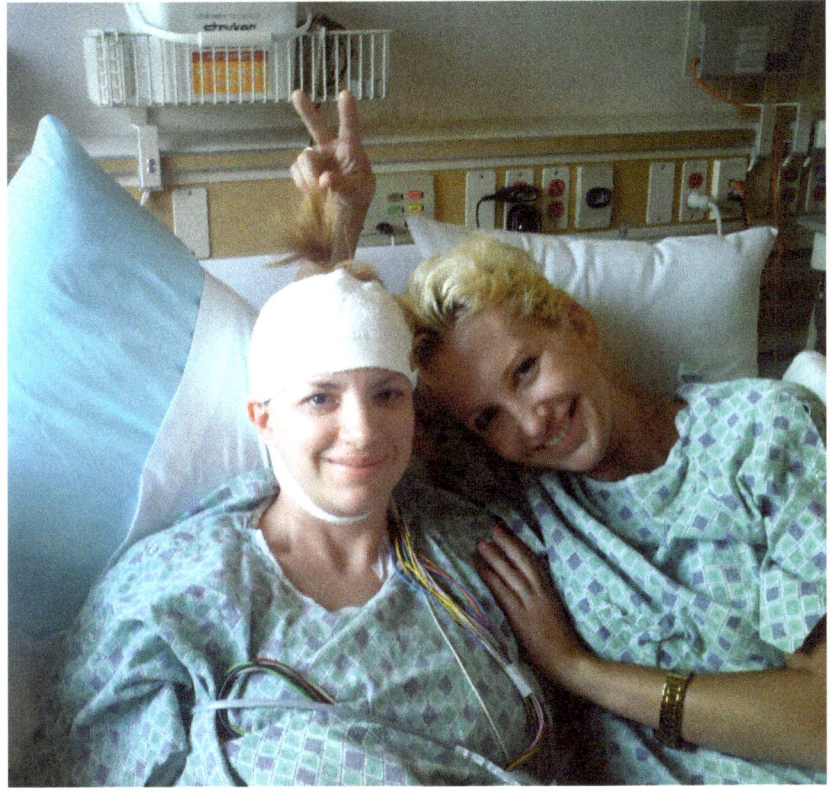

Seizure monitoring with my bed buddy, Krista. Smiling but terrified.

## 9/19/12

I'm still at Cedars. I had my MRI last night, finally, and just barely made the cutoff to get hooked up to the EEG machine, which needs to stay on my head for 24-48 hours. My head is wrapped in a turban of gauze to keep all the wires in place, and it looks great :) I spent the night with my mom in a foldout chair, and Krista snuggled up in my twin bed. It was very comforting. I had two seizures, one at 1:30 and one at 5:30 a.m., better so far. I'm drugged out of my mind, but as the doctor said, no news is good news. Hopefully I will get to meet with him this morning.

The best-case scenario is that my tumor is dying very rapidly and shedding dead cells so fast that it is irritating my brain and causing swelling. Worst-case scenario is that my tumor is doing something bad, like becoming more aggressive. He said even if that happens, there are things he can do. So much for the vegan breakfast I requested. I got pancakes, sausage, and Rice Krispies with milk.

I'm really hoping to go home today, missing my kids terribly.

Xo Katie

## 9/20/12

I had eight seizures yesterday. We met with my oncologist this morning, and he didn't look exactly pleased when he came in. He said, "We have two big things," one being that my tumor was enhancing or lighting up more than it did before, which could mean one of two things: one, that it's dying and shedding so fast that it's irritated and inflamed, or two, that it's becoming more aggressive and growing. He is leaning toward the first one. He rescheduled another MRI for tomorrow morning that will show whether there is blood going through the tumor or not. That would be bad. I will keep you posted on those results tomorrow.

I met with a neuro-psychologist this morning who gave me an extensive questionnaire to fill out. There's a possibility that the trauma I had from my initial seizures after the surgery and this latest seizure in the restaurant have caused me so much anxiety that it is actually triggering more seizures. I have a meeting with him in the morning to go over the results of the questionnaire and the evaluation. I'm hoping that it is the anxiety, because I can control that. I just had another writing this post.

If I don't call or write, please don't be offended; my anxiety is just through the roof.

Xo Katie

## Later...

I'm finally home, 24 hours later than expected, but I'm home. Two MRIs later and we still don't have concrete answers. I was hooked up to an EEG machine for 24 hours, pushing a button every time I felt a seizure. The idea was to monitor the seizures and see what kind they were, where they were coming from, and to look at the tumor to see the status of it.

Regardless of the results, my oncologist Homeboy is strongly urging me to try another chemo pill called CCNU, which he thinks would have good results. It's only one pill every six weeks for six sessions. It can have side effects that affect your lungs as well as leukemia, just as the Temodar did. That is rare. I am reluctant to take any more drugs that have side effects of any kind at this point. If the MRI shows no blood to the tumor, then we can take some time and think about it.

The seizures are another issue. They were definitely triggered by the swelling and effects of the radiation, but the anxiety component is huge. I met with the neuro-psychologist from Dr. X's team today, and he was wonderful. He said that the EEG did not show that these small seizures were coming from the tumor, so not a physiological event, but more of a sensory response based on the past trauma and anxiety I feel whenever I get the sensation that I may have a seizure, which happens hundreds of times a day. Lucky has seen one now, so he is not scared by them.

My work now needs to be getting back to the place I was a few weeks ago where I was living fearlessly and not afraid of having a seizure every five minutes.

What I need now is to focus my attention on positive thoughts, my kids, and things like school and day-to-day life. The reason I have gone into so much detail now is because I really can't talk about it in person, texts, or on the phone; it actually raises my anxiety levels.

I will continue to post any and all updates, but I had a seizure just writing this. In addition, my left hand is virtually paralyzed. The swelling of the tumor and up to eight seizures a day have taken a toll, so there is a lot I cannot do. My lovely friend Vivienne brought me an awesome doll today called "The Dammit Doll," and its saying goes like this:

Whenever things don't go so well,
and you want to hit the wall and yell,
Here's a little dammit doll,
That you can't do without.
Just grasp it firmly by the legs and find a place to slam it,
And as you whack the stuffing out,
Yell, "dammit, dammit, dammit!"

I will put it next to my Little Katie Kick-Ass doll that was made for me.

I want to say a special thanks to my friend of almost 35 years, Krista, who dropped everything and slept in my tiny twin hospital bed with me so that Micah could be home for the kids. And also to my mom, who was there on a cot every night, listening to our fits of the giggles. It sounds crazy, but somehow we can always find the funny!

Xo Katie

## 9/23/12

I'm having a rough morning. Good news is that I went 24 hours without a seizure. That's the longest since 9/11.

The bad news is everything else. Every time I have a seizure it knocks out my hand for hours. With so many seizures lately, my hand is paralyzed all the time. It is so frustrating, I can't even tell you. I burst into tears because I can't put Haven's shirt on. No one understands. Micah thinks that because I know eventually it will come back (weeks, months?), it shouldn't be that upsetting. It feels as though the world should stop because my world has stopped, but it just keeps going and going. Not a great day, can you tell?

Xo Katie

## 9/24/12

Three seizures today, not enough rest. The good news is that I was able to mentally ward off many others. There usually comes a point, though, where I don't have the strength to keep it from coming, and it's often as I am lying down about to fall asleep, making it a little hard to relax. I'm eating a giant frozen yogurt now brought to me by my hubby. Because I NEEDED it.

I am a prisoner. I am a prisoner in my home and I am a prisoner in my body. And there isn't a fucking thing anybody can do about it. I have a warden and a stalker. I am a prisoner in my mind because I can't say what I really want to say. Nobody listens to me anyway. When I say, "I can't talk about this anymore; it's making my anxiety go up," they keep talking. When I need something from the store, they decide arbitrarily for me if I really need it or not. I am reduced to child status. Yet I still have a stack of bills in front of me, and I have to fold socks using my teeth. I have a sick baby again, who only wants me. I didn't even get to rest in the hospital. How could I possibly rest here? I got so angry at Micah tonight for not helping me open the mail that I went outside in the backyard and started throwing the patio furniture. I was in a complete rage. I want to kill someone, hurt someone, destroy things.

Micah called it "rearranging the furniture."

This has been such a miserable day. I won't bore you with the details too much, but my doctor has tripled my steroid medicine to see if it helps with my hand and the swelling around my tumor. Unfortunately if my hand does improve, the steroids are going to make me want to strangle someone with it. It's a lose-lose situation.

Supposedly my doctor never got the two messages I left on Friday, so I was left to worry all weekend as to whether my tumor was becoming more aggressive or not. So after two calls to his office this morning, one from me and one from my father, I finally got a return call. My MRI showed a little bit of blood flow, but what they would expect from someone who is responding well to the treatment. BUT, they can only be about 70 percent sure that that's what it's showing because of all the swelling.

So naturally he wants me to try out this other chemo pill called CCNU, just in case. I will meet with him Wednesday to discuss it. This chemo can have serious side effects such as major pulmonary issues that can manifest years later, as well as leukemia, which he has seen happen.

As a result of me feeling like an adult trapped in a child's body, I have to please beg everyone to stop offering me advice. No more "you shoulds" or "Can I offer some advice?" or "You need to try..." Please stop. I am completely overwhelmed and I don't want to hurt or offend anyone's feelings, but you have to understand that I am in complete survival mode right now. I cannot even take care of my basic needs let alone work on raising my consciousness level! I am still reading and appreciating books. I just have to do it at my own pace. Just give me a few weeks to pick myself back up and then hopefully I will be back in fighting mode.

Xo Katie

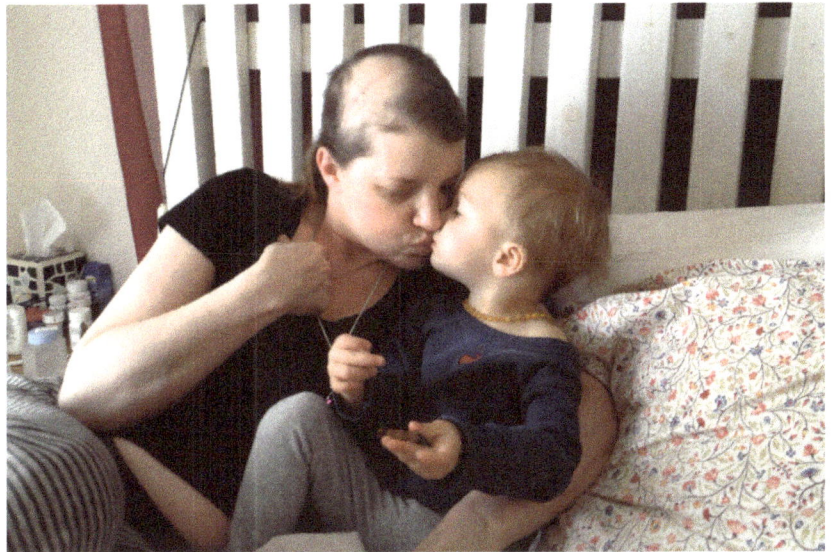

Haven visiting me in my bed. I'm missing out on her life.

## 9/25/12

Feeling a little bit better today, mentally at least. I got some stuff done with my mom's help, two naps, some laughs, and one seizure.

I'm back down to my normal steroid med, so I don't feel like killing someone anymore. I have a doctor's appointment tomorrow. There are gonna be some big decisions to make, very stressful, but I have decided to be rational and not make any decisions based on fear. Tired, love to you all, thanks for the support and understanding my mood swings.

Xo Katie

## 9/26/12

Big day, an important doctor's appointment. It gave me a stomach ache all day. So...some good news, some more good news, and some news left up to interpretation that could be great or terrible. UGH.

My MRI is showing a lot of inflammation, and that's to be expected. The doctor told me before the radiation that this MRI is a baseline and I shouldn't put much weight into it, that the inflammation could even look like growth. Unfortunately, that was also when I was expected to be continuing on the Temodar (chemo). Since I had the allergic reaction and had to stop the chemo, now he is nervous. My tumor is "enhancing" or lighting up much more on the scan, which could signal extreme necrosis—meaning the tumor is dying and shedding dead cells at an extreme rate—which would be the best response they could hope for OR, and this is a big OR, the tumor has "flipped a switch" and has suddenly become very aggressive and dangerous to the point where you wouldn't want to even wait a month before doing something. He is 75 percent sure that things are fine. He felt even more relieved after seeing me in person because my hand has gained a little function since he saw me in the hospital, and my hand is basically the biggest indicator of how the tumor is responding. If I continue to get function back, then it's just inflammation and we are in good shape; if the hand gets worse, we need to act fast.

My choices are to get another biopsy and test one of these areas that are lighting up, not a popular choice by me, immediately start the other chemo pill called CCNU, and do four cycles (six months) of this. A viable option; this chemo has more serious side effects, but it can also have better long-term outcomes than the previous chemo, assuming I need it at all. The third choice is to do nothing, wait three weeks, repeat the MRI, and see if I have any improvement in my hand. He doesn't expect that the next MRI will show improvement—that can take months—but if it doesn't look worse, and my hand improves, then we know we are going in the right direction.

So, like I said, the good news is that he is 75 percent sure things are fine, my hand is better than he thought it would be, and I didn't have a seizure today—first time in two weeks! The bad news is that 25 percent of him is very concerned. This is such a hard decision. But again, deep in my heart I believe everything is fine, more than fine, and I refuse to make a decision based on panic. Whenever I've done that in the past, it has not gone well. Whenever doctors have tried to scare me with statistics, they have been wrong. This is a huge life-or-death decision, that's how he is presenting it to me. At the last minute he did say that if it is the worst-case scenario, there are things in his back pocket he can use at his disposal, but obviously we don't want to get to that point. I am heavily leaning toward waiting three weeks to see if my hand improves and if the MRI stays stable. I get to reduce my steroid by half in a few days. I know my family will be happy. Stressed and psychotic is not a good combination.

I'm back! Although I may be getting Haven's cold :(

Xo Katie

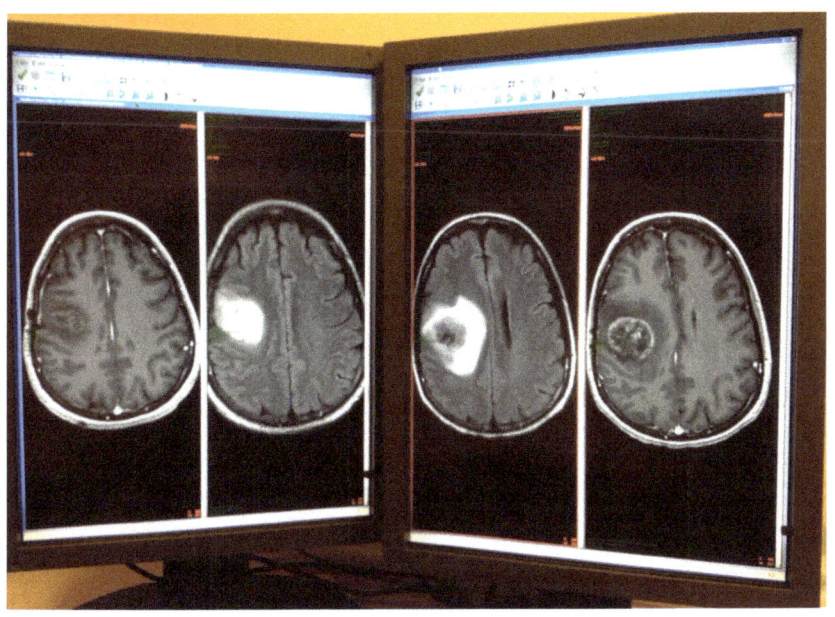

Before radiation on the left, after radiation on the right. Dying or growing?

## 9/27/12

I had a seizure this morning almost right when I woke up, but it had been about 36 hours, which is the longest stretch so far. My hand got temporarily worse, but it's doing well now. I've been working on it all day. Trying to touch my thumb and pinky makes me break out in a sweat! It's so hard, but I did it tonight and couldn't do it yesterday. Yay!

Lucky has gotten so blasé about my seizures now. He says, "Are you having a seizure, Mom? Okay," and walks away.

Now time for some levity because we all need it.

Yesterday my friend Cheri was babysitting me, and we were on my bed when I started having a seizure. Right then Lucky came in and decided to start rifling through my end table drawer (I tend to keep my chocolate stash there). Anyway, he pulled out something that a six-year-old should not have any knowledge about and said, "What's this, Mom?" Now I am literally in the middle of a seizure and can't speak very well and I am trying to practice "mindfulness" where I take deep breaths, focus on sounds like the air conditioner coming through the vent, watching the ceiling fan, to calm myself and reduce anxiety. Obviously this all went out the window. I quickly grabbed it and shut the drawer. Knowing he had found something, but having no idea what it was, he had this funny smile on his face. Thankfully the seizure was short-lived, and Cheri and I burst into laughter; we could not stop. It was such a ridiculous moment. So much for having any dignity left in my life. At least Cheri and I joke that it's okay because she's an OB/GYN! She said that she's never seen someone laugh during a seizure before!

Xo Katie

## 9/28/12

For someone who has never asked anyone for help before, I think I'm getting pretty good at it. Whaddya think?

Xo Katie

## 9/29/12

Bad day, five seizures so far. Woke me up at 5:00 a.m. Freaking out.
Xo Katie

## 9/30/12

Better day, two very small seizures, but upped my drugs, so hopefully I will talk to my doc tomorrow. I got a bit of strength back in my hand since I've had fewer seizures, so I'm not panicking as much. Lucky got to go to his first real baseball game today! I'm sorry I missed it, but let's face it, I would've hated it. Planning something creepy and grotesque for my Halloween costume and my bald, scarred head. It shouldn't be too difficult.
Xo Katie

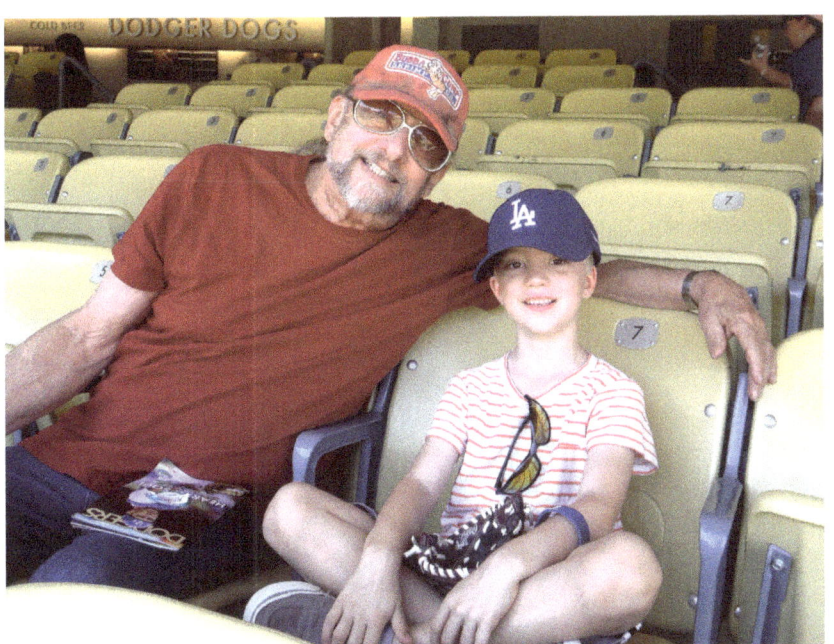

Lucky at the game with my dad and Micah

## 10/1/12

I can't believe it's October already. I can't wait to start decorating. My arms, hands, and shoulders are bruised from bumping into walls; sadly the only thing that has improved is how proficient I have gotten at opening things with my teeth.

It's amazing how sensitive the brain is and how easily my thoughts can control my seizures and anxiety. I can no longer watch TV shows or movies that trigger my fight-or-flight response, no crime shows or scary movies of any kind. I will immediately have a seizure. So I am watching many old reruns of *Friends, Seinfeld,* and *Roseanne*. My life has become so small. I wonder if I will ever go to a theater again, out to dinner, dancing, the gym, parties. I can't imagine it. It's so depressing.

Xo Katie

## 10/1/12

**Song of the day**
**"Little Earthquakes" by Tori Amos**
It feels like this song was written for me. Seizures are my own private earthquakes. Will it be a 3.0 or a 9.0? I never know.
Xo Katie

## 10/4/12

It's been such a depressing day for me. I feel my joy slipping away. No progress in any way. I am now under direct orders from Betsy to only think about the things I do have and not to dwell or even think about what isn't working or what I don't have. So here it goes:

I have:

A wonderful husband who supports me wholeheartedly and always tries to help me think positively, and who makes me laugh.

Two beautiful, healthy, smart, and loving children who make me laugh every day.

Wonderful, supportive parents and in-laws who would move mountains for me and take all of my suffering away if they could.

Amazing and supportive friends and a community of people who help us SO much.

An amazing school full of great people.

An abundance of food, clothing, toys, and love for my whole family.

A house with a lovely yard for my children to thrive in.

Freedom from worrying about things that don't matter.

The best doctors who really want the best for me.

My right hand and two mostly working legs.

A little bit of hair growing back on the left side :)

An outlet like this where I can tell my feelings without feeling judged.

A brain that acts up but still works.

Good books that inspire me.

Fall weather.

Holidays.

Music, and

Internet shopping.

Thanks to Betsy for this exercise. It does help.

Xo Katie

## 10/5/12

I've decided that my hand will improve every day, my tumor is shrinking and swelling less every day, and these mini "events" I have are meaningless and it's just a dead tumor trying to get absorbed by my brain in an enclosed space, without much place to go, and a poor lymphatic system.

Xo Katie

## 10/7/12

The front yard is 80 percent decorated thanks to Micah, Lucky, my mom, and Haven (I helped out a bit). I'm trying to become okay with the phrase "I don't know" and surrendering to that. It goes against my nature but I need to try. Betsy and I are working on getting me to be able to flip her off. Not even close yet, but everyone should have a goal.

Haven woke at four this morning and was calling for me, and the anxiety of not being able to care for her brought on a seizure. I cried out of sadness at the situation.

Xo Katie

## 10/8/12

I am debating whether or not to continue to wear hats and things. I know I will have to put up with some amount of staring as I don't look like a "typical " cancer patient. When you see someone with no hair and no eyebrows or eyelashes, you can be pretty sure they have gone through chemo or have alopecia; you don't feel the need to stare. But when you see someone with hair from the ears down, eyebrows and lashes and a six-inch scar on their head, you either think, *Wow, bad accident* or *I hope that's not contagious*.

The book I've been reading is about recognizing your own magnificence and seeing yourself as a perfect person, loving yourself wholeheartedly. I have never really liked the way I look; in fact most of my life I have thought of myself as some kind of freak, just like the people who have body dysmorphic disorder, where people can tell them they look normal, even good, but they never believe it. People said I was pretty, but I never felt it. If I could get noticed by a popular, attractive guy, then I felt I must have some worth. I felt so intimidated and inferior. I felt the best about myself in my early twenties, but even then, not good enough. I needed lots of attention from guys to make me feel accepted. I always felt like my dad preferred my sister to me, so I guess I wanted a guy who would *choose me* over anyone else, which would mean I was worthy, special. That's probably only one of many reasons. Then came the children, and my body changed. I started looking older, etc. I definitely never saw myself as perfect or magnificent. I definitely never accepted myself, let alone felt accepted by other people. So now, here I am, looking even more like my worst fears, completely stripped of my identity, and I don't even recognize myself in the mirror. No long, blonde hair to hide behind.

In the most beautiful testament to love, my husband has told me and my mom that he doesn't even notice my hair, that he only sees me. Lucky has never said anything except expressed wonder as the hair fell out and has never suggested any embarrassment. He has even said he thought I was "cute" when he learned what that word meant. Haven has only ever said, "Boo boo head?" and "Mommy okay?" because she sees my scar. My husband and children only see me. So who else should I care about? If I can't finally accept myself as a person of value, not because of how I look, then I am not really accepting myself or loving myself still.

I have had to stop and restart writing this three times because of the anxiety it brings up in me. For sure I will get stared at, for sure I don't feel pretty, for sure I will feel self-conscious that people are trying not to look, but I can't help it. So do me a favor if you see me, whether it's at my house, at school, or at a store or whatever, just get a good long look, ask questions. I don't mind. It's better than having someone pretend to not be looking. It looks weird, I get it. It's going to look weird for a while; hair doesn't grow back fast from radiation, and my head has been burned. But maybe this is the greatest opportunity ever to strip it all away and see if I can accept myself. At least until winter comes, because a bald head does get cold :) Update: I just got back from Target with Micah, no hat! It felt good. I actually think people are staring because I walk like a drunk person, not because of my head :) Anyway, it's a first step.

Xo Katie

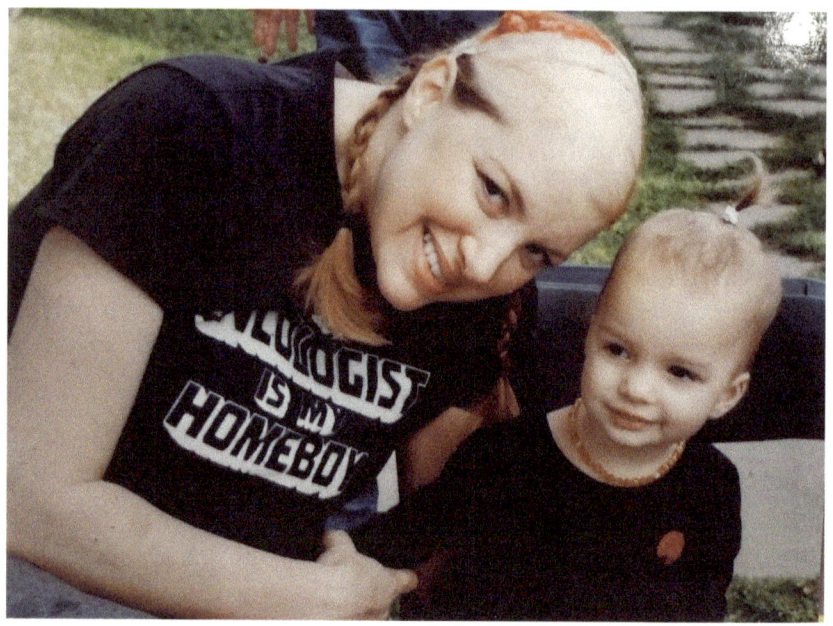

No hat. I think Haven has more hair than I do!
(Part of my Halloween costume is showing).

## 10/10/12

Doctor's appointment today. It's hard not to get anxious when you feel like someone holds your life in their hands and they are watching every move you make to judge whether you are worse or better. No pressure. Realistically he probably won't tell me much today, but I have an MRI next week. That's what I was thinking about at 11:00 p.m. as I tried to fall asleep and had a seizure. Sweet dreams.

Xo Katie

## 10/11/12

I couldn't post yesterday because I totally got freaked out after my appointment and started Googling—what a terrible idea. I can barely walk now, I'm dragging my left leg so badly. We won't have any definitive results until my MRI on the 22nd, so this is all about best-case scenario, worst-case scenario, and what's in between.

Okay, best-case scenario: Radiation is working great, the tumor is dying, and the resulting swelling and enhancement on the MRI is normal and will slowly go down, and I will see improvement in my hand and MRIs every month. Worst-case scenario: My tumor has flipped some switch and become a much more aggressive malignant tumor such as grade-four glioblastoma multiforme. Terrible option. Not that likely based on what I started with, but a possibility nonetheless.

In-between scenarios: something called "radiation necrosis." What this means is that the radiation was too much of a good thing. My tumor could be dying at such a fast rate that my brain, with its very limited lymphatic system and inability to clean away all that dead tumor, is swelling and causing the loss of function in my hand and seizures. Doesn't sound that bad, but it is. First of all, radiation necrosis and grade-four brain cancer look the same on an MRI, so they would have to treat both. They could do a biopsy to rule out grade four, but that's brain surgery again with all of the risks and side effects that go along with it, plus you are still only getting a piece of the tumor. You don't know if what you are getting is representative of the whole tumor. Secondly, radiation necrosis can cause permanent damage if the swelling lasts too long, and the healthy brain gets damaged. This could actually go on for years after radiation. It can be fatal. There is a drug to treat necrosis called Avastin. It's supposed to be very effective, but it can have major side effects like stroke, holes in the GI tract, etc. If it is grade-four cancer, then I would immediately go on the chemo CCNU.

Again, the issue is that both look the same on a MRI, so they could treat me with both drugs.

Major negatives to both. They are both dangerous drugs, with no guarantees.

If my MRI on the 22nd looks the same or even a little better as far as swelling and enhancement, then we assume it's normal swelling and do nothing, even start reducing my steroids. If it looks worse, then we start drugs immediately. Again, my hand is a good indicator of how the swelling is doing, and there hasn't been much improvement there, if any. I also still have some palsy in my face. Obviously we hope this is all a normal, great reaction to radiation and not overreaction.

I took Lucky and Haven to school today and didn't wear a hat. Of course it was the coldest day in a long time! I am overwhelmed by the support and love I got. Thank you, friends. One dad gave me a big hug and said, "You're the bravest person I've ever met." I appreciated that so much. Had an itty, bitty seizure right in front of Lucky's class. I think my nerves just got the best of me.

Xo Katie

## 10/14/12

I am thankful today for:
Good food from loving friends.
Much-needed help today from Krista.
A good talk with my mom.
Cuddles in the morning from Lucky, my wonderful, loving boy.
Playing with Haven (and I may be biased, but I think she is the cutest, smartest, sweetest, easiest, funniest, most perfect girl in the world. I can't wait to watch her grow up).

Xo Katie

## 10/16/12

Hi. I have a hard time going on Facebook anymore, or watching TV, or reading magazines. I get jealous of people with "normal" problems. I wish I didn't feel that way. But I will accept myself as I am and know that one day all will be well again. I think and hope that I will forever be changed and not care about who lost weight or who's engaged or how big their ring is. How about you?

I had a seizure at 5:00 a.m., but I didn't even wake up Micah for the first time, just focused on healing and rode it out. Little earthquakes.

Xo Katie

## 10/16/12

### Later...

Had a little freak-out tonight. Gotta be honest: I'm really scared. This whole MRI thing is scaring the bejesus outta me. This not knowing is making me nuts. My hand, "the indicator" of how I'm doing supposedly, is not doing any better. I'm trying to not put any expectations or fears on the results, but that's easier said than done. It's hard when your son wants to play with you and show you the new game he's learned, and I have to tell him I can't do it. It's hard when your baby cries because the nanny is leaving because she spends more time with her than I do. How can I reconcile these things in my mind? It breaks my heart. I cried really hard tonight. My mom was here to hold me and kept telling me it's temporary, but nobody knows that. I want to believe it and I'm practicing, but the reality of the situation is hard. I want my life back. I would give up all my hair permanently to be able to play with my kids and go places with them, to change Haven's diaper and put her new little hairs in a ponytail. The nanny got to do that first, not me. Feeling sorry for myself right now, and stressed. I guess I need to do a gratitude list.

Here it goes:

I am grateful because my arm works and I can still carry Haven and give Lucky hugs.

Micah is working a lot this week, and work is good, even if it stresses me out to have him gone.

for a fridge full of amazing food donated by amazing people.

I have a family who are making themselves crazy to get here to help me.

I have the Internet—seriously, what would I do all day without it?

I am grateful for the health of my family and friends.

Xo Katie

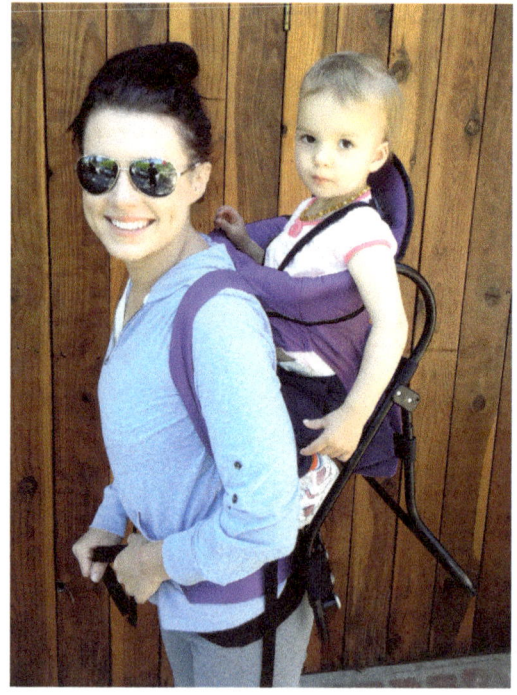

Haven and Hannah

## 10/17/12

It's been an emotional day. I cried all over my poor friend who was sitting with me. Called my doctor and told him I was having a nervous breakdown. There wasn't much he could say, but he did tell me that he has seen people who got temporarily worse after radiation, but ultimately ended up doing better long term because the radiation worked so well and didn't have necrosis. He says he's seen that a lot. I am going to hold on to that thought to get me through to Monday.

I'm a blubbering idiot. TV makes me cry, nice things people say make me cry, a text from Micah saying he misses me causes me to burst into tears. Man, I love him. I can't even sleep anymore unless I'm touching him. He's my rock. A great husband and fantastic daddy. I'm hoping to wake up feeling good enough to take Haven to her class, even though it exhausts me. I love to watch her play; she's such a riot. Tonight when I put her to bed, she asked for Lucky to come in and give her kisses and hugs. He was so honored, he gave her about five hugs and kisses and said, "You're the best little baby." I am grateful to witness that tonight.

Xo Katie

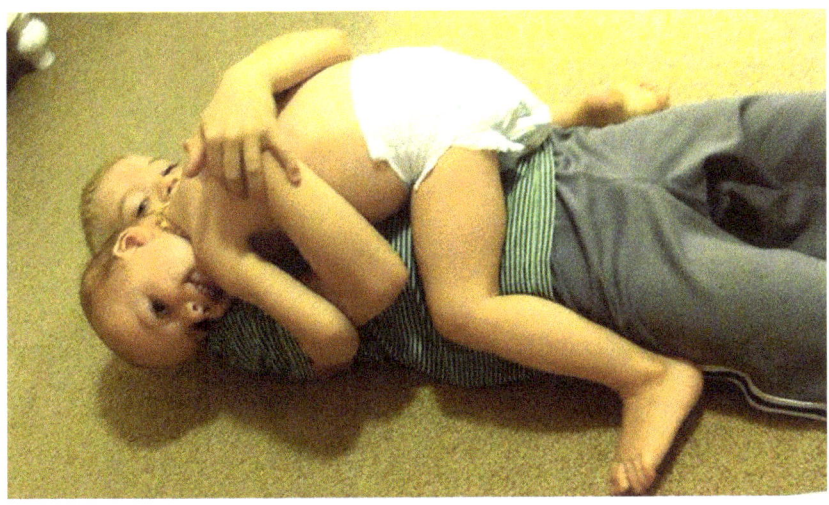

Brother love

## 10/18/12

It feels like I've been hit by a truck. I'm so tired. Drained.

## 10/20/12

Hi. I've been busy. Getting ready for our neighborhood Halloween party in the 'hood. I'm planning to do something gory and in bad taste with my head tomorrow. I can't really pass up the opportunity. I love Halloween!

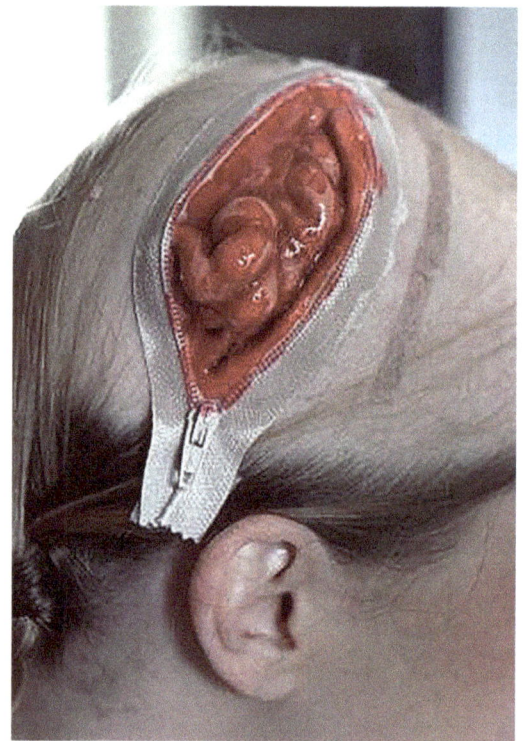

It's not real! Happy Halloween!

As I've said, it's been a tough week, getting closer to MRI Monday, and I'm trying to stay CALM, and not have any attachment to the results, knowing that whatever they are, everything will turn out fine. My life has been filled with medical obstacles, and I have always overcome them. This will be no different. I started a new book called *The Power of Now* by Eckhart Tolle. Not an easy read I have to say. It's about trying to stay in the moment. Ironically, while reading it my mind starts to wander! I read a few pages, then feel the need to take a nap!

Healthwise I am status quo, seizures, maybe two or three a day. Stress has been making them last longer. Had a two-to three-minute one this morning, and it left my lips numb. My hand is still knocked out. I saw my neuropsychologist yesterday. He poses some interesting questions. I said to him, if I knew that my hand would be better in a certain period of time, like six months or something, then it wouldn't bother me so much because there would be a light at the end of the tunnel, and he asked, "What if they told you that you wouldn't get it back?" I had to think about that. I said I would probably go through a period of depression, and then I would start finding ways to cope. What choice would I have? There are people in this world who are worse off than I am, for sure. I have everything I want under one roof. I would find a way to cope. With that said I am getting tired of dragging my hand around behind me; it is constantly getting bumped and bruised, and yesterday I accidently dragged it across the top of the hot toaster. I need to be more aware of what it's doing.

I've done a few errands this weekend. I wish that going out in public didn't make me so anxious. I just can't shake that memory of being in public and having that big seizure. That memory is still so vivid. So just going out gives me the actual sensations that I'm having a seizure. I try to calm myself, but then I spend my whole time trying to shift my mind instead of enjoying the moment. Hence the new book!

Xo Katie

## 10/21/12

I was able to take my kids to their Halloween parade. I even did my costume. Lucky wanted me to walk with him, and I was able to hold his right hand with my left. That definitely goes on my gratitude list today. Even though my MRI is tomorrow, I feel less anxious than I did a week ago. I am living in the moment, distracting myself with things that need doing and things that bring me joy. I am at peace with whatever happens tomorrow because it has already been decided, and worrying about it now will do me no good.

I am optimistic anyway, as always. I love the word hope. It has gotten me through a lot. I actually almost named Haven Hope because I felt like when other people thought I should stop trying to have her, I never even came close to giving up hope. Thank God I didn't, because she is pure love, even more than I could have hoped for. Dream big.

Xo Katie

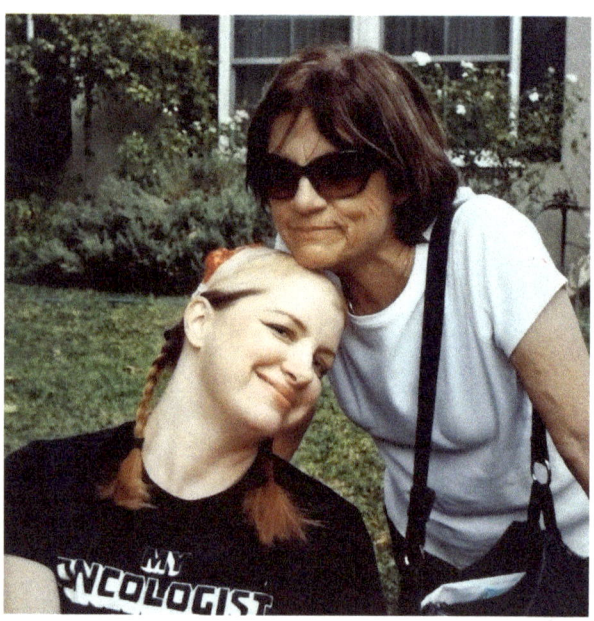

At the Halloween parade with my mom

## 10/22/12

Okay, I know a lot of people are on pins and needles, so I will give you the scoop.

Unfortunately, not too much change except that it (tumor/swelling) has gotten a bit bigger. It is pushing my brain off center. Not what we hoped for but not surprising. Basically we are faced with the same dilemma we were facing a month ago except for the fact that my hand is getting worse, which is concerning my doctor. The fact is that we may never know without a biopsy whether or not this is tumor growth or "pseudo-growth," which just means that the radiation did its job, maybe too well. The biggest problem is that this swelling is putting so much pressure on the motor area of my hand and face that if left to resolve on its own, which could take up to a year, it could cause permanent damage in my hand and face and maybe my leg. Not a scenario I can live with, so we are left with choices. Get a biopsy and see if this is tumor growth or necrosis. If it's growth, then we would know to just attack it with a different chemo and that's it. OR, we assume it probably isn't tumor growth but still do chemo anyway. At that point we would have covered all the bases, which my doc is encouraging me to do. In addition, to get rid of the necrosis and restore the use of my hand and prevent permanent damage, I would also take Avastin, which would get rid of all swelling and necrosis, shrink the tumor significantly (according to him), and restore all function in my hand within a matter of days. Sounds pretty amazing. Then you have to weigh the possible side effects. The chemo is generally well tolerated (I've heard that before), maybe some nausea, maybe some more hair loss, it's hard on blood cell counts, and can cause leukemia.

Avastin can cause strokes, pulmonary problems, and holes in your GI tract. Usually the Avastin side effects happen with the first dose, so within a couple of weeks. The good news is that I could get off all these other drugs: steroids, seizure meds, anxiety drugs, and get my hand and life back. Possibly very quickly and my tumor could shrink "significantly." After an hour and a half of talking with the doctor, we decided to go with both drugs.

I can't take the chance of losing my hand permanently, or worse, the whole left side. I've been living like a prisoner in my house with round-the-clock care for six weeks and it sucks; it's not much of a life. We feel the risks are worth the payoff of getting my life back and quality of life with my family.

If my insurance approves it I could potentially start this week with a four-hour infusion of Avastin. Also, I would start the CCNU (chemo) pill that same day. I don't feel pressured or like I'm basing my decision on fear. It feels right.

Xo Katie

## 10/23/12

I am going to take a break from talking about this decision today. I hadn't had a seizure in 24 hours before yesterday, and since we left the doctor, I've had five, three in the middle of the night, one really long one. I'm exhausted and stressed. I'm doing research and looking into a possible second opinion at UCLA, just to be extra sure. Very hard choices. So I may not answer calls or texts today. I'm going to try to get back to that place of calm and trust. Thanks for understanding.

Xo Katie

## 10/24/12

Still trying to wrap my mind around my decision. If you have called or emailed and I haven't responded, it's because it's too hard to talk about. The stress was getting to me.

I made an appointment for a second opinion Monday morning at UCLA with their neuro-oncologist just to clinch the deal and help me feel even more confident in my decision. I was helped and reminded today by my friend and hypnotherapist, John, that many things in my life have gone well for me, many times even better than expected, and that I am not always the person who gets the rug pulled out from under them, not always the person who things go wrong for. I am blessed in so many ways, and I have made many good decisions in my life. I consider myself to be the luckiest unlucky person there is, if there can be such a thing.

I need to start trusting myself more. Doctors aren't perfect, drugs can be unpredictable, but what I can trust is my ability to think and make decisions for myself. I still feel like I'm making the right decision. After these last two weeks of not being able to use my hand, and watching it get even worse, I can't risk losing it anymore. I was asked what I would do if everything works as well as we hope, and I know I would spend as much time as possible with my kids, doing things with them, taking them places, creating memories, enjoying my freedom, my independence, my privacy. Living without anxiety and fear for the first time in months would be heaven. I honestly can't even imagine it at this point, but I have all the hope in the world.

Xo Katie

## 10/26/12

I'm more tired than usual today, only one seizure since yesterday, and of course it happened as I was filling out my paperwork for my doctor's appointment at UCLA. It's so clear that they are stress related, and nothing stresses me out more than talking about this fucking tumor and these drugs. I'm feeling good about going ahead with the plan, even before the second opinion. I am noticing that I am getting weaker on my left side, my arm and maybe even my leg, as I notice

I'm tripping more and shuffling more, and I am afraid I will need a walker or wheelchair soon. It makes the decision easier.

I know that I am capable of making good and right decisions, and I think this is one of those that will turn out even better than I hoped. When I go back and analyze the decisions in my life that have turned out well, or even better than expected, they were all based on love, love for myself, not fear. "Oh, if I don't do this something bad will happen." They were all made with the idea of moving me forward and getting me to the next stage in my life, fulfilling dreams. I fell asleep last night thinking of as many of these choices I made as I could and realizing that there were even more than I thought, that not everything in my life has to be difficult before it can be good, before the dream is realized. As my dad would say, "You fell into a butter tub," meaning things worked out perfectly for me.

Everyone should spend time tonight thinking of ten things that worked out perfectly for them, whether through hard work, luck, or just good decision-making. I was so stuck in this thinking that even though everything always turns out okay, I was destined to suffer first, but upon reflection it's simply not true. Sometimes I made bad decisions (and learned from them), sometimes I got lucky, sometimes I made really good decisions, and sometimes I worked really fucking hard.

Xo Katie

## 10/27/12

Second opinion is set for Monday at UCLA, so good timing. I had a big seizure yesterday, the first one of its kind since the restaurant. Thankfully I was home. My children are so amazing and sensitive. Haven instinctively knows when I'm having a seizure, and comes over and touches me and says, "Mommy okay?" and Lucky will come and give me cuddles and kisses. I stopped taking all of my supplements on Monday because I felt disappointed that they hadn't reduced the inflammation, and the doctor basically said, "Don't bother."

Xo Katie

## Later...

More thoughts: Someone very smart and dear to me asked an important question: Do you feel that you've made any mistakes or bad decisions in this process? A hard question. Ultimately when I thought about it I had to say "No."

Every decision I made was based on research and the best information from my doctors. I trust them, still do. So then, going back to the first "event," which we felt unprepared for, where the rug had been pulled out from under us, the surgery.

What if we go back and instead think of that situation as the first stepping stone in a process that will lead me to being healed, maybe in a way that will be even better than if the tumor had been removed? We don't know the greater plan here. Every step leads to somewhere. All of these rugs being pulled out from under us could be magic carpet rides! Woo hoo! Just like my turbulent and potentially dangerous, precarious pregnancies, I got way more than I could have dreamt of in my wildest dreams. My babies definitely rode in on magic carpets! Why limit myself to "standard treatment" when my body knows it can do better than that. My doc says the CCNU chemo, even though it can be harder on blood counts and have dangerous, but rare, side effects, ultimately people on it do better long term; they live LONGER. So maybe being allergic to the other one will serve me better. Maybe reacting too strongly to the radiation, then getting rid of the necrosis with Avastin, will shrink the tumor to the equivalent of scar tissue!

Before, they were only saying 20 percent shrinkage. So I will stay

open to the adventure, because that's really all any of us can do.
**Song of the day: "Magic Carpet Ride" by Steppenwolf**
Xo Katie

## 10/28/12

Feeling very fragile right now.

## 10/29/12

Okay, I'm going to try to get through this. It's been an exhausting but good day. First, Dr. Cloughesy at UCLA felt like what I was experiencing was most likely a normal response to radiation, not tumor growth (mainly because I have that great IDH1 marker that makes my tumor so much less aggressive). He even felt like I have probably had it since I was 15 or 16 years old! 30 years! That's nuts! He also didn't feel like this was radiation necrosis because real radiation necrosis doesn't present itself this soon after radiation; it normally starts months or years later. Great news! So what we are left with is "a tumor that's on its way out." We all looked at the MRIs together, and he confirmed that it did not look like the tumor was growing or getting more aggressive (yay!) and it did not look like radiation necrosis! Just a good response from the radiation with admittedly a large amount of swelling that is causing neurological issues. He felt like there was still the option to do nothing but wait for the tumor to continue to die, which could cause the swelling and issues to get temporarily worse as it peaked, and then it would probably slowly go down. The problem with this option is that it could take months or a year, and in the meantime I could lose function permanently, and in the meantime my quality of life sucks because I still can't use my hand, my leg could get worse, and I have to stay on steroids. I would probably still have seizures and need continuous care. Not a good option for me.

He didn't feel that the chemo was necessary because he didn't feel that it was tumor growth, but he also didn't think it would hurt, and that it was a reasonable thing to do, especially since I didn't get to finish the other chemo.

He felt that the Avastin was worth trying, but didn't have the enthusiasm that my other doc does. He said basically that it will either work within the first two to four weeks or it won't. I would probably know within the first two weeks. He did think it would reduce the swelling, but wasn't as encouraging that I would regain function in my hand, at least not fully, but that once the swelling was reduced then physical therapy would help. Both doctors agreed on that. They also agreed that physical therapy at this point would be useless. Once some swelling goes down I can start tapering off the steroids. I asked him if he felt Avastin and CCNU were a reasonable course of action, and he said yes. He also felt that I had a lesser chance of having the negative side effects, like a stroke, because "you are young" (yay!).

So basically we got the green light from him, as well as the great news that he thinks my tumor is not growing or acting dangerous. A good day.

Xo Katie

## 10/30/12

Hi. Everything went well today. It was a little stressful morning trying to get out of the house by 6:45 a.m. so we ended up leaving without me having taken any of my regular meds, no seizure meds or steroids. We had to make the hospital and doctor's office scramble to get them for me. After some blood work was done and cleared, we were good to go and then had to wait for the pharmacy to get the Avastin and "premeds" ready.

The premeds consisted of Aloxi, an anti-nausea med for the CCNU tonight, and 10 mg of the hard-core steroid Decadron. I'm already on eight milligrams a day, so now it's 18, good grief. Then the Avastin was ready and they hooked me up. It took about 90 minutes from that point. Nothing exciting, I listened to my iPod and read my book. I am feeling some minor, positive changes. I can hold my left and right arm out in front of me with my palms up. I couldn't do that yesterday. My arm feels "lighter," less like dead weight. I can move my fingers a bit. Looking forward to seeing what develops in the coming days, but looks positive for now. Starting the CCNU tonight.

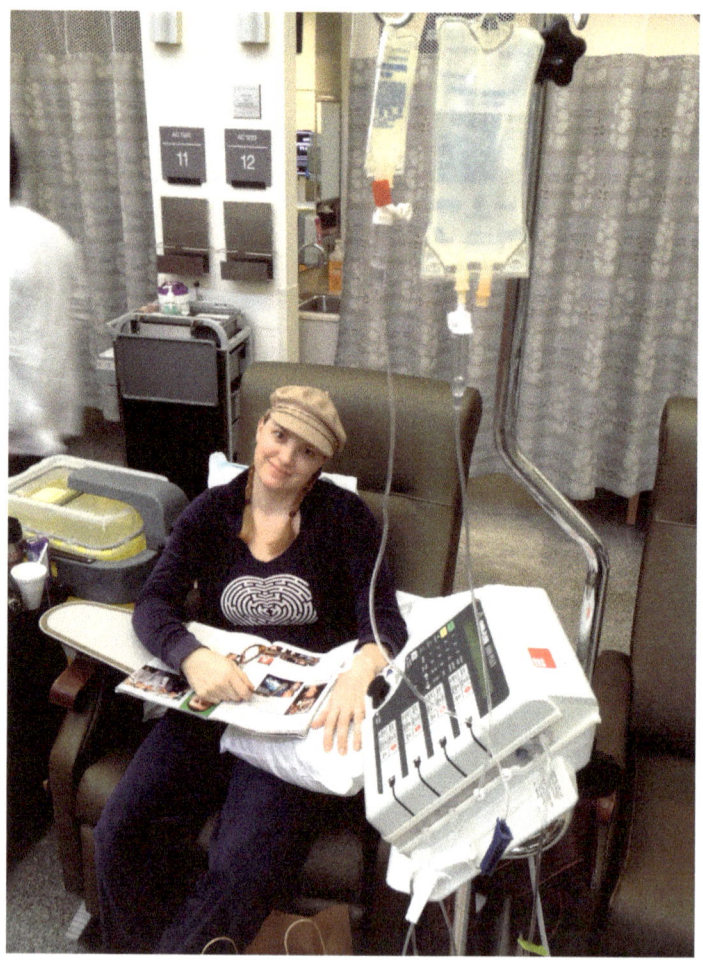

Hooked up to Avastin and CCNU

Hopefully I can start tapering off the steroids soon. I can't really describe the feeling of being on Decadron. I can understand why athletes take them, though, because they make you feel as if you could actually tear someone apart with your bare hands just because you can't find your pen :). Sometimes I feel like my head might start spinning around, then just fly off. The rage is so scary, you can't imagine it's possible. It's a really unpleasant feeling. In addition you are ravenous and craving all the foods that are the worst for you, like carbs and sugar. Plus you get this round "moon face" just to make you feel worse, because being angry and bald isn't bad enough; you can add round and bloated to the list.

Xo Katie

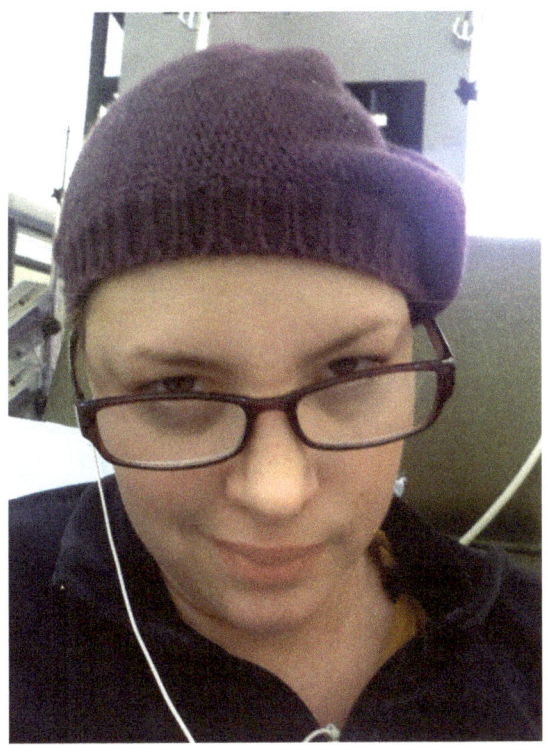

IV Avastin, not doing well, losing function on my left side and crooked face, hoping this helps.

## 10/31/12

So blessed to have been able to do everything I wanted to do with my kids this Halloween. We decorated, went to Lucky's All Hallows Eve at school, went to the pumpkin patch, carved pumpkins (yes, I did, with one hand), got great costumes, went to our neighborhood parade, and went trick or treating tonight. I felt really good and walked about eight blocks. It was a perfect night.

Today I have noticed that I am walking better, not dragging my foot, not bumping into walls, not banging my hand into doors, and I have been able to pick up a couple of things with my left hand. The palsy in my face looks better too, to me anyway. I'm feeling optimistic. I officially started chemotherapy last night. I was so tired today and woke up with a slight headache, but got a second wind this evening. One seizure this morning, but that's it. Can't wait to taper off the 'roids as the heartburn is murder. Excited to see what improvements I see tomorrow.

Xo Katie

## 11/3/12

I haven't posted in a while. I've been busy using my hand! Little bits of progress every day. It's exciting. Lots of times I forget that I can use it, and I have to remind myself to not just let it hang by my side. I'm still dealing with lots of anxiety, still worried about side effects of these new drugs. With every headache I imagine I'm having a stroke. I think my imaginary symptoms and anxiety will be harder to get rid of than this tumor. I can't believe it's November already. Thinking about actually being able to host Thanksgiving is exciting, and brings new meaning to the term "Thanksgiving."

Xo Katie

## 11/4/12

I'm definitely feeling the effects of the chemo, just generally wiped out. I feel slow and I know I am stumbling over words; my voice is even strained. I remember when I first started radiation and chemo in July and was complaining to my doctor about this kind of stuff and him saying that I needed to remember that I was on radiation and chemo and that he'd be surprised if I wasn't feeling this way. So I need to cut myself some slack and remember my body is being bombarded right now by some pretty toxic drugs.

I think, because I'm not doing the chemo again for six to eight weeks, that hopefully my body will adjust, and I'll get some energy back before I have to take the next round. Meanwhile I will do more Avastin in eight days.

I've been thinking a lot about the fact that Dr. Cloughesy at UCLA thinks I've had this tumor since age 15 or so. That changes some things for me. It rules out pregnancy hormones as a cause. Micah happily ruled himself out as a trigger, but what's more interesting to me is what it leaves in. For it to start growing at such a young age, you have to break it down to genetics, environment, or factors such as stressors.

As far as genetics go, there isn't a lot of cancer in my family. Both of my grandmas had cancer in their 70's but went on to live 20 more years, that's it. If we look at environmental factors, then there could be a few. I had a uterine birth defect, and my sister had a heart defect.

Not to place blame at all, nobody really knew any better, but I was raised in a home with two smokers, so lots of secondhand smoke. Plus my mom smoked while she was pregnant. And don't forget those three CAT scans to my brain when I was thirteen, a ton of radiation to a growing brain with a thin skull. There have been studies done that show that CAT scans to a child's brain have caused brain tumors and leukemia. My doctor told me that back then in 1982, they weren't even sure that their CAT scan machines were calibrated correctly (even if they were you still get 150-200 times more radiation from a CAT scan than an x-ray), so you could be getting much more radiation to your brain than they thought. This happened at 13 years old and apparently right before this thing took residence in my head.

I'll obviously never know, but it does make me think about my kids and what I can do to protect them. Not to scare people but brain tumors are the second highest form of childhood cancer! I never would have guessed that. Just more to think about.

Xo Katie

## 11/5/12

I am finally able to flip Betsy off! Yay! Being able to raise one finger independently is a big deal. I haven't been able to do it for at least a month. Progress!

Xo Katie

## 11/6/12

I got my baby girl dressed all by myself today, from diapers to socks to a sweater with little buttons! Huge deal. I haven't dressed her in over a month. If I can take care of my children's needs and take basic care of myself, then I am happy. Next Avastin infusion is the 14th.

Xo Katie

## 11/7/12

I'm starting to allow myself to imagine/fantasize a time when my life won't be consumed with all things cancer. It's almost incomprehensible to me that there will be a time when I don't need help, I will be driving again, even just being able to be alone. Will there be a time when I won't be taking medication, really? Once the chemo is done there will be a point when we are just watching things with MRIs every few months and trying not to worry about it in between. That will be it for the rest of my life. I think the majority of the work at that point, even now, will be about my anxiety. Living life without worrying about the "what-ifs." It's what I'm working on with the neuro-psychologist. Man, it's tough. It's so easy to let my mind go to "the bad place" and think about not only what could happen, but I even have anxiety about what could have happened. For example, I get really upset when I think about the week before my surgery when I took Lucky to Disneyland by myself. I think about what would've happened if I had had a seizure and Lucky would've been helpless and on his own. I can really get myself into a tizzy thinking about that. I know it didn't happen, but I can't help but feel fear about that and wonder if I will ever feel safe being alone with the kids, especially in a situation like that. It's a sad feeling.

On a much more positive note, I am still seeing progress little by little every day. I can now touch each finger to my thumb, unimaginable a week ago. My next goal is to be able to type with two hands!

Xo Katie

## 11/9/12

So, I was cleaning off my desk today and found my folder that had all my medical paperwork in it. As I was going through it, I was amazed at all the things I did and all of the people I went to for advice, "healing," herbs, etc. Looking back I can see that everything I did at that time was out of panic. Some of the advice I followed and people I went to now seem crazy to me. Some were outright scams. Obviously at that time I was just in shock and would've done and tried pretty much anything if you told me it would buy me time or shrink my tumor. A lot of time and money wasted. I feel so differently now; I feel less vulnerable, less gullible. Now I listen to my instincts, do my research, listen to my doctors, and get second opinions. Now I work really hard to not operate out of fear or panic. I ended up throwing most of that paperwork and info out, and it felt good.

There is definitely a place for complementary therapies, supplements, energy healers, etc., but I don't need to participate in ALL of them.

Xo Katie

## 11/11/12

Haven't been feeling very good. I couldn't tell if it was because I had a minor cold, or if it's the new chemo, or the Avastin. I only have a few hours a day, usually in the morning, where I have energy and feel pretty good. As the day wears on, even after a good nap, I feel weak, shaky, achy, tired, and just plain bad. I also have bad insomnia. I did a little research, as I'm prone to do, and discovered, as I suspected, that it's the tapering off of the steroid Decadron that is making me feel terrible. Decadron is so hard core. After being on it for only a few weeks, it completely shuts down your adrenal glands and constantly floods your body with the stress hormone cortisol. When you try to get off the steroid, you have to do it so slowly so that your body can adjust and start up the adrenals again. Stopping the steroid suddenly can kill you. I want to get off it so fast that I've been pushing the doctor to keep the taper going, but I think I may have to go slower than I'd like because I am getting headaches that wake me in the night, and I'm not functioning well in the day. At this point I don't know which is worse, being on it or getting off it. Thanks for listening to me vent!

Xo Katie

## 11/12/12

Nine days without a seizure, but what's even better is that today is the first day when I haven't felt like I was going to have a seizure. That's huge. I've had days without seizures, but I would always feel like I was on the verge of one, or I actively had to stop myself or work on calming myself. Today I felt normal. Hoping for more days like this. Also hoping the Avastin on Wednesday does a number on the swelling and I get some more function back. I am still making slow progress but I want it faster. I can see the loss of muscle in my hand and arm. My doc says to wait on physical therapy until a few more infusions so we know what I am actually left with, and because there is still swelling, there is no point to doing it now. People don't realize that the real problem isn't with my hand; exercise won't help. The problem is in my brain. I've had people ask me if I've tried acupuncture, or herbs. Really? I don't want to be rude, but it's brain cancer, not a headache.
Xo Katie

## 11/14/12

I had my infusion today, lots of hurrying up and waiting. Before my infusion they have to run blood work, then get the okay from the doc; then the pharmacy has to deliver the meds. Unfortunately my blood counts were low, platelets about half what they were two weeks ago. FYI: platelets are responsible for clotting, so if they get too low, you can have bleeding internally, etc. They are still not too low, so the doc gave us the green light to do the Avastin because the blood counts are from the CCNU not from Avastin. But it is still a big deal, so now my blood needs to be checked every week, and if it gets below a certain number, I may need a blood or platelet transfusion. This is a common side effect but it usually doesn't happen until the fourth or fifth week, and we are only two weeks in. Yet again my sensitivity to medication kicks in. Just going with the flow. If things do get worse, then they will decrease my dosage and also switch me from an every six-week schedule to every eight weeks.

In the meantime I am going to take supplements like astragalus and shark liver oil to increase my platelets, and I will also be hitting the pipe because melatonin is also good for blood counts and marijuana raises melatonin levels really high.

My doctor was really happy about my progress and how much I've improved. He thinks I will improve even more and that after Thanksgiving I should start some physical therapy.

Xo Katie

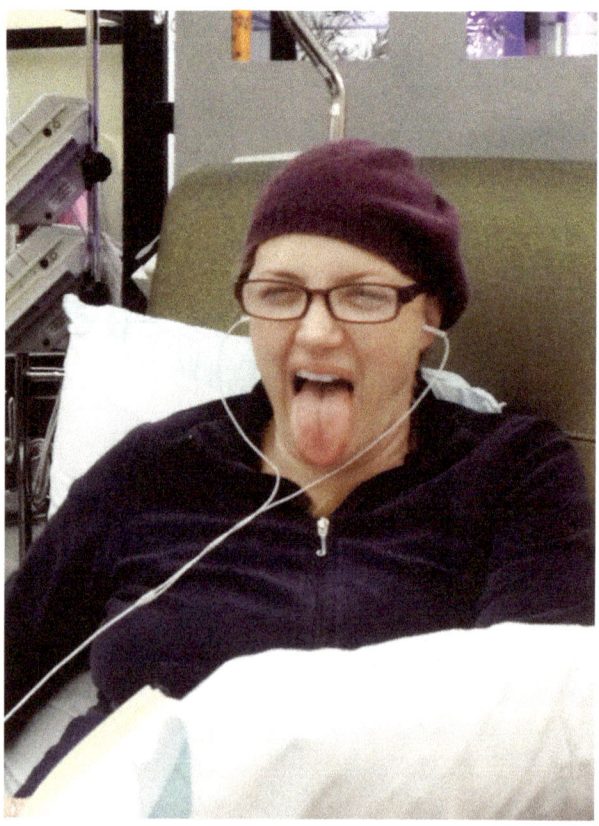

Being cheeky

## KATIE KAISER SMITH

### 11/16/12

I am suffering from an annoying side effect of the Avastin; it is attacking my vocal cords, so it sounds like I am losing my voice all the time, and it can be a strain to talk. My doctor calls it the "sexy Avastin voice" and says it will eventually go away. Right now it just makes talking tiring.

I've been thinking lately about the whole "cancer" label. I have such a hard time with it, especially, as I've said before, since I don't view myself as someone with cancer. I'm not delusional, but I can't get behind cancer awareness campaigns—is there anyone who isn't aware of cancer? What I want to say is "I HAD cancer but I don't anymore." Realistically that could be true. I don't want to use the term remission either. What that really means is that you've been able to keep your cancer at bay for five years; it doesn't mean it won't come back. They don't use that word anyway for brain cancer. They say NED—No Evidence of Disease, because it is considered terminal. You either have an active tumor or a dormant one (NED). Let's face it, a lot of cancers come back, especially brain cancers. It doesn't have to, but I want to think long term. I want to be able to live my life without having to look over my shoulder all the time. Unfortunately, there isn't a lot of data on long-term survivors, meaning 20 years or more, because back then there was no chemo that could pass through the blood-brain barrier, and if you got radiation you got whole brain radiation where they didn't expect you to live long enough to experience the horrible side effects of what that does to you.

That's why I don't choose to surround myself with cancer. There are no examples of what to expect or what to look forward to. I don't want to actively resist it because I believe that what you resist persists, so I need to be comfortable with talking about it. But it's not going to encompass my whole life. Lucky has never even heard the word, and I'd like to keep it that way. It's hard to say, or even write down that I have/had brain cancer. "Oh, I have a grade-three anaplastic astrocytoma, brain cancer." That's a mouthful. I know what people are thinking when I tell them. "Oh shit, she's going to die." "Her days are numbered—her poor kids." It's what I'd be thinking too if I heard someone I knew had brain cancer. Let's face it, it sounds terrible. But there are definitely worse things to have, not many, but my prognosis is good. It's bad, but it's not as bad as it sounds. At least it doesn't have to be.

Sorry to ramble on, just some stuff I was thinking about.

Xo Katie

## 11/19/12

Yesterday Lucky was at my friend Paige's house playing with her son Logan. They were talking about their neighbor's cat who is very ill. Logan asked if the cat had gone to heaven yet. Paige said no, and explained to Lucky that the cat had something wrong with its heart and that its heart was not working right. Lucky thought for a moment and then said, "That's not what my mom has." Paige said he was right, that it's not what I have, and assured him that the doctors were making me better. When Paige told me this story, I started crying. That he would even think that made me so sad. I wish so badly that this wasn't a part of our lives and that neither one of us ever had to think about me not being there for him. I read an article about Rosie O'Donnell, whose mother died when she was 10, and she says she barely remembers her. That scares me. A lot. If I died, Haven would have no memories of me at all, and even Lucky would struggle to remember me. My doctor said that we are lucky and that he had a friend who died suddenly of a heart attack at 40. He said I have the time to take photos and videos and to write things down for the kids, and I should take advantage of this time. That's so sad but also good if you think about it.

These are the hard facts. Haven is a baby. I don't know if I will live long enough for her to remember me. This is in the back of my mind whenever I am with her. We all know I am a "glass half full" kinda girl, but I can't pretend that I don't think about this shit. On the plus side (cuz I always like to close with a plus side), I am typing this with two hands (one is very shaky), and I braided my own hair last night. It didn't look very good, but I did it nevertheless. Baby steps.

Xo Katie

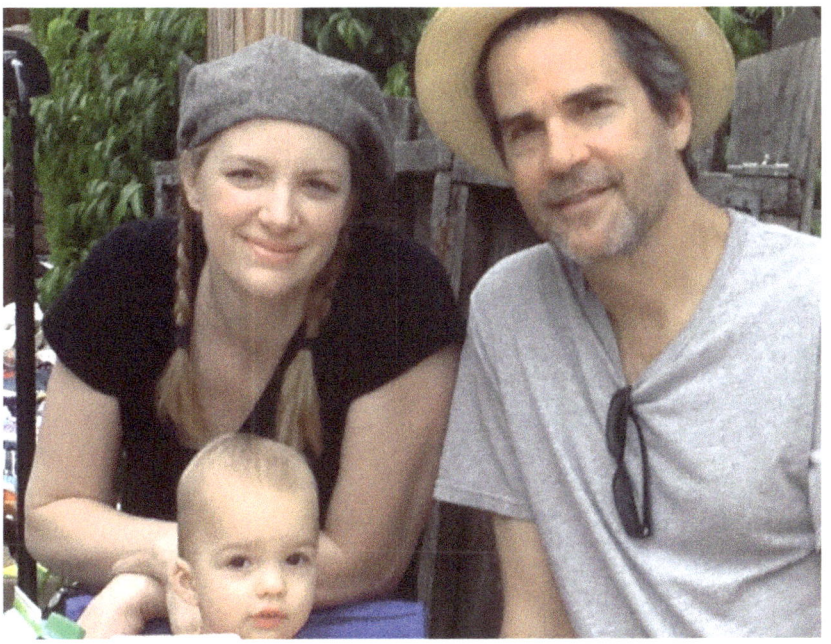

Catching memories on film

## 11/21/12

I'm thankful for so much this year. If I didn't have this thing in my head, I'd say I was leading a charmed life. Blessed with amazing family and amazing friends. I don't know what I did to deserve such amazing friends and family. This may turn out to be the least stressful holiday season ever for me. I definitely appreciate things more considering I had no idea how I would be right now. I was heading toward being in a wheelchair, and now I am about 80 percent back. It's a miracle. The blood work I had yesterday came back great; my numbers are up, so no blood or platelet transfusion for me this time! Yay! I've been taking supplements that are meant to help blood counts: shark liver oil, astragalus, and melatonin. I guess they worked. I am so thankful. I'm thankful for no seizures for two and a half weeks. I'm thankful for the quarter inch of hair I have now. I have a hairline again! I'm thankful for modern medicine and my doctors and complementary therapies.

Special thanks for making my holidays less stressful: Renee B, Melanie W, and Arch and Julie S. I don't know how to say thank you enough.

Xo Katie

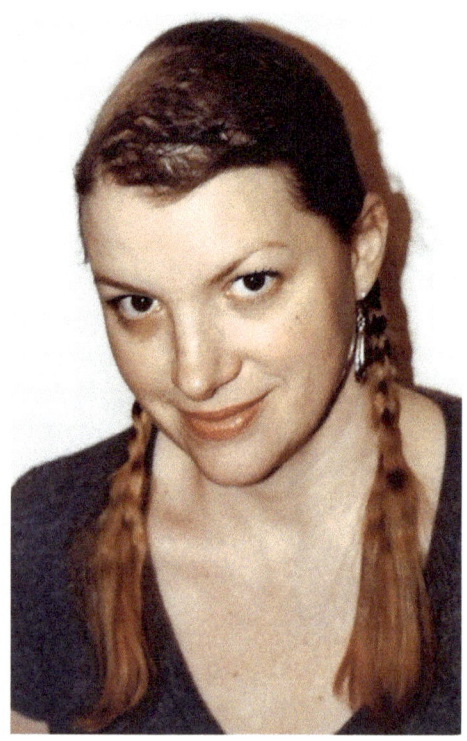

I have a hairline again!

## 11/23/12

Hope everyone had a nice Thanksgiving. Ours was excellent and I've already had three meals from the leftovers. So happy that I was able to fully participate.

My boy turns seven tomorrow. He makes me so proud. What a sweet, loving, smart, and funny boy. Seven years ago I was eating Thanksgiving dinner in the hospital and feeling more thankful than I ever had before. This is going to be a short post because I want to write in Lucky's journal tonight. He has three full journals and Haven has one. It's hard to be disciplined enough to write regularly, but I try. I think it's important, especially now. I'm glad that I have because it would be really hard to try to play catchup now. Don't let it pile up, get those digital photos printed out! My two cents for the day,
Xo Katie

## 11/26/12

Now that Thanksgiving and Lucky's birthday are over, I'm excited to gear up for Christmas. I'm excited to be able to fully participate, planning our Christmas card, the kids' portraits, and wrapping gifts (all by myself!).

My friend Andrea asked me a question recently, and I told her I would think about it and post about it. I had told her once, a while ago, that raising kids was like being pecked to death by chickens. She asked me if I still felt that way. The answer is: sometimes. When I am feeling that way, I try to remind myself to be in the moment and stop thinking about all the things I could be/should be doing, try not to lose my temper or my patience as much, and remember what's really important. I'm definitely not perfect, though, and I'm definitely the stricter parent, or "The Hammer" as we like to call it.

I do lose my patience and my temper, my mind does wander while building Legos, but I make more of an effort to appreciate all these times and take a mental picture of each moment. I feel that if I act too differently or spoil my kids like I want to, then they would know something was wrong. I want them to feel safe and secure, to feel consistency. Me, being myself, is one of the best gifts I can give them.

It's too bad that it takes something like this to help me realize how precious even the mundane can be, especially when none of us are guaranteed a long and healthy life or the chance to see our children grow up. We just don't let ourselves think that way; it would be hard to maintain that anyway. There will hopefully be a point when even I start to forget. That would be a bit of a blessing.

Xo Katie

## 11/28/12

I lost a very special pet today, my cat Panda. I actually didn't lose him. He was taken out of my yard by a Pit Bull and a Rottweiler and killed as my babysitter chased them screaming. They ran, with my cat in the Pit Bull's mouth, back to their yard, where they dropped my now dead cat and ran back into their open gate. I am so heartbroken. He was 15 years old, and I had him since he was four weeks old. He was a beautiful Himalayan mix with gorgeous blue eyes. I loved him very much and he didn't deserve to die like that. I can't stop thinking about him and his last moments.

Xo Katie

## 11/30/12

So I have decided not to tell Lucky about Panda. Tonight Micah accidently broke Lucky's "favorite plate" (who knew?) and he cried for 20 minutes in his bed. I feel like he's so sensitive right now. I think Panda just ran away for now and I'll deal with it later. He needs some distance between me being ill and losing another beloved pet.

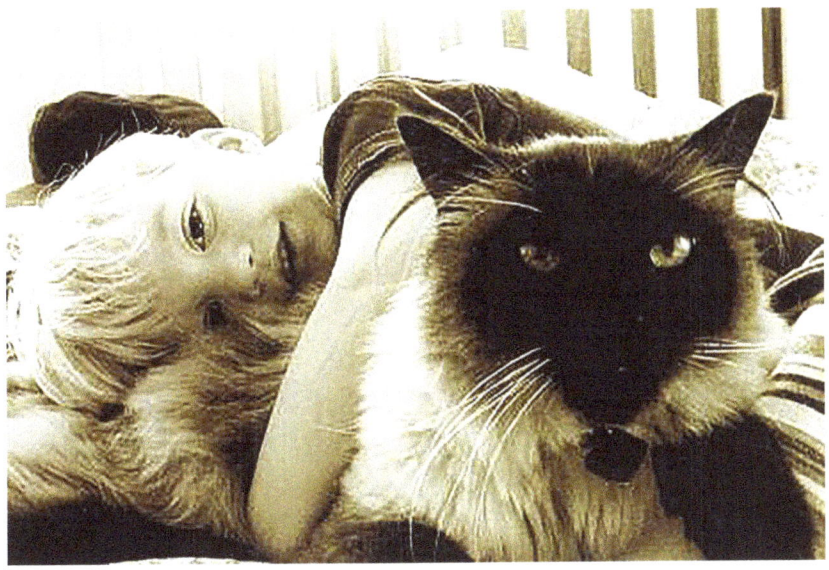

Lucky and Panda

I am getting another infusion of Avastin next week. I have seen some more improvement in my hand since the second infusion. I can type faster and more proficiently, but my hand is weak. Many times when I go to use my hand, like pushing a button or carrying a plate, my hand will shake and tremble. I am also almost off the steroids. I only take one milligram a day now, and I notice that my hand is weaker for a couple of days after we cut down on the dose, probably because of some "rebound swelling." I think that in a week or two, I will be done with it, hopefully for good. I have gained about 15 pounds because of it and can't wait to be done with it.

I am seriously debating whether or not to continue on the chemo. I will have an MRI in two weeks, and depending on what it shows I will make my decision. It is so hard on the body, and I don't want to take something so toxic if I don't need it. My whole body hurts, but it's very strange. I have pain in just my middle finger and in some toes, pain in my hips and knees, and it hurts to stand up out of bed in the morning. I will continue with the Avastin for a little while and then, based on the MRI and possibly another consultation with the UCLA doctor, I will decide whether to continue the chemo or not.

Looking forward to taking my kids to our school's winter faire tomorrow and the start of celebrating Christmas. The Advent calendars are coming out tonight as well as the Elf on the Shelf. I love this time of year. One month ago I had no idea how I would be at Christmastime, and I am so grateful I am functioning and able to do more and more every day.

Xo Katie

## 12/6/12

I had my third round of Avastin on Tuesday. It's been six weeks and my doctor is thrilled with how my hand is doing. He remarked on how "fluid" it was. I'd say my hand is about 90 percent back. It trembles sometimes because the muscles have atrophied, but my doctor says it's just weak. I am down to one milligram of Decadron (steroid) every other day. I will stay on some seizure meds, probably for a long time; then I can drive in a couple of months, hopefully. I will have an MRI in two weeks. My doc expects considerable change :)

Xo Katie

## 12/8/12

Misery loves company. Unfortunately that's a true statement. There is something comforting about someone else going through the same thing you are. When someone says to me, "I know someone who had a brain tumor," I always ask, "What kind is it? How big? Did they get it out?" I'm almost disappointed if they did. I haven't found anyone yet who is in the exact same situation as I am, and it's very isolating. Maybe it's different with other kinds of cancers, but with brain tumors there are so many different kinds and so many different scenarios that it's unlikely I will ever find someone who is going through the same experience. When I hear of celebrities getting things such as thyroid cancer or multiple sclerosis, I think, *I wish I had that*. I'm actually jealous. Even though their situations are different, it makes me feel better to hear about them. Not that I would wish this on anybody, I wouldn't, but it's going to happen, and it makes me feel not so alone. Does that make me a bad person? It feels like it does.

Xo Katie

### 12/15/12

I was going to write last night about how depressed I was because I have a red rash on my face and we don't know why, and then I saw the news and heard about all those children at the Sandy Hook school in Connecticut and decided I have nothing to complain about. My children were fast asleep in their beds. I went in and kissed them and covered them and tucked them in instead. I prayed for those parents and went to sleep.

Happy birthday to my husband Micah today, a great husband and father.

Xo Katie

### 12/17/12

I had my MRI and Avastin infusion today. Long day that started with an 8:15 a.m. MRI and ended at 5:30 p.m. with my infusion. The MRI looked good :) The swelling has gone down 35-50 percent, and the tumor has shrunk 15 percent. Doctor Rudnick was very happy. He said things are definitely moving in the right direction. He thought that if I hadn't started this treatment, I wouldn't be alive right now; at the very least I wouldn't be walking. We plan on taking my MRI back to UCLA to see Dr. Cloughesy to get his opinion as well. After the next MRI in two months, we will start weaning off one of my seizure meds. Right now there is still a chance I could have a seizure. I'm having a lot of dizziness, and he thinks it's definitely from the seizure meds.

Well, that's my update. If you don't hear from me, it's only because no news is good news. I'm trying to live my life as best I can considering I still can't drive and still need supervision, especially when I'm with my kids. I'm enjoying doing Christmas things and looking forward to a good holiday with my kids and family. Hope you are too,

Xo Katie

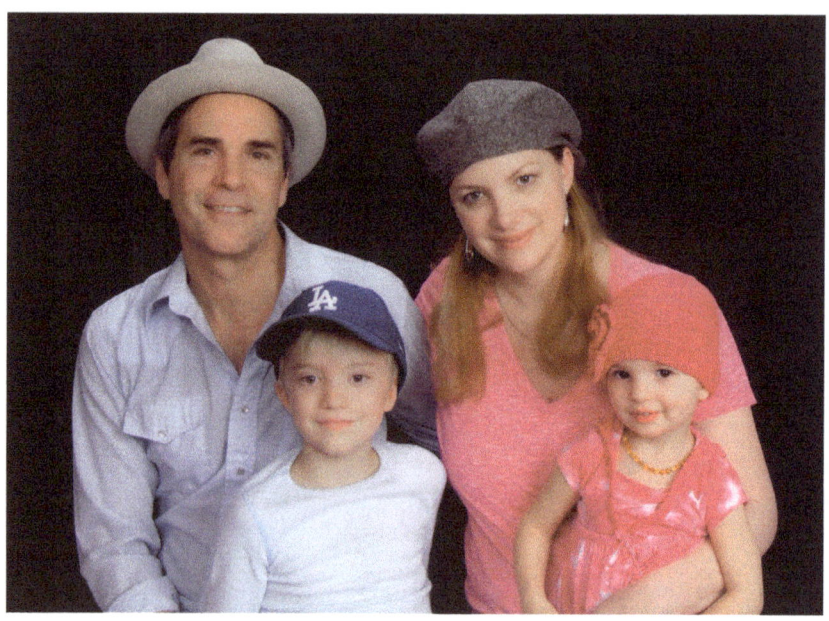

Yearly family photo, we decided we should all wear hats!

## 12/18/12

I don't know why I am not feeling as happy or satisfied with the news yesterday as everyone else seems to be. I think I was hoping for more. I know I was. I also wasn't expecting the doctor to tell me that I might have been dead by now if I hadn't opted for this treatment; that was never even mentioned. I am starting to wonder if anyone ever really "beats" brain cancer or if they are just buying themselves time. I find myself thinking, *Well, when I'm dead...* Whether it's two years from now, five years, or 15 years, I am just assuming that at some point this disease will get me. I don't want to think this way, but I also don't want to delude myself. I consider myself an optimistic realist.

When I'm in an optimistic phase I think, *Well, of course they are developing new, state-of-the-art treatments as we speak, so I just have to stay alive long enough for them to find a cure. Brain cancer is one of the most deadly cancers, so they throw a lot of money and research toward it, and they will find a cure for sure.* I relish the moments when I am preoccupied and I get an hour or so when I don't actually think about it.

I want Dr. Cloughesy to see my latest MRI and get his opinion on my prognosis. He was so much more optimistic and sure last time. I'm desperate for someone to give me assurance that I will be here to see my kids grow up, but I know no one can do that for me. When I hear from someone that they had a dream or a vision or a feeling that I would live a long time, it makes me so happy. I believe in those things, so I hang on every word. The thing that can make me spiral into depression is hearing about someone my age who just died from cancer. Or someone I went to school with who died from cancer and left three young children. These stay in my mind longer than they should. I want to be that exception.

Xo Katie

## 12/19/12

Thank you for the positive messages. They bring tears to my eyes. I love you guys.

## 12/22/12

Haven't been feeling well the last few days. I'm pretty sure I have a sinus infection. My whole face hurts, and I have had a throbbing headache for days and days that's only getting worse. I haven't had a sinus infection in 15 years, but the chemo makes me more prone to infections, so maybe that's why. Also my stomach is hurting really badly, probably from the chemo. I am nauseous and have barely eaten all day because it feels worse after I eat. I had the doctor on call paged and got a prescription for antibiotics. Hopefully I will wake up without a headache tomorrow. Supposed to go to a Christmas party tomorrow. It would be nice if I could actually eat.

You know I like to end on a positive note: I was home alone with the kids today as Micah came and went on multiple errands. First time I've been alone with them in months.

Xo Katie

## 12/25/12

MERRY CHRISTMAS EVERYONE

Hope you all are having a great holiday. Mine was pretty great. I feel better and my kids had a great day—that's all I care about.

I have decided, or I'm going to try, to not focus on the things I may never get to do, but instead I want to focus on all of the things I still have left to do. Everyone has things they want to do before they die, and we all think we have all the time in the world. I want to make sure that those things get accomplished. Making that shift made me feel better.

I got an amazing gift today from Krista's mom, Judy. It's a family heirloom, a needlepoint that says, "Yea, thou shalt see thy children's children." I burst into tears when I saw it. It meant so much to me. I took it as an omen.

Xo Katie

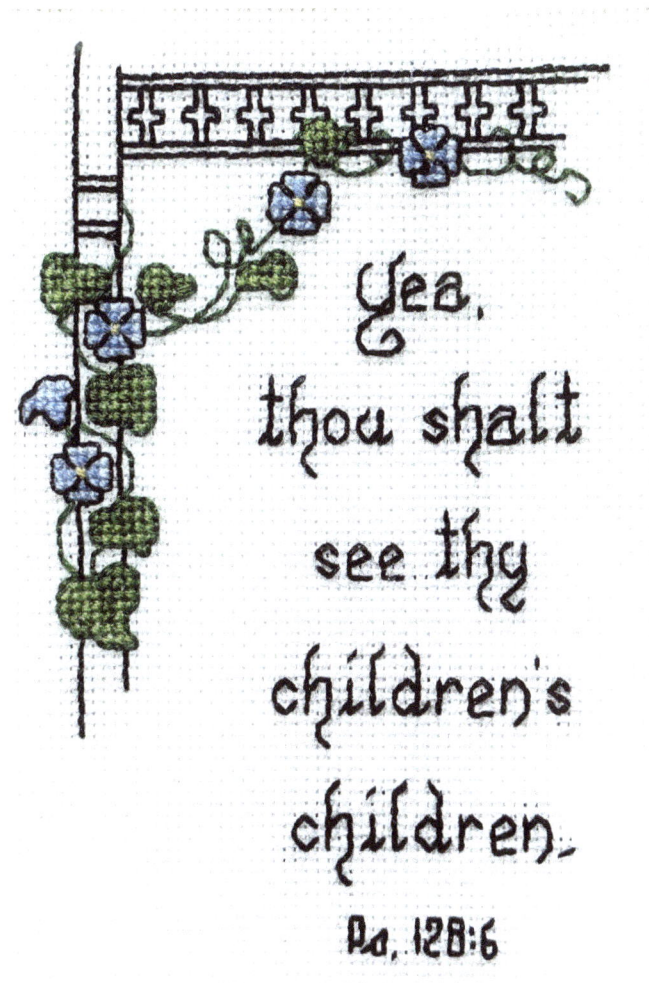

The perfect gift

## 12/26/12

I did good today. I almost bought one of those books where you can record yourself reading a book to your kids. I thought it would be nice for them to have me reading to them when I'm gone. Then I said, "Fuck that, I'm going to read to them in person."

Xo Katie

## 12/31/12

My New Year's resolution is to enjoy the present and not worry about what's around the corner. Definitely my biggest challenge and life lesson. I was having a freak-out meltdown tonight, and thank God Krista answered her phone at 11:00 p.m. on New Year's Eve to talk me down and remind me of this. Why is this so hard? I am so worried about not being here for my children that I am not appreciating the time I have with them.

My mom bought me a wig today. When I tried it on in the store, it looked so much like my old self that we both started crying. I want that Katie back. I've never seriously asked "Why me?" I figured the reason would reveal itself eventually, but I don't know how to live like this. How do you live with constant fear? I feel like I've been taken hostage.

Hence the resolution. It's not going to be easy, but I am going to try my hardest. What are your resolutions?

Happiest of New Years. Can't say I'm sad to say goodbye to 2012!

Xo Katie

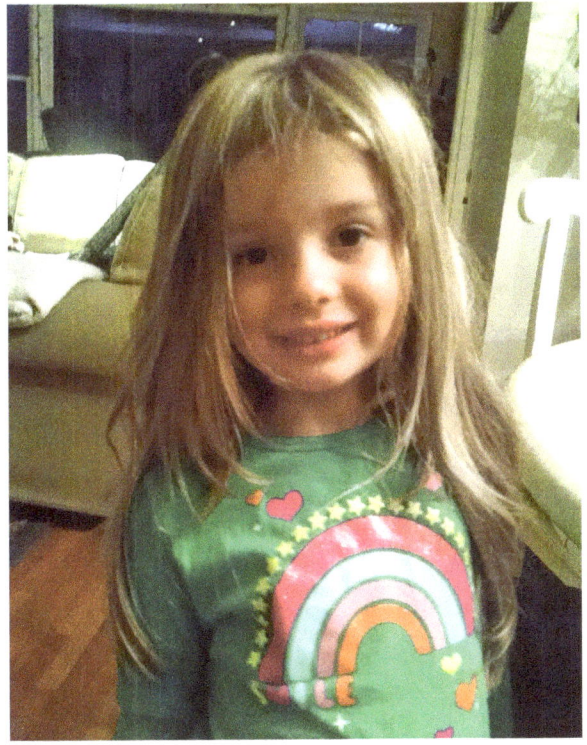

Haven wearing my new wig

## New Year! 2013
## 1/5/13

    I was in a rough place for a bit, but I'm coming out of it. STILL battling a sinus infection, which is frustrating, but considering the fact that I am immunocompromised, it could be worse. I had another Avastin infusion on Tuesday. It affects my voice, which makes it uncomfortable to talk, especially on the phone because I can't project; plus for some reason I just can't stand talking on the phone. I used to do most of my talking on the phone while I was driving (sound familiar?) and I haven't driven in eight months, so talking on the phone just takes me away from my kids and things I need to be doing at home. I also met with my doctor and asked him some important questions. I asked him why he said I wouldn't be here now if I hadn't started this medicine and why, If it was that serious, why did he give me a choice? He said he was alarmed at how rapidly I was declining and that it wasn't necessary that I start both medicines, but I needed at least one. Doing both was the most aggressive choice.

I also asked him a question that had been weighing on me. I asked him, "How does a brain tumor kill you?" I really didn't know and I needed to know. People don't realize that breast cancer doesn't kill you. If it did then having a mastectomy would be the end of it. Breasts don't kill. What happens is that by the time the cancer is found, errant cells have traveled to another part of your body that is crucial for survival, like your liver, lungs, or brain.

I wish that removing the cancer solved everything, but it doesn't always. So I needed to know what would happen in the worst-case scenario. I like information. I don't want to be surprised.

He said that the cancer would spread throughout the brain, and most people get sleepier and sleepier until one day they just forget to breathe. He said it's not a painful death. Could be worse. Now I can put that behind me and not think about it anymore. I plan on being around for a long time.

Xo Katie

## 1/7/13

Today I went to UCLA to see Dr. Cloughesy again to get his opinion on my latest MRI. He said the MRI definitely looked better, and he felt that what looked like remaining swelling may in actuality be scar tissue. There was definitely swelling before, but it's hard to tell now what is remaining. If the next scan doesn't show any shrinkage, then it is probably scar tissue; if it shrinks more, it is swelling. He said if it shrinks down to a very small tumor, then it might be reasonable to consider trying again to remove it. People who have their tumors removed have a better prognosis.

He mentioned again how my tumor, with the gene mutation I have (IDH1), is the "best tumor to have." We asked about new treatments that might be around the corner for me. He said there is work being done on a new medication for people with the IDH1 mutation specifically, which is good for me, and it will probably go into clinical trials in a year. I could only qualify, though, if my tumor is growing, so at this point it's better if I don't qualify and let other people be the guinea pigs.

I asked him what my prognosis is as far as life span, and he said it could be anywhere from 7-20 years. He said they don't know why it's seven for some and 20 for others. I wasn't surprised by this information because I've done the research from day one. Not that I'm happy about it—at the longest I would only be 61! Unacceptable. Micah was shocked. I saw it in his face. When we left the doctor's office, Micah was in a daze, and I said, "Now does it seem real to you?" I kind of felt he had been in denial. I was secretly glad that he could feel the sense of horror that I had been dealing with. I think I know why some people have a longer life span—positive attitude, healthy lifestyle, and support system.

Xo Katie

## 1/10/13

It's strange how my diagnosis has affected my relationships with people. I have made new friendships with people who I probably never would have met or hung out with, and now I feel such an affinity and love for them. They are strong when I can't be and they hold me up. They support me and don't ask anything in return because they know I don't have much to give right now. Then there are the people who are supposed to love you the most, and they can't handle it. Some are in denial and expect things to be the way they always were and some are scared because it hits too close to home; maybe they think it's contagious, or they think, *If it could happen to her, it could happen to me.* I've made many more friends than I've lost, but the loss still hurts. I had lunch with a friend today who used to be a client of mine and she said, "I don't think we'd be having lunch together right now if this hadn't happened to you," and that's probably true for a few friends. I'm grateful for these friendships. Definitely a positive thing that's come out of this. One of my mentors, Kris Carr (a cancer survivor), says, "The cream of the crop will rise to the top."

My goal, as I've said, is to bring joy into my life, which can sometimes include making hard choices. I have no choice but to be selfish right now, for the first time in my life, if I am to save my life. My true friends understand this and know that I do care about them and that I know the world doesn't revolve around me.

Xo Katie

## 1/11/13

Barfing. Cool.

## 1/15/13

I'm going in for an infusion tomorrow, and I plan on giving my oncologist a laundry list of my aches and pains and other odd symptoms. I fully expect him to say it's to be expected and there's nothing he can do about it. The doctor at UCLA recommended that I stay on this chemo for six rounds. I'm only halfway through my second and already can't imagine doing this for nine more months. As the saying goes, "I'm sick and tired of being sick and tired."

I can officially drive at the end of the month since we plan on me staying on the anti-seizure medication. I am tapering off of one seizure med (Vimpat) but staying on another (Keppra). If I go off both, I can't drive for six months. Even though I will be able to drive, I won't be driving the kids for a while. I have a lot of anxiety about it. Driving myself is one thing, my kids are another. My hair is starting to grow back. I lost it from the top downward, and now it is growing back from the bottom upward. The sides and hairline are the longest at about one inch, and the top is about a quarter of an inch. There is a large bald spot surrounding my incision, and I was worried it would never grow hair, but it is just starting to sprout there. Yay! It's amazing how it improves my outlook.

Xo Katie

## 1/16/13

No Avastin today. Platelet count is too low. I need to be careful not to injure myself. No contact sports, so I have to quit the wrestling team :) and if I hit my head I need to go to the ER.

Xo Katie

## 1/17/13

Lying in bed with Haven. We were hanging out outside when I had my sixth seizure today. I've taken a huge step back. I'm back to taking Ativan multiple times a day whenever I feel one coming on, and I just took one now. My hand isn't working well, and it scares me to death. I can't go back to that place.

I'm very nervous about my appointment tomorrow, I have been stressed because of the kids being sick, and not getting enough sleep when Haven is up five times a night, her birthday and Valentine's Day coming up and hoping she would be well enough, getting our taxes done, etc., and sometimes taking my meds a couple of hours late. I pray to God that's the answer.

Xo Katie

## 1/20/13

I had a lovely day having brunch with friends and a family bike ride around the neighborhood, my first time on my bike in probably a year. A little wobbly but it felt good.

Tapering even further off my Vimpat seizure med. Clearly it's messing with me because I have seizure hallucinations all day long. Meaning I feel less protected so I keep getting the feeling that I'm going to have a seizure—or am I? It feels so real. I think I will stick here and not lower it for a while until I feel more confident.

Xo Katie

## 1/24/13

This is the first day I have felt decent in a while. Most people know the common side effects of chemo, but there are many more minor side effects that are just plain weird. They don't tell you everything you might experience because you may not get any of them, and there are probably dozens. Some of my common side effects are: nausea, upset stomach, loss of appetite, tiredness, no more period. (Too much information?) Sounds like heaven, but I have perpetual PMS. Not good, ask Micah.

Some of the stranger side effects are:

Because chemo attacks rapidly dividing cells like cancer and also hair follicles, nails, and mucus membranes, I have pain in my nose, my fingernails and toenails are curling inward on the sides, sort of like ingrown nails, I can't tolerate anything even remotely spicy, and my toothpaste makes me feel as if my mouth is on fire. I have joint pain, especially in my knees, and the top of my right foot hurts all the time as well as my right middle finger and right shoulder, no idea why. I have a headache every day.

I'm going to ask my doc about taking a break from the chemo. It

depresses me to feel bad every day. I can't eat the healthy foods I want to eat because they make me sick to my stomach. I can't exercise, I can't take my supplements, and I'm in pain. I want to take a few months off and get strong. I'm not even halfway through, and it gets worse each time. We'll see what he says...
Xo Katie

## 1/25/13

Thanks for the support! I appreciate all the nice comments. It actually could be a lot worse, so I'm lucky. I have been smoking more pot, and it does help somewhat. I have driven a couple of times, just a few blocks to Target, etc. Going to drive a little farther today.
Xo Katie

## 1/28/13

Had my MRI yesterday. I will get the results today and another infusion of Avastin. My platelets went back up to 108,000 from 23,000, so we are good to go. I'm nervous to see the MRI. The story of my life from now on, I guess.
Xo Katie

## 1/28/13

Good news! The tumor (or Mr. Zero as I like to call it) has shrunk some more. Not a ton, but enough so that my doctor is very happy. Overall, since June, it has shrunk more than 50 percent. It's weird how they calculate the percentages because last time he said 15 percent and this time he said less than 10 percent, but he actually said it's more than that when you take into account the whole 3D tumor instead of just the image on the MRI. It's still lighting up and that lighting up worries them because cancer lights up, but so do calcifications, and an old tumor like mine could likely have calcifications. But they can't tell the difference. The glowing bit could still be some swelling or scar tissue. He said this MRI was really important because a lot of people will have an initial good response, but then sometimes it stops or even starts to get worse, and it's this second MRI that really proves the meds and radiation are working. He says as long as the tumor keeps responding to the meds, he wants me to stay on the Avastin, at least as long as I'm on the chemo. I'm not going to get a break on the chemo, but because my platelets took such a hit last time, he is going to reduce my dose by 25 percent and says not only will I not feel worse but I should start feeling better. He said he pushed me at first because he wanted to take advantage of the combo and see the response. But now we can back off some. If he's right and I don't feel worse, then I will just plow through it until June.

By the way, Micah has a new nickname for me. Since my surgery there is a portion of my head that is still numb, hence my new nickname, Numbskull.

Xo Katie

## 2/3/13

I'm starting to think it's the Avastin, not the chemo, that's making me feel so bad. I haven't done the chemo in six weeks, but I did the Avastin a week ago, and the headaches, body aches, and stomach problems are back. Yesterday was horrible. No amount of Advil could help me, and I could barely keep my eyes open. Ended up taking a Vicodin and going to bed at 8:00. Woke up feeling better, but the headache returned by 11:00. Took a two-hour nap. I'm supposed to take the chemo this week. UGH. Hopefully things won't get worse. If it is Avastin, then I should feel better by the end of next week, we'll see. I hope so. My baby turns two a week from Friday!

Xo Katie

## 2/4/13

Got a kid home from school with the stomach flu. Nothing more pathetic than his sad little face crying after throwing up for the sixth time. I'm so nervous about this bug spreading through our house that I've turned it into a hazmat scene, sanitizing everything. I'm trying to stay clear of him, very hard to do, and keep Haven away, even harder. She keeps saying, "Lucky okay? Lucky, okay? He's better now." She's so worried. My main concern is that if I get sick, how will I keep my seizure medication down?

Friday afternoon Lucky took the train with his grandma down to Riverside to spend the night at their retirement community. Saturday Micah, Haven, and I drove down to pick him up. I watched a woman, who had to be about 90 years old, knitting. Her hands were so agile. Looking at these women with their high-waisted polyester pants and orthotic shoes, I was somewhat jealous. Their lives were behind them; they'd made it. Their children were grown, their grandchildren were grown. They got to see it all.

Life always seemed so precarious to me, but even more so now. I am amazed anyone makes it to old age.

Saturday was a hard day. I felt worse than I had in a while. Terrible headache I couldn't get rid of, stomachache and complete exhaustion, couldn't keep my eyes open. We came home from Riverside, and I had to take a Vicodin and went to bed at 8:00. For sure it is the Avastin. I looked up the side effects: headache, backache, and body aches are all among them. Haven't taken my chemo pill yet, supposed to this week, but I'm going to see if I can put it off one more week (went eight weeks last time) until I feel better.

I feel okay now except for a stomachache. Maybe it's psychosomatic :)

Xo Katie

## 2/6/13

Lucky is still sick but getting better. So far we have kept it contained thanks to bleach and antibacterial soap and crazy diligence! Unfortunately I have had to stay pretty clear of him, although we played some card games today. Haven misses playing with him a lot. He pretty much just lays on the couch and has been watching a lot of TV. Hopefully back to school tomorrow or for sure by Friday.

I've been spending some much needed time in my garden doing weeding and seeding. What a mess. It's been three years since my yard's had any love because I was pregnant, then had a newborn, then my diagnosis. It's overwhelming. It felt good to do yard work. My goal is to have it done by Easter.

I took Haven to her class today. She's so funny. A typical conversation:

Her: "Have gum."

Me: "You'd like to have some gum?"

her: "Have gum, Haven have gum."

Me: "Maybe later we can have some gum, not now."

Her: "Have gum. Have gum now. After lunch have gum. Have gum maybe. Chew it, no swallow gum. Gum. Gum. Gum. Gum!"

Okay, Rain Man.

Geez. Now replace gum with Stinky Bunny (the little blanket she chews on), chocolate, lollipops, playing in the car, etc. I love every minute with her.

I got my medical records in the mail today. I always like to have a copy for myself, and it came in a box! Not an envelope, a box. It's an inch and a half thick. Just tearing into it now. Fun stuff.

Xo Katie

## 2/7/13

So at five a.m. Lucky comes into our bed and says he has something stuck in his throat. Turns out it was vomit. All over my bed. So exhausted. A whole day of Micah and I doing nothing but cleaning again. Going to nap now...
Xo Katie

## 2/10/13

As hard as we tried, and we tried really hard, Haven now has the stomach flu. Friday she picked up one of Lucky's cups and quickly took a sip before we could stop her, and that was all it took. Yesterday afternoon it started, and it went on all night every hour or so. I am so tired. So begins another day of massive cleanup.

I guess it's true that God never gives you more than you can handle because yesterday Lucky was miraculously better. It took him six days. Haven's birthday is in five days, six days from when this started. Already she is bouncing back quicker. Even at its worst she was so dainty and civilized about it. She never cried and was so sweet. She called it "choking." I guess it's true what they say about the difference between men and women when they are sick. Sorry, guys.
Xo Katie

## 2/14/13

Happy Valentine's Day! We had a rough night with Haven; she was up five times with her stomach hurting and three not so pretty diapers. Today is day six and that's when Lucky got better, so I have high hopes for her birthday tomorrow. I got some sweet valentines from Lucky and am going to lunch with Micah today. Hopefully

I'll get a nap later. With both kids' birthdays on or within a day of a holiday, it's a lot of work. Once one thing is over, it's immediately on to the next.

I was supposed to start my chemo pill last week for round three but didn't because of the kids being sick; then I had blood work done that showed my platelets were down from 110 to 85, so we are putting off chemo for another week. The platelets need to be over 100. I'm glad actually because I didn't want to feel sick for Valentine's Day and Haven's birthday. Worked out perfectly, as always.

My hair is growing a lot, even in the incision area, which is where the main beam of radiation went in. It is very sparse there but starting to poke through. The rest of my hair feels like what I describe as "kitten fur." Micah says it's more like stuffed animal fur.

Xo Katie

## 2/16/13

Shortly after I posted the last message, Valentine's evening, I had a massive seizure. It started very suddenly around 7:30. I had just sat on my bed, and it felt like I was hit by a semi-truck. It literally knocked me over. I had just enough time to yell for Micah, who ran in in full panic mode. This was no ordinary seizure, this was a grand mal seizure, full body contortions and contractions. I couldn't be moved, my left arm shot straight out in front of me as stiff as a board and made hammering motions, my right arm twisted behind my head, and my legs were rigid and twisted. Micah was afraid I was going to fall off the bed, so he tried to lift me but couldn't. I yelled for my Ativan, but he couldn't find it right away, which sent him into a panic, because at the same time he was frantically calling all of our neighbor friends to see who could stay with the kids if we had to go to the hospital. Meanwhile I'm saying "I can't breathe, I can't breathe, hold my hand!" as I'm hyperventilating. He needed to leave my side to open the front door for our neighbors and the paramedics because I told him to call 911; after six Ativan it wasn't stopping. It would seem like it was dying down and then I would panic, and another would immediately start. It was a nightmare I couldn't wake up from. Imagine being in a straitjacket with a gag in your mouth and a plastic bag over your head. The bag has a tiny hole in it, so you breathe furiously to get that air. Meanwhile, my friend Paige was on one side of me and Betsy was on the other, telling me that I was breathing fine, but in my mind I was suffocating to death. This went on for at least 15 minutes. This kind of seizure has been the scariest thing I've ever been through, and I never wanted to experience it again, and here I am.

I lost two days of time. I remember nothing except the ambulance ride. I don't remember getting out, I don't remember the hours I spent at the hospital or the entire next day, Haven's birthday. I think I have some brain damage. I have had to go back and re-type these words too many times to count. The saddest thing for me is that I missed Haven's birthday. I was there, I just have no memory of being there. The effect of all the Ativan I took wiped me out so badly that I literally remember nothing. I am heartbroken. I spent so much time planning and sewing and creating her little woodland fairy theme, and I missed the whole thing. And we hardly have any photos. That makes me want to cry.

We are hoping it's just the decrease of my seizure med and not that things have gotten worse. Remember we pushed the Avastin and CCNU later as well. Appointment on Monday and Avastin too. I've had two smaller seizures today, my hand and arm only. The biggest drag is the loss of mobility in my hand and not being able to drive.

Xo Katie

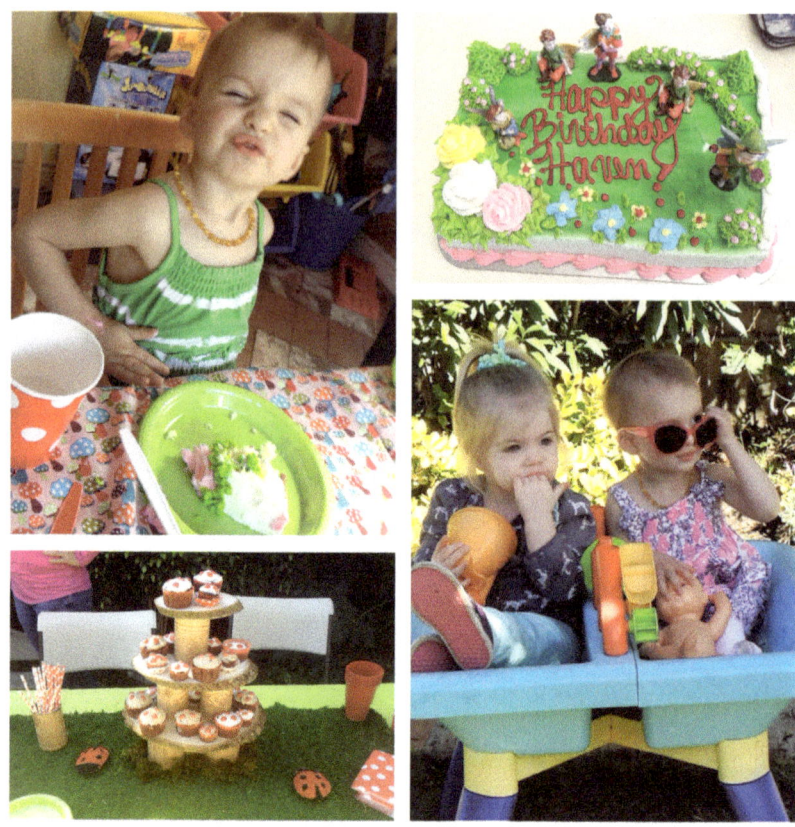

It took me 10 years to find these photos of Haven's second birthday, the only ones we have.

## 2/18/13

Had my appointment today, no bad news. The doctor pretty much felt the same way that we do, that the Vimpat med was decreased too fast and that my brain was still irritated. He feels that my anxiety and the subsequent panic attack that comes with a major tonic clonic(grand mal) seizure is what makes me feel as if I can't breathe. And that a lot of these smaller seizures I have throughout the day are anxiety driven as well. Like I said before, it's traumatic stress disorder. I will make an appointment with a specialist in the field. I have had at least 10-15 seizures today; there were about nine I was able to talk myself down from, and the rest required some Ativan. I feel like a zombie most of the day, but it helps with the seizures.

Just like in the past, the further I can get from a seizure, and the fewer I have in a day, the more relaxed I will get.

The "good news" is that I don't lose consciousness, which I would prefer actually, but then I could fall and hurt myself. It's also supposedly good that my limbs don't become completely rigid. I don't know why. Anyway, if the doctor was overly concerned, then he would have scheduled my MRI immediately, but he kept it for three weeks from now, which is a relief. He did not feel that it was anything bad regarding the tumor or it getting worse. Thank you, GOD.

Xo Katie

## 2/21/13

Sorry I've been out of touch and not answering texts or emails. I am having a really hard time with this latest setback. I find myself in a bad depression with the idea of starting over and having to build myself up yet again. Compound that with the fact that I am having 10-20 seizures a day, mostly small but you never know where it will lead. I am drugged to the gills, but it doesn't seem to matter. My best analogy is this: You've been hit by a 9.0 earthquake, your home is devastated, you are buried under a pile of rubble, and you can barely breathe. You can't call for help because your chest is crushed, and you can't move any limbs. As soon as it ends another one starts. You panic, sure you will suffocate to death. You hear people talking, but you can't yell for help. Close your eyes and try to imagine this. Somehow you are found and you survive. Now come the aftershocks; they can be big, a 6.0, or small like a 2.0, but it doesn't matter. Every time the earth moves, you have a full-fledged panic attack, adrenaline soaring, fight-or-flight kicking in. You can't breathe again, you are going to die, you can't yell for help.

Now try living that way, taking care of your kids, making breakfast, cleaning your house, paying your bills. You can't be alone because who will rescue you? I had to walk away while changing Haven's diaper and let my mother take over because I started to seize. It can start while I'm chewing. I have to spit my food out so I don't choke. I wake every morning to a seizure.

Even this doesn't adequately describe how horrible it is, and you will never know unless you've experienced it.

The difference between now and in October was that we knew why I was seizing then. As of now they don't know. It could be that my tumor is shrinking and that's irritating my brain. I was told that one drop of blood can be enough to cause a seizure. Hopefully the MRI in two weeks will tell us something. In the meantime I am very low. I feel like I am crawling out of my skin. I'm back to around-the-clock supervision and two-hour naps every day.

Xo Katie

## 2/22/13

I have to brag on my daughter for a moment because these are the reasons I keep putting one foot in front of the other. My daughter is not only smart but incredibly sensitive and intuitive. I have always believed that she is the reincarnation of my grandmother Mea (pronounced Mia); hence her middle name is Mea.

Remember, she just turned two last week. This morning I was having a mild seizure. I didn't even feel the need to announce it because I felt I could breathe through it. I was sitting at a dining room chair with my head hanging down so no one could see my face twitching. Haven ran into the bathroom where Micah was getting ready and said, "Mommy's calling you," which sounds a lot like

"My calling you" with "Stinky Bunny" hanging out of her mouth, so he said, "You're calling me?" and she repeated two more times, "Mommy's calling you."

When he came out of the bathroom, he could see me and knew exactly what was happening, and he said, "Oh, Mommy's calling me." I never called for him or said a word.

Xo Katie

## 2/26/13

I am actually teaching Lucky that you can use the power of your mind to make things happen. I have been doing this for years in little ways like with board games and such, but now when he sees me having a seizure, I practice breathing through them and I tell him, "Watch this" and then I say "stop" and the seizure stops. He says, "How do you do that?" It rarely works, but the one time he was watching it did!

I have spent the last few days practicing taking slow, deep breaths and leaning forward instead of on my back; that way it doesn't feel like my tongue is filling my throat. Many times I can stop a seizure this way, but once in a while this wave comes over me, and I just know it's going to be "the big one." This happened on Friday. I was home with my mom and was sitting on the floor cleaning Lucky's room. I called for her and told her to call Micah (who was on his way home from CVS getting my meds), then call 911. Micah, in a panic, also called all of our neighbors.

During the whole five-minute seizure, I was able to breathe. I never felt like I was suffocating. I didn't need to go to the hospital.

P.S. I have stopped and started this post four times because of anxiety. I have an MRI in the morning and will probably finish this after. Too nervous.

Xo Katie

## 2/27/13

I'm going to post a quick message because I'm back to the place where just talking or thinking about seizures will bring one on. Plus the last two days have been very exhausting and overwhelming. Triggers for me are tiredness, anxiety, stress, and overstimulation.

I had an MRI today which showed very little change, some minor shrinkage and possibly some small hemorrhages. Most likely I have become tolerant to the medications that I have been on, and they are not working as effectively. In addition to the medications I am already on, the doctor is adding a new seizure drug called Depakote. Hopefully this will be the answer because I feel as though I am back to square one.

I know people want to visit, but I just can't handle visitors right now unless they are just here to sit. I will put it out there on this board when I need help, so thank you. The farther I get away from seizures, the less anxiety I will have, and that will help a lot. Just be patient with me.

Xo Katie

## 2/28/13

I have a group of amazing moms (and dads) working on a fundraiser for us of very lofty proportions. Everyone taking time out of their busy days to help us. This is just the tip of the iceberg. Books, cards, flowers, plants, fruit, gift cards, three months' worth of food delivery service, energy healing, fresh green juice every day, massages, acupuncture, prayer circles, prayer blankets, holy water from the Vatican, prayers at the Wailing Wall, handmade dolls, gifts for my kids, offers to clean my house, free haircuts (ha!), many lunches and dinners out, and DVDs to keep me entertained, and many fundraisers that have kept us above water for months, and donations above and beyond. Most importantly prayers and inspirational words, a warm hug with a big smile. THANK YOU!

Love from the whole Smith clan,

Xo Katie

## 2/28/13

I have much to say but don't know if I'll be able to get it all out.

This has been a rough road back from a place I thought I wouldn't see again. I'm sad and depressed that although I was here for Haven's second birthday, I don't remember it. It's depressing that I once again need to be watched 24/7 and have lost all privacy, and freedom, not just of my body, but of my mind. I feel crazy again, on edge all the time, like I'm crawling out of my skin. You know I like to use analogies, so here's another one.

This is how it goes all day: You feel sick to your stomach all day, you've got the sweats, your mouth is watering, you keep telling yourself you are not going to throw up because you know that if you start, you won't be able to stop, maybe even end up in the hospital from dehydration. You are so exhausted from trying NOT to throw up that you finally throw in the towel—and it's even worse than you thought.

I swear Haven is psychic. This afternoon I was home with Micah, my mom, my friend Julie, and our babysitter. I started feeling a seizure come on, so I just sat down on the living room floor and kept my head down. No one noticed and everyone went about their business. Haven went into my bedroom and got my lockbox of meds and brought it out and handed it to me. She's so frickin' smart. I want to eat her alive.

Xo Katie

### 3/1/13

In a deep, dark hole and trying to claw my way out of it.

### 3/2/13

Better day, thanks for all the love. Spent some time outside weeding yesterday. I'm going to find my iPod and listen to some music. I always forget how much better I feel afterward. I also need to remind myself to live fearlessly.
Xo Katie

### 3/2/13

Don't know what I did today actually. Didn't garden, didn't listen to music, barely went outside, didn't cook. Napped. Wow, that was my whole day. Sad.
Xo Katie

### 3/3/13

Morning doctor's appointment tomorrow. I refuse to leave without answers. I will not continue on this way; it's inhuman. So depressed.
Xo Katie

### 3/4/13

I had a horrible dream last night. Normally a bad dream is enough to send me into a seizure and wake me up, but not this time. I was dreaming that I was walking into a bathroom with a normal bathtub, and as I turned the corner I could see a little lifeless body floating face down in the water. I grabbed the baby and knelt down next to the tub. I started to give her mouth-to-mouth and chest compressions and soon she was spitting up water and breathing again. I was shaken by this dream, and the message that was coming to me, either from Haven directly or from my grandmother was this: Things may look as bad as they can get, but you never know what's possible. You have the power to turn it all around. Was I the baby and I am saving myself? Hmmm…

Obviously for me this has been a dismal week, and things have seemed pretty bleak. I've got some pretty severe depression, anxiety, and panic, and none of that even includes the actual problems of the brain cancer and the seizures. The doctor today is waiting to see if my blood levels on this new medication, Depakote, has reached a "therapeutic level" in my blood. Once it does then there is very little chance (notice I didn't say none) that I will have another massive seizure. These could be because I'm undermedicated, but we also know they are triggered by anxiety, stress, anger, or any kind of upset (I'm fun to live with). It could also be the shrinking and small bleeds. Basically we don't know. His feeling is, everything looks good; let's get the meds right so I don't have any more big ones, which will calm me down and calm my brain down; work on my anxiety with my hypnotherapist and the neuro-psychologist; and go from there. I know there is still a very physical aspect, though, because by the end of the day, whether I'm stressed or not, and I nap every day, there is a feeling of "unwell" that comes over me like a wave, and I can't push it away. It becomes like a volcano when I try to squash it down, and no matter what, it comes bubbling up into a seizure and usually requires two Ativan, which is a decent size seizure.

One of my doctor's final statements to me was "I never said this was going to be easy." Clearly. I ruminate a lot on suffering, the idea of suffering. I don't think in the big scheme of things I have really suffered that much. More mentally than anything else. I have had some pain and discomfort, but mainly I suffer with my thoughts. I think because I am positive and spiritual, an eternal optimist and hopeless romantic, I can endure the rest. What are you? How would you manage?

Xo Katie

## 3/7/13

I woke up at 4:30 a.m. to a boy with a stomachache. Good God, not again. We went into full vomit mode—towels, buckets, gloves, etc. Nothing. Then Haven wakes saying, "My stomach hurts, throw up." Nothing, so far so good.

I have to brag about Micah for a bit. I don't give him enough credit. With help from my mom he practically runs this whole ship. The other day I heard Haven giving him a long explanation about who knows what, and he said, "Here, pull up a chair and let's talk about it." He was so patient with her. Sometimes I worry about how my kids would be without me, but moments like these help me feel better.

Feeling down again.

Xo Katie

## 3/10/13

It's always something, I'll tell ya. In trying to get the dosage of my new med Depakote correct, I may now have "Depakote toxicity"! The signs are extreme tiredness and confusion but much worse is the extreme restlessness. It actually feels like bugs crawling under my skin. I want to rip my skin off or break stuff. I'm going insane. All I can do is take more Ativan, which makes the transformation to total zombie complete. I've been sleeping for three days straight. It sounds kind of funny but it's maddening. So after paging my doc, we are toning down the Depakote some. I hope it works fast. I actually told Micah that if I start talking about killing myself to take me to the hospital. So don't ask me how I'm doing or how my weekend was. It sucked.

Xo Katie

### 3/14/13

I can't believe it's been one month since my seizure. It feels like only a week. The drugs can create amnesia, and I believe that's what's happening. I seem to have lost weeks. Lucky has been sick and very stressed out. He has a sinus infection, but more importantly he is worried about me. I talked to my neuro-psychologist about it, and he said that I shouldn't over-talk it but just be there for him and love him, tell him that everything will be okay, because it will, and constantly tell both kids that I love them. Kids just need to know that they are loved. We are back to having 24 hour surveillance on me, and I really appreciate all my friends who have volunteered to sit with me and bring us food. You are lifesavers. I told my psychologist about what an amazing support system I had and how I had almost a different person to drive me for each day of my six-week radiation, and he said he'd never heard of anything like that. He couldn't believe it.

I'm finally starting to feel more normal, or normal like I did in October, not normal like I felt in December. Now the work begins on how to get back to where I was, only now we have no swelling to blame. We have nothing to blame, which is almost harder.

Xo Katie

### 3/16/13

I just want to reach out to everyone who responded to my cry for help. I was in a desperate place and I got a lot of encouragement. A friend told me recently that she doesn't call me because "I don't want to burden you." Please burden me.

I know no one can really understand what I'm going through, but it's going to be a lonely place if everyone goes running for the hills because they don't know what to say. I may cry, but that's okay. I need to—a lot. It makes me feel better. You are not making me sad or causing me to think of my situation. Believe me, I think about it all the time anyway. It's nice to have someone to cry with. I get lots of cards from people saying, "I was just thinking about you and wanted to tell you." I love that, but you can call and email too. I may or may not respond depending on my energy level or mood, but it doesn't hurt to try. It's nice to hear from old friends too.

Today I sat in my backyard with a friend from junior high and watched Haven play. Then she drove me on a quick errand to Target. Perfect. Slowly getting used to the "new normal" again. I like my new neuro-psychologist. He has helped me already and he has a kind nature. Plus he thinks I tell an "entertaining story," so you gotta love that. Don't know if I mentioned that I did about eight hours of neurological testing first, awaiting the results on how I compare to similarly educated people in my situation (ha ha!). Anyway, thank you to my loyal friends and family who have stepped up, yet again.

Xo Katie

## 3/17/13

For my dad, Happy Birthday:
"'Come to the edge.'
'We can't. We're afraid.'
'Come to the edge.'
'We can't. We will fall!'
'Come to the edge.'
And they came. And he pushed them. And they flew." —Guillaume Apollinaire
Xo Katie

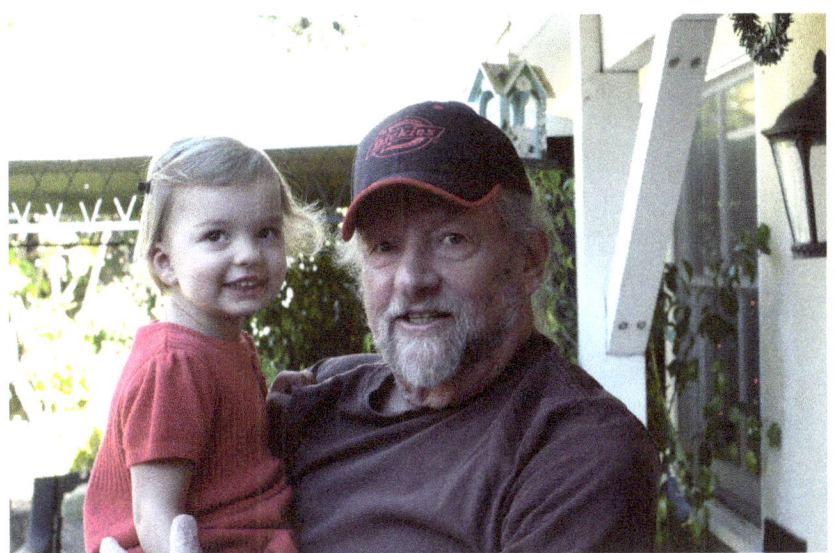

Haven and my dad

### 3/18/13

Turns out my Depakote levels aren't high enough. It's a game of trying to find the right number. Once it's stable it tends to stay that way, but it can take some time to get there. Obviously we want to avoid those toxic levels that made me want to rip my skin off, so it's a fine line. The good news about Depakote is that it supposedly has been also known to shrink tumors. More bang for your medicinal buck. My mantra today is "Every day in every way, I'm getting better and better."

Xo Katie

### 3/20/13

I talked to someone yesterday I hadn't seen in a while and he said, "Wow, you are so positive. I get such good energy from you." That was a big compliment but also accurate as I feel positive most of the time. I know there are people out there who don't call or email because they are uncomfortable and don't know what to say. Face your fear, get uncomfortable. My favorite quote today is by Eleanor Roosevelt: "You gain strength, courage and confidence by every experience in which you really stop to look fear in the face. You are able to say to yourself, 'I have lived through this horror. I can take the next thing that comes along.' You must do the thing you think you cannot do."

"You must do the thing you think you cannot do." My favorite part.

Xo Katie

### 3/21/13

Of course Micah is working all day tomorrow, and my mom, who was supposed to spend the night and days, is sick, my ride for my doctor tomorrow fell through, I had to find a ride home from school for Lucky, no sitter for Haven on Fridays…and when I freak, Micah freaks because he doesn't want to see me get upset. So he called in the troops. The Grandparents Sippi are driving up from Riverside and spending the night, so I am covered tonight and tomorrow. Bless them. I cried when Micah called them because I don't want to put them out, but I was also crying because of the way we have to live. We had gotten so comfortable and were feeling so good. I was driving! Then blammo! How do I ever let myself get comfortable again? What if I had been driving? What if I had been home alone with Haven? In a swimming pool? On a ride at Disneyland? I can think of 1,000 situations that could be life-threatening to me or someone else if I were to be taken by surprise again. How do I live like that? I NEVER feel safe! There is a stranger lurking in my house ready to cause me harm at any given moment. The best part is that I get to remain conscious during the entire horrifying ordeal.

Quote of the day: "The difference between being on an unknown journey and being lost is simply a matter of perspective." (Unknown)

Xo Katie

### 3/24/13

I got to go with my family to a kids' birthday party today. First really normal, fun thing we've done together since February 14th. I got to see some good friends I haven't seen for a while. Also no seizures, so far. Lucky lost his other top tooth. He is an official kid. I'm grateful I get to see that rite of passage, a toothless smile. Now I hope I can remember to put something under his pillow tonight.

Quote of the day: "The positive thinker sees the invisible, feels the intangible, and achieves the impossible." (Unknown)

Xo Katie

### 3/27/13

A fun day and a hard day all at once. I wish I could be there for other people the way I've always been. I don't like this side. To have to be so vulnerable in front of others, to air your dirty laundry with your spouse and have to have someone else braid my hair. It's embarrassing. And there's nowhere to go. I can't even go for a simple walk by myself. To be so tired I can't play with my children, or read to them, or put them to bed because all I want to do is collapse. Yeah, yeah, it's all temporary, yeah, at least I'm here, I know, I know, but you're not here. I am. I want my life back. No quote today.

Xo Katie

### 3/28/13

Already uplifted this morning. The weather went from 40 percent chance of rain on Easter to 10 percent! Yeah! I'm so happy.

Xo Katie

## 3/31/13

Hi friends, HAPPY EASTER!

A holiday where I don't wind up in the hospital is a good holiday. I've been AWOL for a while, mainly because I've never felt worse in my life. The last couple of weeks have been hard, but I went through a phase where I felt acclimated to the new drug, Depakote; then they raised the dose, and things just got worse and worse. The last couple of days, I felt so miserable that I called my doctor and told him I wanted to jump out a window. I was hysterical. I said I couldn't live like this. My whole body hurts, my skin hurts, my head hurts. I can barely stay awake for two hours at a stretch, and then I nap for three hours. Life is passing me by. I can't see living this way.

Yesterday when I called my doc crying, he told me to just stop the Depakote.

I had a new drug called Zonegran that I had been taking for seizures for two days, and he said that was long enough to be able to go off the Depakote.

I spoke with his assistant, who told me that the side effects of this new drug are tingling in the fingers, dizziness, and, for lack of a better term—her word, not mine—"stupider." So I've got that going for me. We have proven, though, over the last few days that my wit is indeed intact.

I had a very lovely, if not frantic, Easter. I still was not feeling well when I was assembling baskets and hiding eggs last night, and I was so tired, but it all worked out. My kids were adorable, and my family and friends were great. I have an infusion tomorrow and hopefully a lot of rest today.

Xo Katie

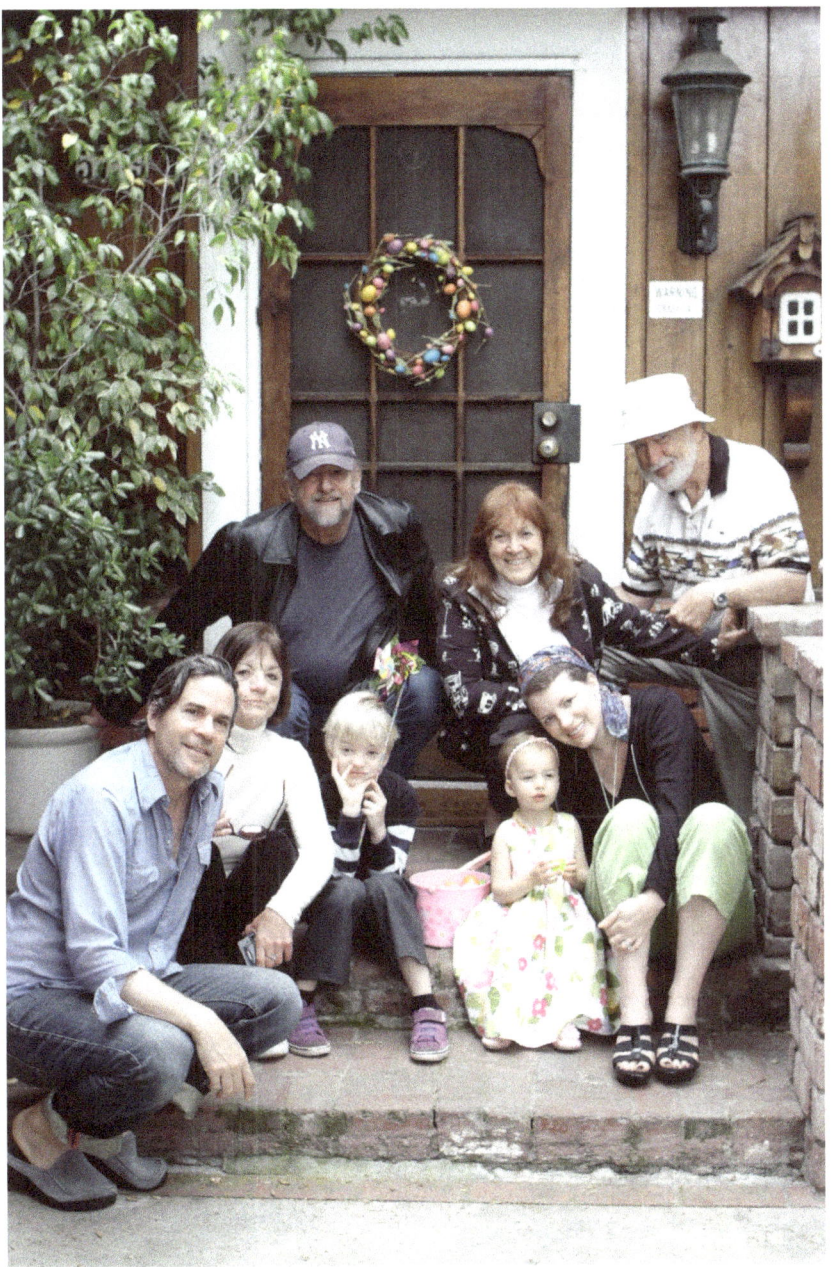

Easter with the whole family

## 4/4/13

Hi. I haven't posted for a while. I've been feeling like crap. Tons of anxiety and stress. The toll this takes on your body is nothing compared to the toll it takes on your relationships. I wrote an angry letter to Micah in my journal today. I will never give it to him, but I needed to write it down. Illness can bring out the best and the worst. It's really hard on the best of relationships. In college I took a class called Marriage and Family Relations. It said that marital satisfaction plummets when you have small children. Add to that a major illness and major medical bills, and you're looking at major stress.
Xo Katie

## 4/5/13

Here is yet another example of why everyone, especially me, needs to be their own advocate for their health care. Today I am pretty sure I realized why I had the seizure on Valentine's Day. After MRIs and consults and second opinions with no answers, I had an epiphany. The doctor I saw at UCLA asked right away if I had missed any doses of my medications. I hadn't, but I didn't remember that my Cedars doctor had been tapering me off one of my seizure drugs, Vimpat, for the previous month. I was so out of it after the seizure that I don't even remember meeting with him. Doctor Cloughesy said that 85-90 percent of people with seizures can control them with only one medication called Keppra, and the rest of us have seizures that are harder to control. That's me, of course. I went five months, though, without a simple focal seizure on Keppra and Vimpat alone. Without knowing that I needed both meds, my doctor at Cedars tried tapering me off Vimpat, and then I had that big one. Obviously I am dependent on both Keppra and Vimpat for now. For the last two months, I have been so depressed and walking on eggshells, wondering when the next Big One will hit because the doctors couldn't give me any reason why the last one happened. My fear and anxiety were ruling my life. I had months of freedom taken away from me, and I was terrified and drugged.

I called Doctor Cloughesy at UCLA and gave him this information, and he definitely felt it was not only significant but that I should feel relieved because this was most likely the cause. I also called a seizure specialist who I had seen previously, but he is booked for a while. I talked to his nurse, who also validated this theory. I still have anxiety, but there is a sense of relief that is unbelievable. Hope that I can get that freedom back. Thank you, God.

Xo Katie

## 4/10/13

My anxiety is so much better since remembering about the tapering of my meds. The anxiety isn't gone, but it's definitely decreased. For those who are interested, there is a two-day brain tumor conference at UCLA May third and fourth with many interesting topics. Three doctors I have seen personally, including Doctor Cloughesy, who I am considering switching to, will be the main speakers.

Xo Katie

## 4/13/13

Hi. I haven't posted in a while. Honestly I hate to admit it, but I have been virtually paralyzed by anxiety and panic. It's as if my day is a series of panic attacks one after the other. I collapsed at the Target checkout counter yesterday with Micah and Haven. I felt as if I was having a seizure for sure, popped three Ativan in my mouth, then calmed myself and realized it was nothing. My heart was racing, I was sweating, but no seizure—a panic attack—so I spit the Ativan out. It was like that all day long. It was physically painful. I had appointments with my neuro-psychologist and my hypnotherapist, which helped a lot. Twice in the afternoon I was able to stop an actual seizure by saying out loud, "This is panic," and it would stop. My panic can actually cause a real seizure if I let it go. But it is constant and exhausting, and the more I talk about it, the worse it gets. I have to practice my calming techniques. I have never felt like this before, but if I take too much anti-anxiety medication, I become like the walking dead.

Xo Katie

## 4/14/13

Appreciate your health, appreciate your mind because you don't realize how much you need and miss them until they're gone. I've never felt so awful in my whole life. I can honestly say this is the worst so far; I feel as though I am losing my mind as well. The list of medications I'm on is a foot long, and worse than that I feel like I'm losing faith in my doctor. I had him paged tonight, but I feel like he's talking in riddles to me, and it just confuses me more.

I have to tell a story again about my amazing two-year-old. I was giving her a bath the other night and I was feeling bad and weary. I had my knees up and my forehead resting on my knees. My arm was covering my eyes. She said to me, "I'm right here. Do you want to talk to me?" and she was looking right at me. I teared up and said, "Yes, I want to talk to you." Then she went about her normal chatter. She blows me away.

Xo Katie

## 4/15/13

I long for a day when I just feel normal. When I'm not crawling out of my skin again or full of anxiety, or panic. When I can tolerate the sounds of my children's voices. When I can go to a kids' birthday party without having to go into the bathroom to have a crying breakdown because I'm so overwhelmed by all the people. I'd like to go a day or two where my kids don't see me crying. I will see the UCLA doc Wednesday. Can't wait. On the plus side I got called for jury duty, but I think I have a lifetime excuse. Cancer has its privileges. Thanks for all the support and prayers. I need them so badly.

Xo Katie

## 4/17/13

Hi. We went to UCLA today to meet with Dr. Cloughesy, the neuro-oncologist. I feel confident that I am going to make the switch over to UCLA. He also believes it was most likely the decrease in my seizure medication that caused what will be forever known as "the Valentine's Day seizure." He said that it could have been irritation from the radiation, but those are usually much smaller. He said that people who continue to have seizures don't have them because of the tumor itself. My tumor could disappear and I could still have seizures because they radiated not only the tumor but the healthy brain around it, and it's the irritation of the healthy brain that causes the seizures. Great.

Xo Katie

## 4/24/13

Hey, so I had my MRI on Monday. Not much change in terms of size, but everything looks stable and that's good news too.

Xo Katie

## 4/28/13

Every day I think, *I need to post something*, but then every day I am either too busy or too tired or feeling bad. Quite depressing. Rallied today and took Haven to the merry-go-round and to dinner with friends. It's hard to realize that I don't have the energy to keep up with her or run after her when she takes off. I'm so tired.

Xo Katie

## 5/1/13

Hi. Long time, no post. We saw the epilepsy specialist yesterday. It was a good meeting, and we left feeling like we had a plan and some answers. He was bummed that it was decided to start weaning me off the Vimpat without consulting with him first. He would have kept me on the same regimen for two years until I was more stable and then he probably would have chosen the other drug, Keppra, to wean me off of first—and very slowly. The plan now is to take one Klonopin every morning and two every night. I will be dopey but not anxious. He also didn't underestimate the trauma that having a 15-20 minute seizure while fully conscious had on my psyche. He thought these breakthrough seizures could be panic/anxiety combined with the memory my brain has of that trauma. He said once my anxiety calms down and I get used to the Klonopin, I can start driving again. One thing at a time.

Xo Katie

## 5/2/13

I'm pretty upset right now. I have to write or I won't be able to sleep. It seems that maybe I've created such a high standard for myself that nobody can cut me any fucking slack. Anyone else with brain cancer would be treated differently than I am. I have no doubt about it. I still have to be perfect, no matter what. I have to put on a happy face and pretend I don't feel like complete shit or am drugged out of my mind, or having a panic attack and just barely holding it together. In the last eight months I have done everything for our parents birthdays, Halloween, Lucky's birthday, hosted Thanksgiving, Christmas (including the concept and execution of the Christmas card and family portraits), Valentine's Day, Haven's birthday, and Easter. I have bought every family member's gifts (months in advance) and wrapped them. I also made Valentines and heart-shaped sandwiches, planned and executed my kids' birthday parties (two days out of the hospital), created four huge Easter baskets, shopped for Easter outfits, dyed eggs, filled 200 plastic eggs, and I am also the damn tooth fairy and Elf on the Shelf!

Can't I get a break? Can I make any mistakes? I'm not old enough to be the matriarch of this family. I cannot hold it all together. Give me a break. I'm not perfect. And before you say it, I have not brought it all on myself. If I didn't do it, then it wouldn't get done, and I would never disappoint my kids like that. I have a limited time with my kids, and I want them to remember these times.

Yesterday we met with a doctor who couldn't tell me how long I would live. When I said, "Five years?" he said he couldn't say. So all I'm asking for is a little slack.

Xo Katie

## 5/4/13

Hi. Today Micah and I went to the brain tumor conference at UCLA. It was informative at times, boring at times, excruciating, infuriating, and maddening. I had an opportunity to ask the neurosurgeon I met with a year ago, Dr. Linda Liau, how my functional MRI could be so off base. Meaning why did Dr. X say he could remove 95 percent of my tumor and then say he couldn't remove any of it? She seemed surprised and said she never really sees that; it would be highly unusual, but a lot depends on who is reading the MRI. We also had a half-hour meeting with another neurosurgeon, her associate Dr. Yang, who was great. He was very upfront. We told him about my surgery and the seizures during the surgery. He said he would never stop a surgery because someone was having seizures. Many people have seizures during surgery, at least 30 percent. The anesthesiologist is responsible for controlling those, and they should be prepared—anytime you touch and stimulate the brain, the patient will have a seizure. He said if he couldn't stop the seizure, he would have someone just hold the head still and continue! So now we are wondering why Dr. X stopped my surgery. We knew my tumor was in my peripheral motor area and that I would have a temporary deficit afterward, but then he completely turned it around and said it was in my motor area. How could he be so wrong? We are dumbfounded and pissed. Our plan is to take all of our records and MRIs to Dr. Liau and get her opinion. Dr. Yang also said that he thinks there is a high probability that I will have to have another surgery in my lifetime. There is a good chance my tumor will grow or change at some point; it could be a few years or decades, we won't know. He was very pro acupuncture and juicing, though. We liked him a lot, even though his news was depressing. Now we are questioning everything we've been told about my surgery. UGH. Was it for nothing?

Xo Katie

## 5/6/13

I'm going to Newport Beach with a friend this Thursday for two nights and am very excited to sleep in and just relax. I am going to miss my family so much, though. It makes me anxious to leave the kids. Bought a new book that hasn't arrived yet, called *Mind over Medicine* by Lissa Rankin. I'll give a review when I'm done.

Xo Katie

## 5/11/13

Hi. I'm on my first vacation in years, away from the kids and Micah too. I am in Newport Beach with my friend Dana. It's so beautiful here and relaxing. We spent the whole day shopping, mostly for Mother's Day gifts, only to come back to the house and get into a huge argument on the phone with my mother. Happy Mother's Day.

I try so hard to not let these things get to me, but it's just not in my nature, so I feel like my vacation has been ruined. I can't stop thinking about it, even though I know that no one can make me feel a certain way. It's up to me and how I let it affect me. I'm going to try hard to salvage my last day and enjoy some quiet time on the beach. Why does everything seem so difficult? Why am I so vulnerable to people making me feel guilty? It eats at my soul, and that's so bad for me. My grandmother used to say, "Thank God for my friends because without them I'd have no one." It used to piss me off, but she was probably right. We weren't there for her like we could have been. I regret that. I was selfish and self-absorbed. Something needs to change, and it's not going to be my family, so it has to be me.

Xo Katie

## 5/12/13

I'm back from my trip and feeling pretty good. Called my mom and worked through it enough to enjoy my last day, took my nap on the beach, and got the okay to take the chemo, finally. I really want to wait until after my benefit, though, because otherwise I'm afraid I'll feel too sick. I am really looking forward to it. The outpouring of love is unreal, so, so grateful. Looking forward to seeing my kids in the morning. I miss them.

My new regime of Klonopin in the morning and two at night seemed to work better last week. Around nap time I feel pretty bad and then around 4:00 I start feeling bad too. When I say bad it's hard to explain, but it's almost fluish, body aches, exhaustion, trouble thinking, and that seizure feeling. Have you ever stayed up for 24-36 hours straight? It feels that bad, so now I find that if I take an Ativan at that time, the feeling goes away. Now is that going to become a problem?

Happy Mother's Day to all the wonderful mommies out there.
Xo Katie

## 5/14/13

The benefit is getting outta control, the event of the season! Bands, singers, stand-up comedy, slideshows, a raffle for a $500 gift card, free food, signature drinks, you name it!
Xo Katie

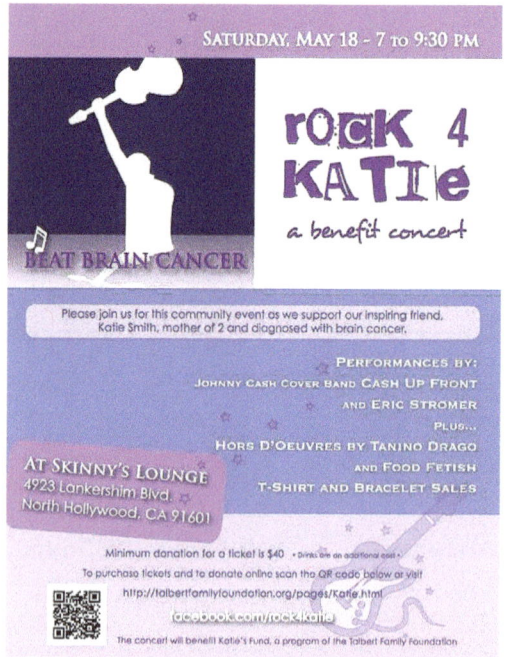

Flier for my benefit

## 5/16/13

We went to Cedars yesterday to meet with the doctor who did my surgery. We wanted answers as to why my functional MRI was so off target and they weren't able to remove any of the 95 percent of tumor that they said they would. We also wanted to know why they would stop my surgery because of seizures. We met with Dr. P (Dr. X was supposed to do the surgery, but apparently he did not), not a warm and fuzzy guy. He explained that the MRI made it look like the creases in my brain were in two sections, one in the motor strip and one in the premotor strip. When they opened up my skull, they saw that it was actually only one section that had ballooned, and the tumor was in the whole motor area. There was no way they could remove any of it; they were even nervous to do the biopsy. He said it can never be removed. If it came down to a life-or-death situation, they would remove it, but my left arm and face would be permanently paralyzed, which he says comes with its own set of problems like blood clots and things. Plus the arm becomes dead weight, which I experienced last fall, and becomes a real pain, so a lot of people will just ask to have it cut off. This guy was a real ray of sunshine.

Anyway, we came out of there with our questions answered but never needing to go back.

Xo Katie

## 5/17/13

I can't wait for tomorrow night. It's going to be very emotional for me. I don't really feel worthy of all the hard work and generosity of so many people, 100 tickets sold so far! Feeling overwhelmed. My friend Kristen Stills has generously donated a guitar signed by all three members of Crosby, Stills and Nash, and all proceeds go toward our fund.

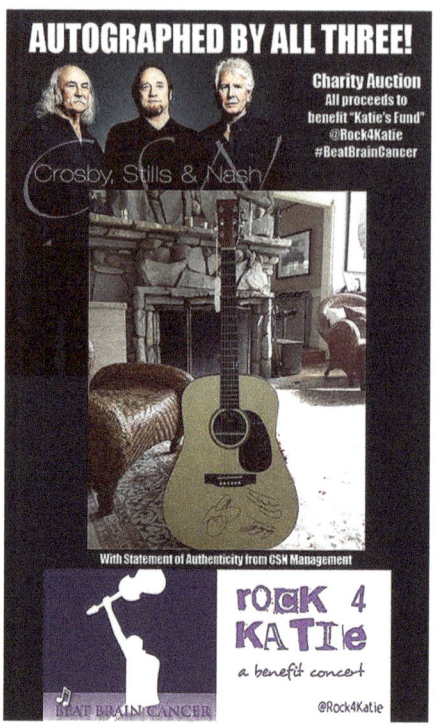

I'm so happy my parents are able to come and that my in-laws are generously missing out so they can be with the kids. If you are coming please come up and introduce yourself. Many of you I know of but have never met, and for others it's just been a long time. Plus I have brain damage :)

Xo Katie

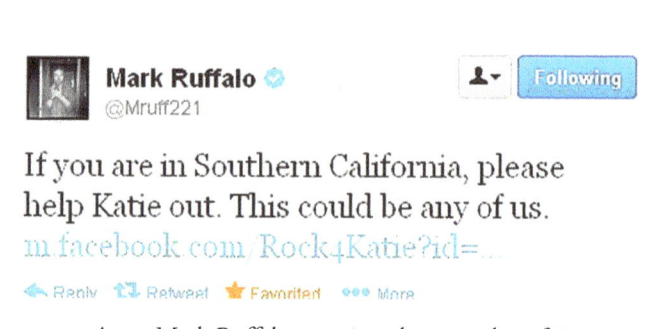

Actor Mark Ruffalo tweeting about my benefit!

## 5/20/13

Hi everyone, our benefit party was a huge success! We far exceeded the minimum we were hoping for! By eight p.m. we had 200 people in the bar! The owners were concerned we might exceed their capacity!

I felt really good most of the time. If I got overwhelmed, then I would just sit and rest for a minute. I actually danced for the first time in over a year and had so much fun. Micah was asked to do a "money dance." He picked four songs to dance to as women (and a few men) pinned money to his clothes. It was pure hysteria, but the best part was how much money it raked in, a whopping $971.00! A special thanks to a special friend who gave $500 of that. I told Micah his new profession was dancing for a living!

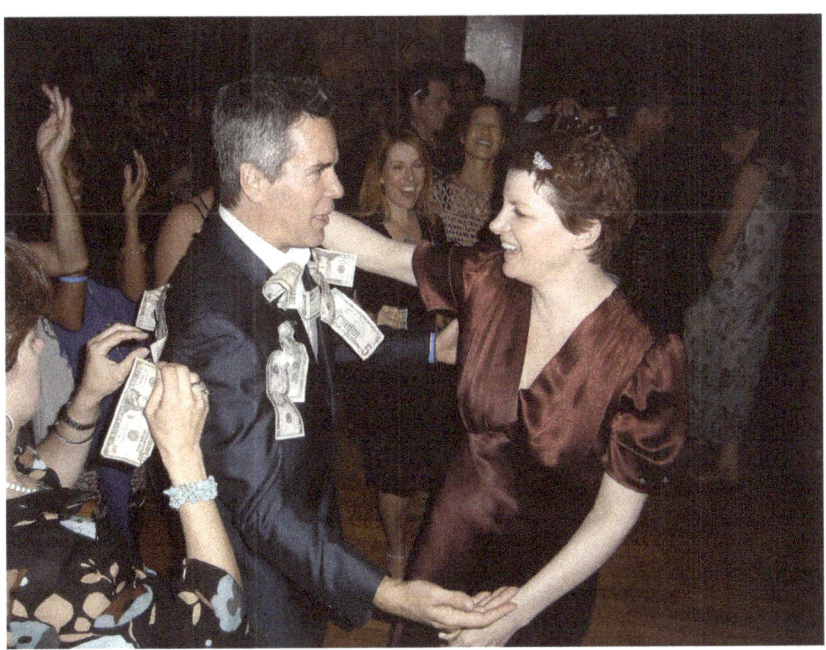

Thank you to everyone who made this dream possible. I don't imagine that many people get to have something like this in their honor, ever. I am blessed with the greatest friends and the greatest school and the most loyal clients.

Xo Katie

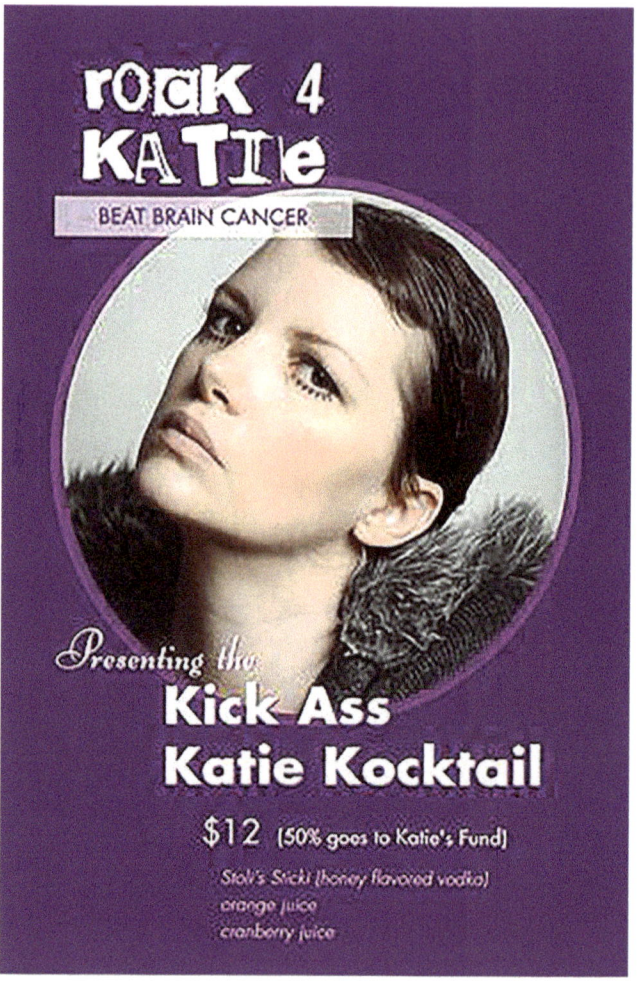

Micah took this photo of me. We thought I should take advantage of the pixie cut since I'll never do it again. Hiding the bald spot on the other side. Very 1960s.

### 5/23/13

Had to write this before I forgot. I put the kids to bed and a few minutes later Lucky came out and said, "Can I ask Mom something? Mom, can you play a trick on me in the night? Like do something funny or put me in a funny position?" As if all I do isn't enough? Now I have to rearrange my kid into funny positions. Kids are so funny. Haven has taken to running through the sprinklers. Every other night they go off at 5:40, and she strips her jammies and diaper off by herself and runs around the yard. Even though she's shivering, she puts up one finger and says, "One more time." Love those babies.

Xo Katie

### 5/26/13

Hi. I've been feeling really dopey lately. Can't stand this new regime of four Klonopin a day. I slept for three hours this afternoon. I hate that. I'm getting nothing done. When I'm not sleeping, I'm wishing I was sleeping. The afternoon felt a little rough, but I made it through a trip to Toys 'R' Us and dinner with two unruly children. My new book has been great for me. I highly recommend it for anyone with chronic illness, pain, or disease.

Today as we were driving to Toys 'R' Us, we saw a group of people riding very strange bicycles, some very long, some very tall. Haven, who is two, said, "When I was a kid I had a bicycle like that." It made me think of those early bicycles in the 1800s/1900s with gigantic front wheels. Micah and I just looked at each other and said, "That's really weird."

She's so smart. I was reading her Spot book, but she was on the floor, not on my lap, and I said, "Spot sat by the pond and watched the frogs."

She said to me, "It's not frogs," and she was right—there was only one frog.

Xo Katie

## 5/28/13

Working with my hypnotherapist, John, has helped me so much. A few weeks ago we were doing an exercise where I (theoretically) ran up a hill where there are obstacles I have to break through, and each one has a word on it. I was running up this hill and got to the last one, and the word was "significance." I started crying. I wasn't quite sure why that word had such an impact on me, but after John left I started thinking about it, and it occurred to me that until very recently with my children and my business, I had never felt significant. I actually felt invisible, undeserving, a fraud. I spent my life pretending to be someone I wasn't just to fit in, to be liked. I felt insignificant. From this realization I felt that illness was my way of feeling significant.

When I was 13 I had meningitis and encephalitis (brain and spinal infections ironically), and for the first time in my life, I felt loved, seen. I was in the hospital for weeks, and people came to visit me and brought balloons, flowers, and gifts. I rode in a helicopter and landed on the roof of Children's Hospital. My grandparents came in the middle of the night. My dad and sister were there, and people were crying over me. While I was in Children's Hospital, I made friends and we ran the place. When I returned to school, they threw a party for me. For that period in my life, I was important. I felt cared for. You can imagine the impact this had on me. I was only a child, but it was clear that when you are ill you are treated special. I don't think I made myself sick, but in the new book I'm reading, the first key is diagnosing why you are sick. I'm trying to figure that out so I can make myself well.

Xo Katie

## 5/30/13

I had a very strange day. I went for my treatment today, but my doctor wanted to see me first, not our usual protocol. Seems he wanted to do a one-year evaluation. Apparently he knew that we had gone to see the surgeon last week, that lovely man who talked about cutting my arm off. Anyway, he has had doubts and thinks that they could have removed my tumor. He isn't happy about the fact that a year later I still have to be so drugged and that I'm not feeling better than this. He actually suggested that I have a consultation with the surgeon at UCLA, Dr. Liau, who I met with last year but at the time UCLA didn't accept my insurance. He wants her to do another functional MRI which shows where the motor areas are in the brain, and see what she thinks. He says it's actually very common for one surgeon to say they can't remove a tumor and for another to remove it no problem. Also, my tumor has shrunk some since then, so things may have changed. He believes that the radiated tumor is what's causing the irritation to my brain and that if it were removed, my seizures would stop.

The fact is that people who have their tumors removed live longer, period. He says that he frequently works with the doctors at UCLA and that he can tell I have lost faith in the Cedars team, not him, but the team, and he has no problem working with the UCLA team. He even said he wouldn't be offended if I met with Dr. Cloughesy (who I've already seen). I did tell him that we went to the brain tumor conference there. He said that my surgery had extenuating circumstances because they could not get my seizures under control; they were coming on top of each other. He said that now they would go into surgery with me on a ton of seizure medication, like I am now, to prevent that from happening again. So there is some benefit to the previous surgery. We learned what to do and what not to do. So basically we are going to meet with Dr. Liau and see if she thinks my tumor can be removed. More brain surgery, that is daunting. I get upset just thinking about it, but if it will add years to my life, there is no choice. On the upside, they won't have to shave my head again :)

Xo Katie

## 5/31/13

I'm reading this book *Mind Over Medicine* and I'm at the part where she reveals her tips for healing yourself, and I realize there are things I need to do, not many as I've accomplished a lot of what I've wanted for myself. One thing I've realized is that living fearlessly, which is what I've been trying to do, is not possible. I can't live fearlessly, but I can be brave in the face of fear. I am brave. This I know without a doubt, and I'm proud of myself. I'm not the person I once was. I also know that I need to forgive some people. I don't need to be right. I just need to forgive and move forward.

Xo Katie

## 6/2/13

Hi. I get many emails and suggestions about different alternative cures, healers, and such. One that gets sent over and over is someone named Stanislaw Burzynski. He supposedly has some revolutionary cure that the doctors don't have, and in order to get into his "clinical trial" there are very strict guidelines. Well, I asked my doctor about him, at the risk of being laughed at, and he said he is basically someone who preys on people by charging them exorbitant amounts of money, no insurance of course, and is using drugs that are already available over the counter and talks about specific diets that I already know about. He's not doing anything revolutionary. There, I trust my doctor. He would tell me if there was something out there that could help me.

Xo Katie

## 6/6/13

I'm looking forward to celebrating our 10-year anniversary tomorrow! Taking off for the weekend, leaving the kids with the grandparents. We're going to the hotel where we got engaged, what a wild ride. I have a wonderful husband. Looking forward to the next 10 years. Hopefully they won't suck.

Xo Katie

## 6/10/13

Hi. I didn't take my computer on our anniversary weekend so I am writing now. We had a wonderful, relaxing time, and sleeping in was heavenly. We stayed at The Madonna Inn in San Luis Obispo, and we stayed in the same room, Cloud Nine, where Micah proposed to me.

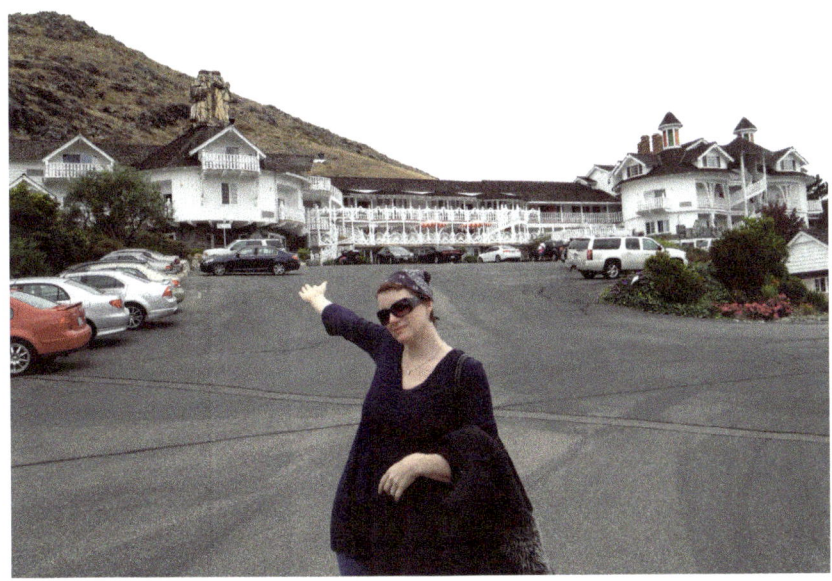

The Madonna Inn

The next day we relaxed at their very amazing pool. I haven't swam in a long, long time, and I have been nervous about it because if I had a seizure while in the water, I wouldn't be able to get out or call for help. Before we got in I said to Micah, "Please watch out for me," and he said he wasn't going to take his eyes off of me. It was so great to be in the water again. We layed out (under an umbrella, but I still managed to get sunburned, something about chemo and not going in the sun, whatever) and ate lunch by the pool. I listened to my iPod and read magazines.

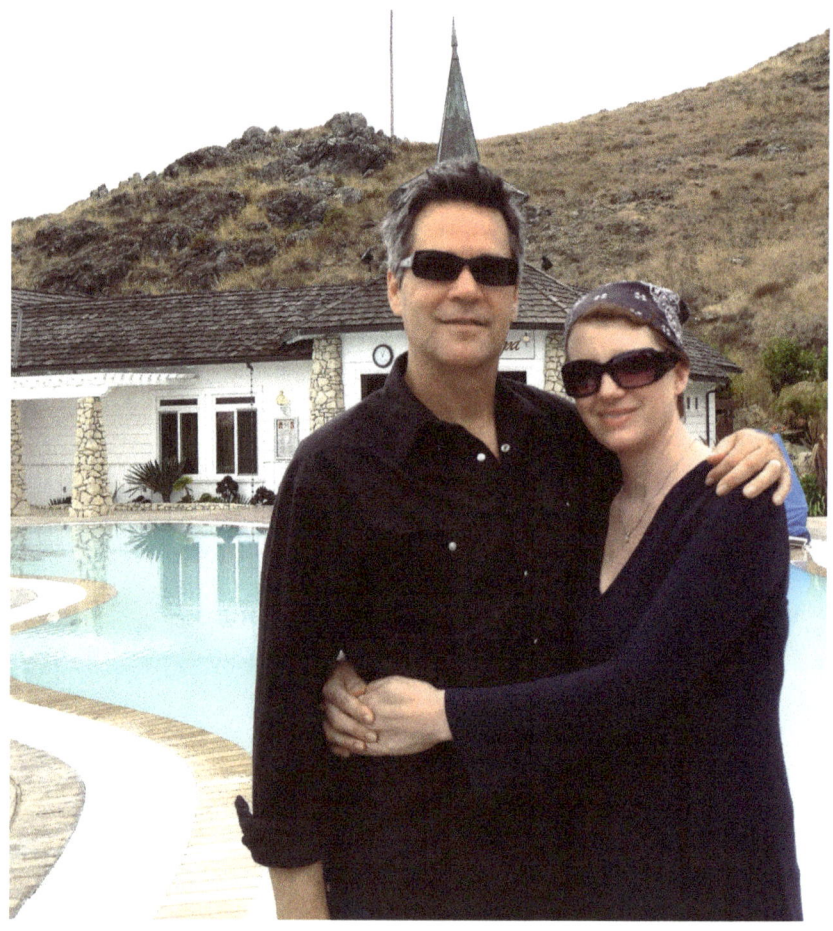

Enjoying the pool

As a gift, I gave Micah a picture frame that I'd had made. At the top it has our names and the date of our wedding. On the bottom it says, "Grow old along with me. The best is yet to be." I have heard that saying before and saw it on a large stone in Newport Beach, and as soon as I saw it, I burst into tears in the middle of this store because I want so much for it to be true. I knew I had to give Micah something with that saying on it. When I gave it to him, I cried again and asked, "Will you grow old with me?" I could barely get it out. Of course he said he would always be with me. Now it hangs over our fireplace.

Xo Katie

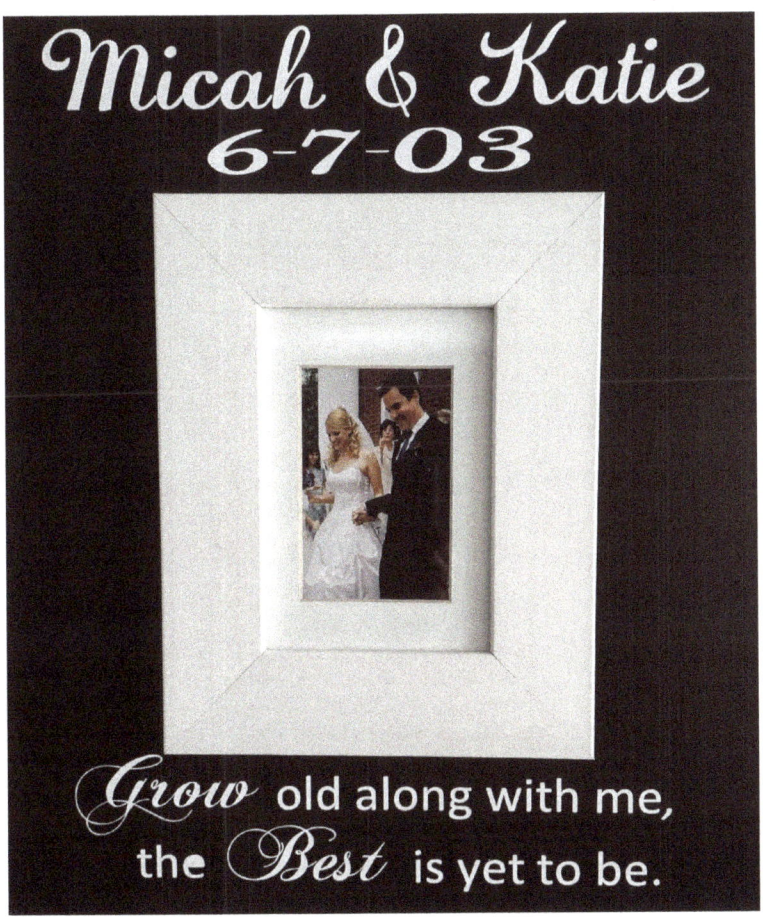

## 6/15/13

Sorry no posts, just a crazy week since we got back. I am taking my kids on a mini vacation to SeaWorld/Legoland before it gets too hot and too crowded. I figured this may be the only vacation they get this year. Hope everyone has a great Father's Day.

When my parents lament the fact that they are getting old(er), I feel the need to remind them that if I make it to their age, I will have outlived my projected life span by 20 years. That stops 'em in their tracks. I hope to live to be 100 and never complain about a wrinkle or liver spot or aching back. I hope we all do.

Xo Katie

## 6/18/13

A very big day. A scary day, an exciting day. We saw Dr. Liau today. She said she thought she could take my tumor out. She said, "I can take it out. I don't see why not." She showed us the latest MRI and how there is a distinct definition line between the tumor and my motor area. Plus, she felt that if it was in my motor area, then I would be having more problems with my hand, arm, face, and leg. Makes total sense. I don't know why that never occurred to me. She also felt it was most likely the tumor that is causing me seizures because it is irritating my "normal" brain. My Cedars doc said the same thing. Dr. Liau felt it was an 80 percent chance my seizures would disappear after the surgery. Because she would be taking out my whole tumor, I would wake up paralyzed on the left side. My arm and hand for sure, maybe my leg and face. It could take anywhere from three days to three months to recover. They will do a functional MRI again; there is no point in taking out dead tissue. The tests will be done in July, and the surgery is tentatively scheduled for August eighth. I can't really believe I am facing another brain surgery. It hasn't even sunk in yet. I will have to process it over time.

Xo Katie

### 6/22/13

I'm trying to gear up for the surgery, feeling overwhelmed already with how much I feel like I need to get done. The stress is already palpable. I don't want to go through this again. I hate being dependent on people. Song of the day: **"Feeling Stronger Every Day" by Chicago**

Xo Katie

### 6/23/13

Sadly, it's amazing how dependent I have become on our sitter Hannah. There were times during our trip to SeaWorld when Haven wanted Hannah over me. It hurts, but then I'm glad, too, because I know in a month I won't be able to care for her at all, and I'm glad she has someone to love. I tear up just thinking about that. I know this surgery will be a good thing, but for Micah and especially for me, I think about all of the negative things that go along with it. Nobody, including me, knows what it will feel like to go to sleep and wake up paralyzed. I do know the devastation of waking up and hearing that they couldn't do anything for me. I do know how hard the recovery is and how hard it is to tell my son that they are going to cut my head open, again. I do know how hard it is leaving my children not knowing if I will ever see them again. I know what it's like to see my parents crying over my bedside, riddled with worry.

My birthday is in a couple of weeks, I'll be 44, and my dad asked me what I wanted. I said I didn't know, because what I really want is to have 43 back. I didn't get to have a 43. Every year counts and I was robbed. I was thinking that out of 44 years, I've had about five good ones. Mostly they were stress free and happy, where I could really enjoy my life. The first one is the first year of my marriage. I was really happy. The three years after Lucky was born and I didn't have to work and just got to hang with him and focus totally on him were great. The day Haven was born was the happiest day of my life. It was the culmination of everything I ever wanted: my husband, my son, and my daughter. I had everything in the whole world—and I got it for just one year.

Xo Katie

## 6/24/13

"If you're going through hell, keep going."
Winston Churchill

## 6/25/13

So today and yesterday were Lucky's first days of camp at his school. Micah and I had to peel him off our legs as he cried and kept running back to us—torture. I knew he would have fun, and I called later and the counselor said he was having fun, but it happened again this morning. This afternoon he said today was better than yesterday, but he still didn't want to go back. I sat him down and asked him what was going on. He said he missed me and just wanted to spend time with me. Sweet, but full of crap. I kept forcing the issue, and I asked if he was worried about me. He asked me if it had been fifteen months since I got my tumor and I asked why. He said he heard our neighbor's friend talking about how his wife had a brain tumor and died fifteen months later. How can people be so stupid. He's a child, not a moron. Let me tell you something: kids are ALWAYS listening.

Since he doesn't know how long fifteen months is, he's been

worried that every day when he leaves I won't be there when he comes home. The seizures are just a constant reminder for him.

I reassured him that that lady had a different kind of tumor and that I've had mine for many, many years. I think he was relieved, but it's hard to tell. I need to make an effort to spend alone time with him. I used to drive him to school every day, and we would have the coolest conversations. I took him to all the playdates and birthday parties. Most of that has stopped. I relinquished many duties to Micah. It also coincided with having a baby, so part of that is natural. It's time, though, for me to start spending more time with him, clearly.

I decided to feel him out and told him that there was a chance that a doctor may still be able to get my tumor out. He actually got a smile on his face.

I asked if he would like that, and he smiled and said yes. He said, "No more seizures," and I said that's right. Phew! I've been so worried about telling him most of all. All he said was "I just don't want to be in camp that day." So funny.

Xo Katie

## 6/26/13

Micah and I got woken up this morning at 6:30 by Lucky extolling the virtues of the Shark vacuum. Seems he had been watching an infomercial for 30 minutes and knew all of the details. He was so excited to tell us that it works on wood, carpet, and linoleum and that if you buy one while the commercial was on, you could get another for free. Hey, it's only $499 in four easy payments! His enthusiasm and memory of detail was amazing, funny, and scary. Exactly why he doesn't watch commercials. One time I heard him laughing, came into the living room, and he was watching TV, and I asked him what he was watching and he said, *"Friends."* Oy.

So I've decided to let my freak flag fly and let my hair go curly. It's getting harder to tame the beast as it gets slightly longer and in this wonderful in-between stage. I don't think I'll be doing that very often as I look like Peter Brady after he got a perm. Then I tied a bandana around my head, and I looked like Lucille Ball, but with a huge bald spot. Lovely.

Xo Katie

## 7/1/13

It's hard not to think of where I was this time last year, health wise. I remember being so fragile just three weeks out of surgery and going to see fireworks and praying I didn't have a gigantic seizure. Now here we are getting ready to dive in again. My wonderful hypnotherapist, John, made a great point today of saying that now that I have discovered I don't need to be sick to be significant, it is all falling into place to make that happen. I have found the right surgeon who will remove my tumor, and I will be healthy again. I think all of the epiphanies I have had over the last year play a part in leading me to this point. Obviously I wasn't ready to take in the messages a year ago, but now I am, culminating in bringing me back to health and a happy ending. That is what I choose to believe.

Xo Katie

## 7/2/13

Out of all of the trials and tribulations in our 13 years together, this is definitely the hardest thing Micah and I have ever gone through. I don't recommend it. Having children complicates things so much. Our lives are all work and no play, but on the flip side, they are my reasons for living. I think the only thing harder on a marriage would be losing a child. Every single day is a struggle. Right now we are in a pressure cooker. We are trying so hard to maintain some semblance of normalcy, but it's just impossible. The tension is thick. I am so stressed and overwhelmed. I am terrified, not by the surgery itself, but by what I will wake up to. The best-case scenario is that I will be temporarily paralyzed; that's the BEST-case scenario. The worst-case scenario is that I will be told nothing could be done. I have been through both of these. Being paralyzed, even temporarily, was a low point in my life. I didn't want to live that way. I know the temporary part. I've also faced the other scenario. It feels like a lose/lose situation, even though I know it's not. I'm afraid if I wake up paralyzed, I will panic. There is no way to prepare for that.

Xo Katie

### 7/3/13

It's funny (not ha ha funny) that girls, now women, who didn't want to be my friend before now are coming out of the woodwork. Whether it was petty jealousy or whatever, they are clearly no longer jealous of someone with brain cancer or they just feel guilty. I watched my wedding video with Lucky the other day and realized how many people are no longer in my life. It's sad because I'm not even sure why.

Xo Katie

### 7/4/13

I'm so grateful tonight for friends new and old. The theme song for the night is **"Good Feeling" by Flo Rida**. Happy fourth and happy 44 to me. If eight is a lucky number and my surgery is on 8/8 and I am 44, 4+4=8, I should be in good shape.

Xo Katie

## 7/5/13

Okay, so I believe in astrology. There you have it. Not the kind in the daily newspaper, but real astrology. My friend told me that Jupiter was entering the sign of Cancer (me), and that means great things for me for a whole year. "Life has not been easy for you over the past three years, but you are in line for a set of lucky breaks that should have you smiling at various points of 2013. Since late 2009, Saturn has been part of the group of planets making Cancer's life difficult, especially in regard to Cancer's home and family life. Lucky you, Jupiter loves being in Cancer! This is the first time since mid-2001 that Jupiter has come to your sign, and now you are in line to receive many rewards and lucky breaks in various areas of your life. In fact, with Jupiter at your side, you will likely find yourself at the right place at the right time, time after time. In truth, all sorts of medical procedures, including ones physical, such as surgery, would likely be successful any time this year. Your twelfth house and first house, both will be emphasized this year and are associated with the healing of your body, mind, or spirit. When it comes to gaining better health, you truly have a very upbeat outlook. Should you discover that you have a health concern at any point of 2013, be comforted in knowing that it is arising at a time when Jupiter is close. *Jupiter will help you find the right medical personnel who understand your condition and who are considered leaders in their field. So while Jupiter in Cancer can't guarantee you would never have a health issue (nothing in astrology is that way) his presence does suggest you will be able to locate a wonderful specialist to help you.*" WOW.

Okay, I do feel better reading this. It makes total sense, don't laugh.

Xo Katie

## 7/11/13

I went shopping today to buy some special toys for the kids for when I'm in the hospital. UCLA actually lets kids visit whereas Cedars wouldn't, but I'm not sure if I would want them to visit or not. I know I will want to see them, but I don't know if I want them to see me. Hospitals can be very scary places. Lucky did come visit when Haven was born, so he knows a little. So I'm trying to get all medical stuff out of the way since all of my deductibles have been met for the year. Today I went to the dermatologist for a skin check. I need melanoma like a hole in the head (see what I did there!). Next up is a mammogram—yay!

Xo Katie

## 7/13/13

My life has become a sitcom, like *Everybody Loves Raymond* or *Married With Children* except for the fact that there is no comedy and no one is laughing, so basically it's just a situation. One non-funny situation after another. I took the kids to a birthday party today at an indoor playground. They had a blast, but I had to take enough anti-anxiety medication to kill a small horse. Yet I still wanted to kill everyone there. I realized I can't be in a room filled with happy people talking about how big their kids have gotten or what new Lexus they're going to lease. I need to be with people whose lives are even remotely close to how miserable I am. It actually helps get me out of my own head, literally, and I can try to focus on boosting someone else up.

I wish my surgery was tomorrow, but I can't believe, cannot BELIEVE that I am having brain surgery again. I'm terrified, terrified of too many things to count. At this point we don't even know for sure if it's on. If it's not I don't know what I'll do.

Stressed.

Xo Katie

## 7/16/13

Today was a better day. I saw my hypnotherapist, and he cracked me up so bad. Who knew that the H.R. in H.R. Pufnstuf stood for "hand rolled"? Makes perfect sense, though. Am I the last person on Earth to know this? Besides making me laugh, he helps bring me back down to Earth.

Xo Katie

## 7/17/13

I will be emailing Dr. Liau on the 26th. We will know then if surgery is on or off. So far Jupiter's been good to me. Here at the Smith house we are preparing as if it's on. I have been cooking and freezing. We have also turned our sunroom into a guest room for the caregivers thanks to the generosity of friends, family, and strangers.

Xo Katie

## 7/20/13

I had a medium-size seizure yesterday, and all day I've felt hungover from all of the Ativan I took. I was alone with the kids, Haven was asleep, and I didn't call for Lucky because there is nothing he could've done. I was on my bed and had my meds next to me, so I took two, then another and rode it out. It's a very lonely experience. When Micah is there he talks to me and uncurls my hand so my nails don't cut into my palm. Also, I know that if he is there, he will know if it gets out of hand and we need more help. I would hate to put Lucky in that position.

Xo Katie

### 7/21/13

I'm going to see Dr. Lissa Rankin speak. She's the author of *Mind Over Medicine*. Couldn't be better timing.

Xo Katie

### 7/23/13

I can't believe how fast time is flying. I had my functional MRI yesterday and it went well. Different from Cedars. Technology is amazing. They had me do some motor functions on the left side, toes, fingers, and tongue, but mainly they focused on the cognitive aspects. They said that even though speech is on the left, it can migrate a little to the right, so they want to make sure they leave that intact. But strangely enough they would have me look at photos of things like dogs, a bench, a tree, and just think of the name—not even say it. I never spoke for the whole hour and a half, just thought about the images. How can they tell I'm coming up with the right response?

Xo Katie

### 7/24/13

I had such an amazing time the other night seeing one of my role models Dr. Lissa Rankin speak in person with my friend Jodi. It's funny, I almost didn't go because I had already read her book, and I didn't see how this lecture would introduce anything new. Boy, was I wrong. As she spoke about her mom's cancer scare, I started crying, and as I was sitting on the floor up front and in this intimate setting, she obviously noticed me. She finished her lecture and then came and sat down next to me and said she needed to acknowledge me and gave me a big hug. I started bawling of course, the ugly cry, and she held my hand and we talked. I told her a little of my story and what I was struggling with. She was so supportive and asked the other 30-40 women to form a circle around me, and she asked to have a healing silent prayer. It was so surreal and special. We talked about my surgery date and how everyone would be thinking about me and sending healing thoughts to me on that day. I was clearly meant to be there that night. She asked for my email, so hopefully we can correspond. A great night.

Xo Katie

## 7/26/13

The news we've been waiting for: From my surgeon: "Hi Kathleen, sorry for the delay in getting back to you, but it takes a while for the physicists to process the functional tractography results from your MRI scan and make the 3D reconstructions. I just reviewed your most recent MRI scans, and I do think that surgery would be warranted. The tumor appears to be pushing on your motor-sensory areas, but not directly infiltrating into them. As such, I do think that it would be possible to remove the majority of the tumor. I can't say for sure whether I can remove all the tumor or not until we are actually in surgery, as I would need to map the motor-sensory areas intra-operatively to confirm the areas that are safe. We can discuss the details and potential benefits/risks of surgery further when I see you in my clinic on August fifth. I should have screenshots of the 3D reconstructions of your brain images by then, so I can show you. Hope you have a nice weekend! Best, Linda Liau."

I'm ecstatic.

Xo Katie

## 7/29/13

I've been trying to get things done, cooking, freezing, shopping, getting our room done, etc. and I've told Lucky. At first he didn't like the idea, but I told him the pros like no more seizures, not having to nap every day, being able to drive, and that he could visit me at UCLA. He liked that. His one demand was that he wanted me to wait until camp was over; he wants to be home. No problem. The eighth is his last day and I will keep him home anyway. I am having more little seizures, no doubt due to the stress. By the way, Lissa Rankin talks about meeting me in her latest TED Talk. So cool! It's called "Is Medicine Killing You?" She mentions me at 13:03.

Xo Katie

## 8/1/13

I feel like I'm nesting, preparing for a baby to come. I've been cleaning the house like crazy, had all the carpets cleaned, cleaned all the couch cushions. The amount of dust accumulated from just closing in our sunroom was crazy. I think that's why I've had a headache every single day, all day. I've been cooking and freezing, buying the kids special presents, and I even started exercising a little. The other day we went bike riding as a family, which means around the block, and I couldn't believe how weak I was! Lots of people are asking me for the lowdown on next week. It's jam-packed with activities. Two birthdays and a baby shower, a pre-op visit, x-rays, EKGs, etc. on Tuesday, a meeting with the surgeon on Monday, Wednesday it's packing and a mani/pedi for sure. As of right now I am her second surgery of the morning. Don't know what time or where yet. Will find out Monday. When I'm in surgery Micah will be posting for me, so check your updates.

Xo Katie

## 8/3/13

I'm getting worried about Haven with me being in the hospital. She has become extremely attached to me lately and gets very jealous when I pay attention to Lucky. Tonight he was sitting on my lap, and she went ballistic. She started screaming for him to get off and came at him, grabbed him by the shoulders, and when he didn't budge, she grabbed him by the hair with two fists and started pulling. She was crazy mad and crying. Of course he didn't move because he was enjoying it, but it did hurt him. It was pretty funny, but I felt bad for her. The next three days are going to be very busy, but it's a good distraction for me.
Xo Katie

## 8/6/13

I had my meeting with my surgeon yesterday, Linda Liau. It was a good meeting. She showed us her 3D image of my brain, so cool. It seems that my tumor is nestled in my motor area. I envision an egg in an egg cup with another egg cup on top. There is an area in between where she will try to remove the tumor, and she feels like she can do it. She is confident she can get at least 90 percent, but as we know, anything can happen. She will get as close to the motor area as possible without taking it out. She reiterated to us how much she LOVES these kinds of tumors and that gliomas have a very individual feel and texture and she can go by feel. Only someone with a lot of experience can detect the difference between normal brain and gliomas. I feel confident in her abilities. Some good news: It appears that my left brain has already started taking over some of the functions of my right brain. That's a really good sign because it means that maybe I won't have as much deficit when I wake up as someone else would. As it is now, we expect paralysis in my arm and left hand, some minor drooping in my face, and weakness in my leg; whether it will be so weak that I can't walk, we won't know until then. I will be at the Ronald Reagan hospital at UCLA in Westwood. The first night I will be in intensive care, no visitors, but after that I can have visitors 24 hours a day and best of all my kids can come! Hopefully I won't look too scary :) Micah will be posting on this page the day of my surgery to let everyone know how I'm doing, so check often.

Right now it appears that I may be the only surgery that day, which means super early check-in. I will try to post tomorrow.

Xo Katie

### 8/7/13

Surgery is set for 1:30 p.m. with a check-in of 10:30 tomorrow morning. Micah will post to let everyone know how it went. Lots of love to you all and thanks for all the love and prayers.

Xo Katie

### 8/8/13

Success!!!!

Hi everyone, it's Micah. They got 90 percent of the tumor out, she had no seizures during surgery, and the initial biopsy of the tumor is that it's grade two! Katie is just waking up and she will be soooooo happy to hear the news. I'll post again soon. Please share this with everyone, and thank you all for your love and support!

Yippie!!!

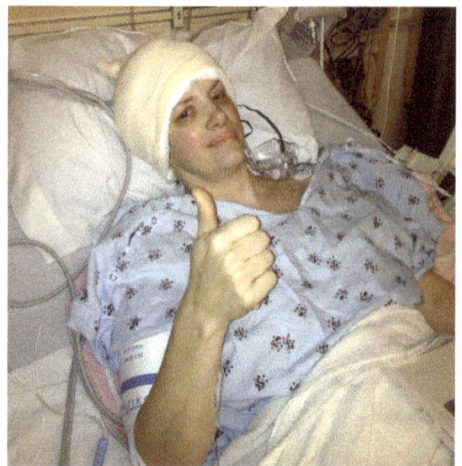 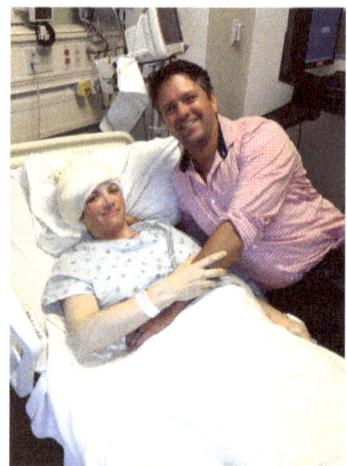

Our friend Dan, the doctor who came to our house to examine me when I first noticed my hand weakness.

## 8/9/13

Hi. It's Micah again... What an awesome day! Katie woke up very fast in recovery and was asking for me. After I was allowed in and told her the good news, we had a good cry together. Then I was able to bring her folks back one at a time for a quick hello since they wanted her to rest. When I came back in she was moving her arm, hand, leg, foot, etc. It was a miracle. Her doc was sure that she would have some paralysis in her entire left side after surgery and that it could take months before she might regain all mobility back. It's surreal to think that she will have a chance to have a normal life again… She needed this so badly. We all needed it. I'm not sure I can even remember what our life was like before this nasty tumor entered our lives. I look forward to getting past all of this and sharing some quality time with my family and friends.

Big Love from Katie's Hubby

## Later...

Hi everyone, here's the latest on my baby boo.

The poor girl has an excruciating headache and thus far no amount of morphine and norco has been able to squash it. She was only able to sleep a few hours during her stay in the ICU, so we spent a lot of time trying to make her as comfortable as possible today.

Now for the good part: she was released from ICU around 1 p.m. and is staying in room 6661 at the Henry Singleton Building / Ronald Reagan Hospital.

She walked today with a walker and a physical therapist, and she did a few circles in her room!

The preliminary report from her post-surgery MRI showed no bleeding and drew no red flags. I'm hoping she will be able to get some quality sleep tonight to heal and that she will get some relief from the pain to enjoy all of the good news.

Thanks for everyone's good wishes and kind words. I hope to try to get back to everyone soon.

Night Night from Micah

## 8/10/13

Hi everyone. It's Katie. I tried to post last night but of course got bumped offline. I was so tired, too, from all of the drugs and trying for an hour and a half with stupid nurses to get a new IV line started. As Micah has told you all the good news, I don't need to repeat. I am so grateful, but all is not roses over here. I think I deserve to kvetch just a little. It's been a much harder recovery this time, probably because they actually did something. BUT, I am in terrible, unending pain. It is almost unbearable at times, like being hit in the head with a hammer repeatedly all day long. It even hurts to laugh or smile.

The first night, the turban they wrapped around my head was

so tight that I was hysterically crying for them to cut it off or at least loosen it. They finally had to page a doctor because I was so upset. I yelled at him when he came because he was telling me that it needed to be tight to prevent swelling. I cried like a wild animal until he agreed to cut some of it. It's not just cloth; it's like a cast.

The first day or so, I had terrible panic attacks. Waking up partially paralyzed, even my tongue is paralyzed, was as scary as I thought it would be. When I eat or have to swallow a pill, I feel I might choke. I can't drink because I can't control the speed of the liquid going down, so they put a thickening powder in my juice to make it so that I don't swallow too fast. I can't move food to the back of my throat to swallow. I got up and walked for the first time yesterday, but my left leg is very weak. I need a walker or at least two people holding me up. I can lift my left arm in the air but can't hold it palms up, and I can squeeze someone's fingers if you put them in my hand, but I cannot pick up anything or let go. Basically I have very little control, if any, over my fingers. My smile is crooked, but my tongue seems better this morning. Obviously when I am on morphine and Vicodin all day, I am a lot weaker and sleepier. My friend Krista spent the first night in bed with me, and thank God for that. We actually kept getting fits of the giggles as I kept cracking jokes all night. For some reason I get so loony when I'm drugged. When I get panicky it's great to have physical contact and someone to snuggle, even if she does occasionally snore.

The steroids make me wired, so I think we slept two hours, not very restorative. Of course, my mom has been here with me too, waiting on me hand and foot, always ready to put the Carmex on my dry lips, and Micah's parents are holding down the fort at home, keeping the kids happy and entertained. I'm hoping they can come to visit me today. I have made a big decision to not go home right away but to head over to their physical therapy unit at least until Wednesday, when Micah's parents leave. I am simply not able to take care of myself. I am also on insulin because the steroids raise my blood sugar, as well as heparin to prevent blood clots. I take eight pills twice a day, not including the IV meds or Vicodin pills, and insulin and heparin shots in my stomach. Fun stuff over here. I think I may be ready for visitors if you can stand the way I look :)

Xo Katie

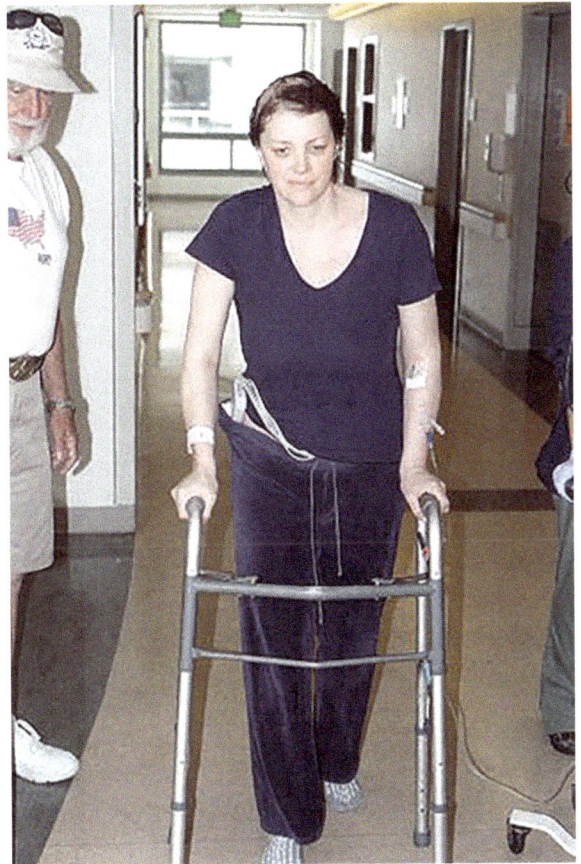

Doing a lap

## 8/10/13

I just got to Skype with my kids.

## 8/11/13

Another day in paradise. Making small improvements, but I am convinced that I need to go straight to rehab, physical therapy, occupational therapy, and speech therapy. As pleased as we were with the movement I had post-surgery, I still have major deficits on my left side. I have a very weak leg, I'm using a walker, I can squeeze a hand but still can't open my fingers, and my speech is slurred. My tongue is coming back slowly. I have made small improvements. I can lift my left arm and now I can rotate my wrist so I can be sort of palms up. That's huge for me; it takes a lot of effort. I am now off Morphine and on Oxycodone. The Morphine would hit me so fast through the IV that the sensation felt like a seizure and I would panic. I asked them to put me on something else. I look like a junkie too. I am a human pincushion. Blood is taken every six hours. They're running out of spaces—Heparin shots for blood clots, pricking fingers and insulin for blood sugar—but the good news is that they are reducing my steroids, so my blood sugar should go back to normal. My pain level is also much better, so even though I look like a junkie, I'm glad to say that I am not.

It hasn't really sunk in yet that I have this thing out and that I have my whole life ahead of me. It's like being pardoned by the governor from death row.

How does one really move forward from here? I know that I want to take the next year to spend quality time with my family and do things that bring me joy. I am going to get through rehab and then take my kids to their first days of school!

The kids came to visit me today. Lucky was a real trooper and so mature. Haven had a really hard time saying goodbye; she cried and begged me to come home with her and read her books. It broke my heart and I cried too. She can't possibly understand why I can't come home. I did a lap around the ward with them and my walker. Lucky thought it was all cool, but Haven just wanted me to pick her up. Something I'm not allowed to do.

Xo Katie

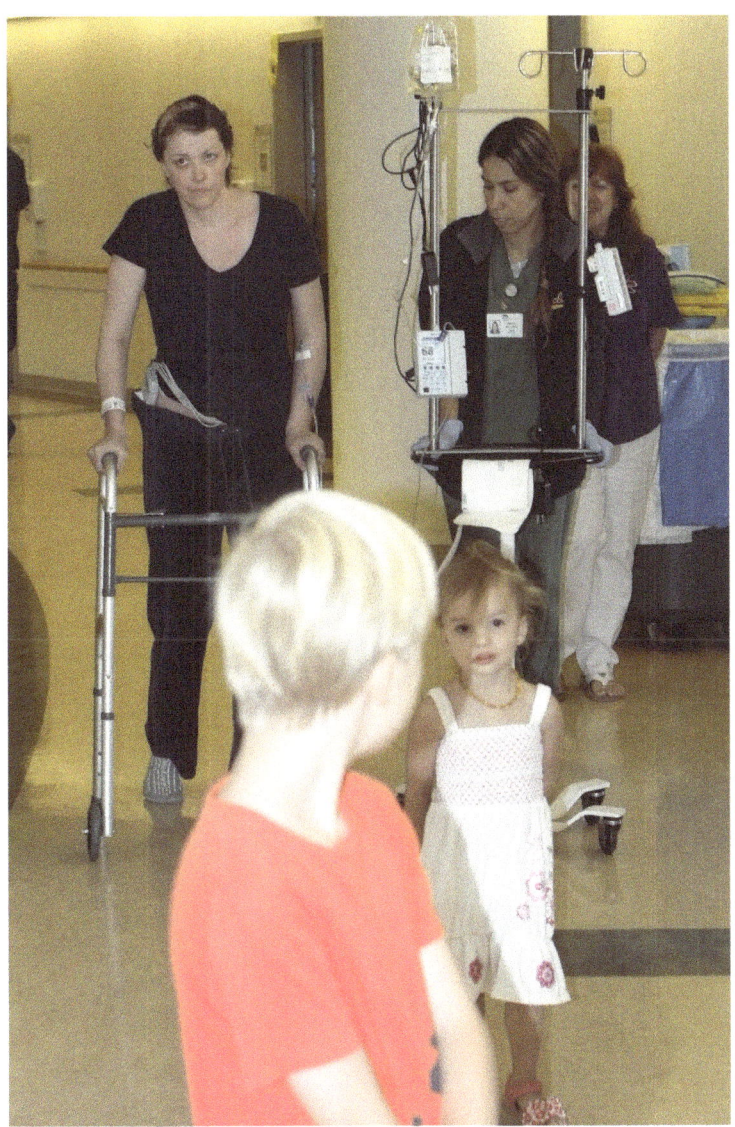

Walking with the kids

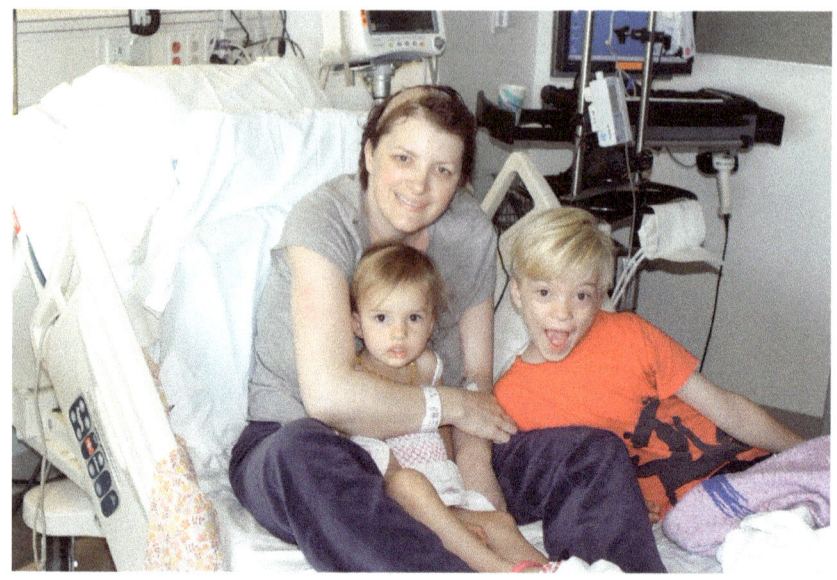

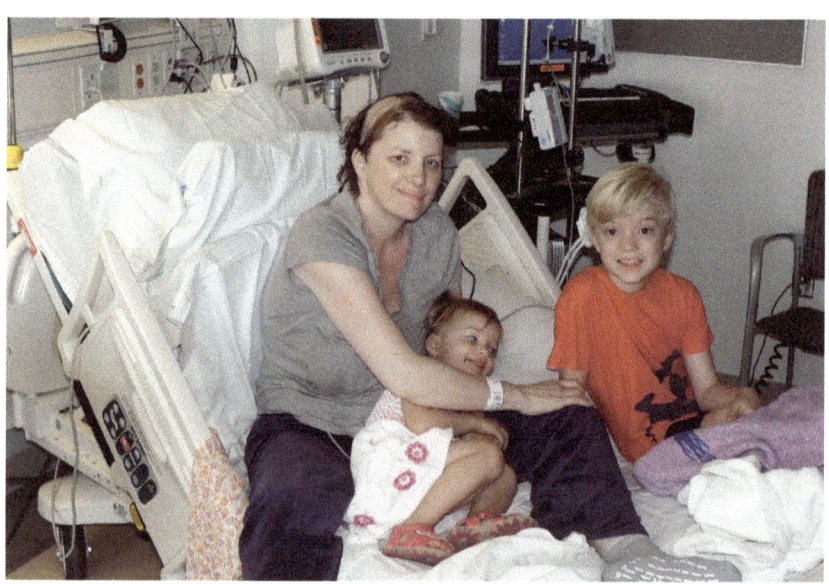

My kids visiting me in the hospital

## 8/12/13

I'm having a blast over here, not kidding; that may be why I'm improving quickly. My mom and I laugh all day. Something strikes us as funny, and we just can't stop. Too bad I usually have food in my mouth, and it all falls out, and I spit and drool. I look like an insane person. I usually end up spitting all over her, which gets us laughing even more. Then I pee my pants and we have to change everything (sorry, TMI), but all you moms know what I'm talking about. The first night my mom said, "Do you want to brush your teeth?" I was in so much pain I said, "I don't give a shit about brushing my teeth." She gave me a look because she's not used to hearing me cuss, and I said, "Give me a break. You can wash my mouth out with toothpaste!" That first night in the ICU, they are not concerned with you getting any rest. That's good, because I didn't. REM sleep ain't gonna happen. In the room to my left, I heard an older man yelling/howling and then the nurse saying, "Sir, please take your hands off your privates." I got fits of giggles for a while after that one; then Krista would start, then my mom. Then it sounded like he was Skyping his grandchildren, and I was thinking, *My mom can barely use her cell phone.* But his wife sounded like the teacher from *Charlie Brown*. Clearly I was hyper aware of everything going on. At 1:30 a.m. housekeeping started cleaning the room to our right. It sounded like they were throwing a party. I asked my nurse to please ask them to keep their voices down, which she did; then she proceeded to stand in front of my door and talk for one hour about her vacation plans. I think we finally fell asleep at 2:30 a.m., and then I heard them moving furniture around next door.

UGH.

At some point I started smelling something really bad, but I wasn't going to point any fingers (because I can't), and then I realized it was my own breath! I should've listened to my mom. Got a fit of giggles over that, and it reminded me of something Micah says, not to me of course, but just as a joke: "What did you have for breakfast? A poo poo sandwich?"

Apparently brain surgery gives me a snorting problem too. With the first surgery, afterward I always snorted while yawning; now I do it while laughing. That cracks my mom up like nothing else. They gave Krista a lovely yellow plastic gown to sleep in, and the nurse told her that she looked like Beauty from *Beauty and the Beast* and I said, "Does that make me the beast?" You can see that I was completely out of my mind that night.

I chose the song "**Delirious" by Prince** as this week's theme song.

P.S. Being transferred to rehab at Northridge hospital tomorrow (UCLA was booked) most likely! Yeah! Closer to friends and the kids' school!

Xo Katie

## 8/13/13

Another restful night in the hospital, not. TMI warning:

Naturally, I got my period yesterday (because I can never catch a break), and because I am on blood thinners my bed turned into what looked like a crime scene! God bless Krista who took care of me, called the nurse, and cleaned up the floor and me! She is truly a best friend! I literally can't get to the bathroom by myself.

As I get better and they wean me off some of these meds, then they alternately need to give me less meds. For example, the steroids raise my blood sugar, so they had to give me insulin. Now my steroids are half what they were, so they don't have to wake me in the night to check my sugar or give me insulin. I hardly take any pain meds, but I am getting those sharp, stabbing, healing-from-surgery pains. I keep asking when I can shower or wash my hair, and they say I can as long as I don't get the incision wet. Yeah, right! I have an eight-inch incision across the whole top of my head. I had a pretty fun night with Krista.

She's a great caregiver. I forgot to mention that her lovely, yellow plastic gown was for the "lockdown" patients, and since we are on the neuro ward, they wouldn't let her walk down the hallways to the bathroom! They thought she was an escaped patient on lockdown! So funny! This morning I balanced on my left leg while picking up something with my right toes, not bad? I do see small progress every day. Can't wait until I can open my left hand; it will make a huge difference. I Skyped with Haven last night. I miss my babies so much. I can't believe I have to be away from them for so long.

Xo Katie

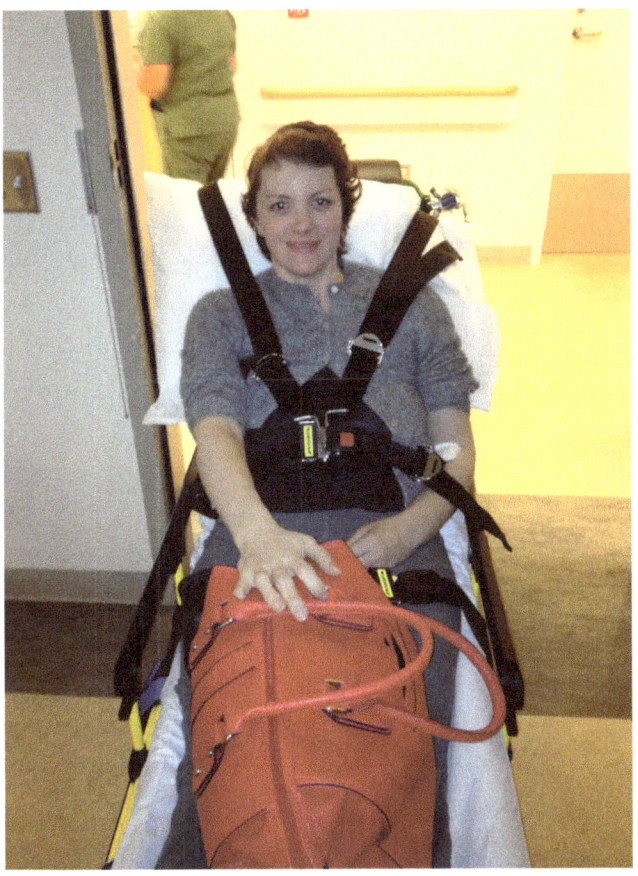

Ambulance ride to rehab

## 8/13/13

Hi. I'm at my new rehab facility and I'm alone tonight for the first time and feeling a little lonely, I must admit. Thought I'd reach out to my friends because I'm missing home and my family so much. I can't believe I haven't held my kids in days. I miss them sooo much. Micah will bring them by tomorrow, but saying goodbye is so hard. I can't even hold my baby yet. I'm trying to remember the long-term goals and not focus on missing them.

I've made a lot of progress in a short time, and that's a good thing. But getting home is the goal. This rehab in Northridge is still a hospital, and it feels like one. I sit in my wheelchair and look in the mirror, and I don't recognize myself. My hair is dark and curly and short. I look like my grandmother except that I have the bald spot still with a huge, scabby incision in the middle, my face is droopy, my mouth is uneven, I can't smile, and I have huge, dark circles around my eyes. I feel like a monster. I cry when I look at my reflection. Who am I? Song of the day: "**Beautiful**" **by Christina Aguilera.**
Xo Katie

## 8/14/13

Finally, a decent night's sleep. I was only woken up once to take a pill. It is not only frowned upon but forbidden to get out of bed by yourself. So even though getting up to go to the bathroom in the night is second nature, you can't do that here. You have to call in the troops. Yesterday I called and a male nurse came in. I'm thinking, *You want me to go to the bathroom with you in here? Are you going to buy me dinner first because I just met you 10 SECONDS AGO!* The degradation continues... Oh, and I haven't pooped in eight days! That's what pain meds do to you! Been up since five a.m. because I wasn't tired and couldn't wait any longer, but now I'm starving, and breakfast doesn't come until eight. Considering eating a Mrs. Fields cookie from a tin a friend brought me.

Xo Katie

## 8/15/13

Hi. Waiting to get to work over here. I'm still making small, sometimes almost imperceptible improvements, but it often feels as though they are not letting me do the things I am able to do, like walk. My bed has an alarm on it, and if I get up without help, it goes crazy. Granted, I am not super stable, but I was walking more at UCLA. My fingers moved a few times this morning—out, not in, which is important. My voice seems better this morning; it was very hoarse yesterday. I'm looking forward to therapy, but so far my improvements seem like they are just related to time passing. One of the main reasons I am okay staying here is because I am still afraid of seizures, and they are keeping a close eye on my meds and making sure they are at "therapeutic levels." I had an ultrasound of my legs yesterday to make sure I had no blood clots, and I am still on blood thinners and steroids. It's lonely here. I'm not used to being alone. I don't like it. I think I am going to put some pressure on them for a little more freedom, though. The kids came yesterday and seemed to have fun and be happy. I NEED to be well by the first week of September for all the school functions and to take the kids to their first days. It's super important to me.

Xo Katie

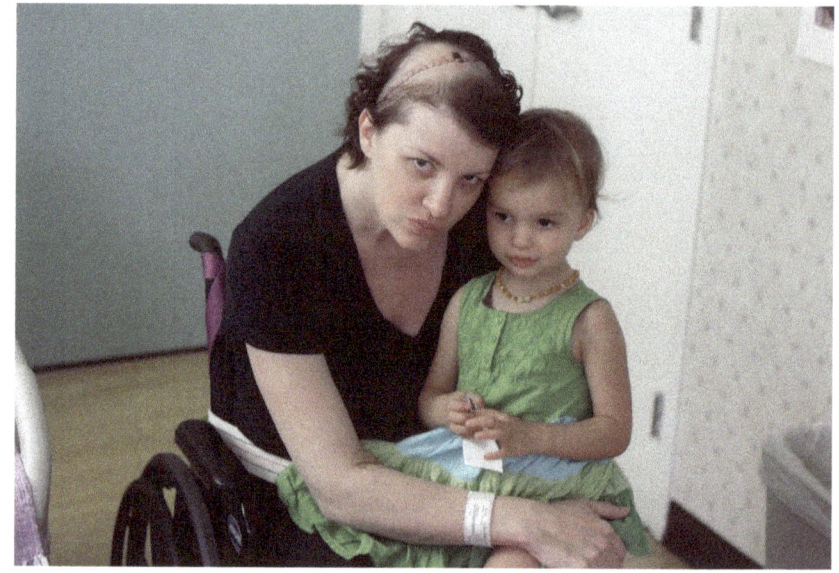

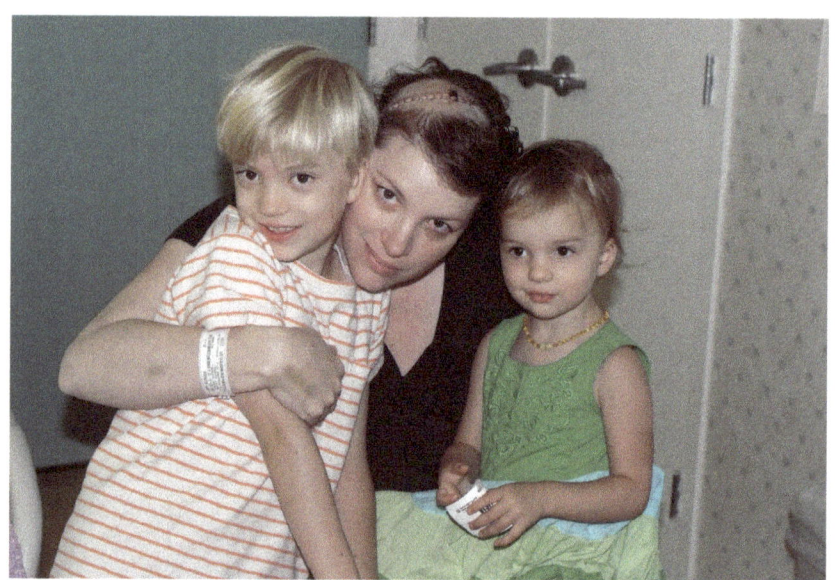

Getting a visit from the kids in rehab

## Later…

Okay, I kind of retract that last post because my physical therapist just finished kicking my ass. I will be sore tomorrow. Off to occupational therapy soon to work on my hand. I also figured out that the key to freedom here is to never get back in your bed. Once you're out, stay out! I am sitting in a wheelchair, but at least I can get around without asking for help. I saw a doctor while I was working out and complained about lack of freedom, and she said that if they report that I am doing really well and walking around on my own, my insurance will kick me out. Got it! I was writing an email to a friend, and I'm going to copy and paste it here because it explains how I am feeling:

"My situation is so odd that I can't even really process it. Everyone is so happy and elated and my family is walking on air, but I feel basically the same. I can't comprehend that I may have a future now, when a week ago I didn't. Especially because I am still in a hospital and I am still dealing with healing from this damn thing. I feel like I have lost my identity, I don't recognize myself in the mirror, I have no job and am not home to be a wife and mother. I still cry every day. I want to go home. Now who am I supposed to be if I'm not the woman with brain cancer? Once I'm outta here I hope to spend the next year reconnecting with my kids. I mentally and physically distanced myself from them, and I don't want to do that anymore. I was afraid to get close. It's going to take a while and lots of time to put this behind me. But I will. Life is beautiful."

Xo Katie

## 8/16/13

I just got back from physical therapy. I got to go outside and walk a few blocks, and it felt like heaven. It's amazing how much you miss the simple pleasures like the sun on your face and fresh air, walking on grass. It feels like I've been under fluorescent lights for a year. The PT said I am definitely better and more balanced than yesterday. I raised a stink this morning because they only had me working with the occupational therapist (hand work) for one hour today, and that was it for the day! A supervisor came to see me, and I went over my frustrations, like working with an intern yesterday who didn't know what she was doing. I said I felt I was wasting my time here. She was very understanding and will fix it for me. At least I get some hand and arm work with the PT lady; she puts me to work, holding a basketball out in front of me and doing squats and pushups against a wall, so I am getting some work on it.

During my OT today they used muscle stimulation, which means they put electrical pads on my arm muscles to make my fingers move. It's kind of a painful feeling and reminded me of what having a seizure looked and felt like because my hand and fingers were moving, but I wasn't doing it. It was the first time I saw my fingers move in a week, so I was happy to see that, and my mom thought it was funny to watch.

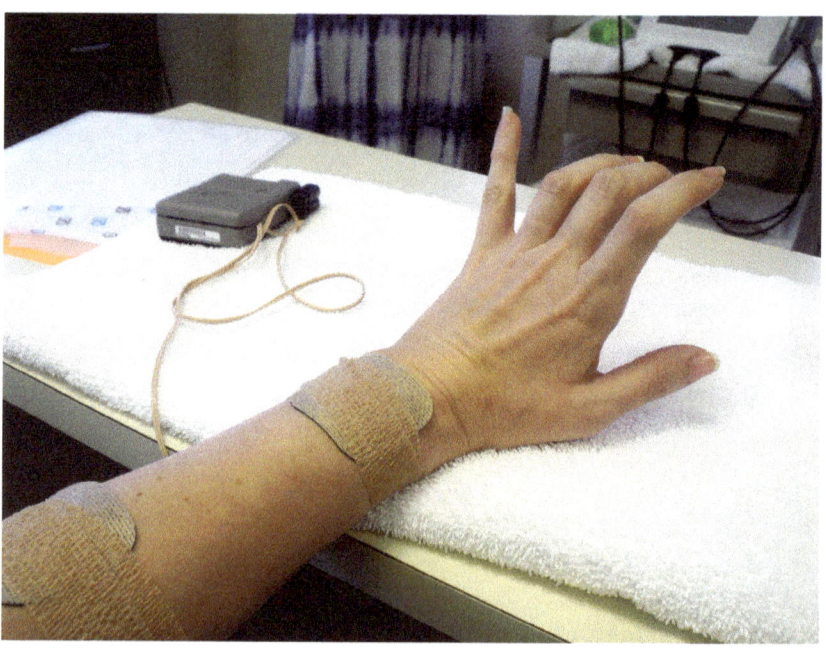

Watching my fingers open

I am not a patient person, very type A, and even though I know I am recovering at a fast pace, it's hard to stave off depression here. I want this nightmare behind me. I know that going straight home would have been a bad decision, but this is so hard. Micah and the kids came yesterday, and as I was coming down the hall, I saw Haven in a little lavender dress. When she saw me she ran into my arms. She looked like an angel, and my heart just melted. The first thing she said was "Mommy, can you come home today?" Saying no broke my heart. Lucky seems like he is handling everything okay, but I just kept pulling him to me and kissing him, trying to connect. Have I said I can't wait to go home?

Xo Katie

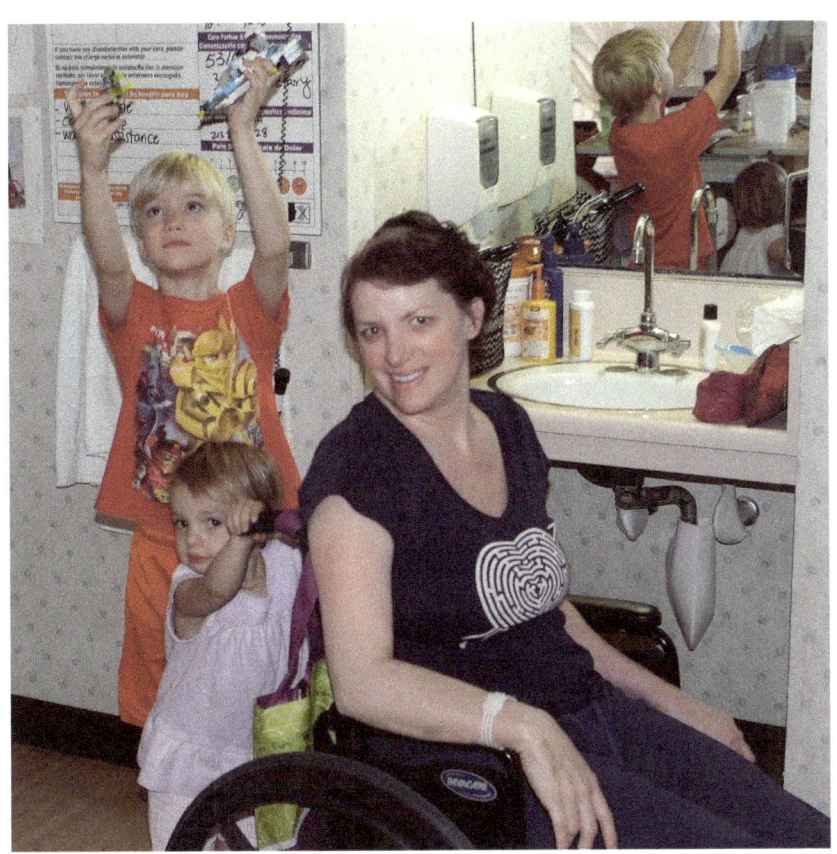

Another visit from the kids

## 8/17/13

Hi. I am home! I checked myself out of that bullshit rehab. I got my schedule this morning and saw that I had only an hour and a half of rehab today and ZERO tomorrow. I end up working on my own most of the time anyway. I threw a FIT and packed my bag, called Micah, and said, "Get me outta here." I cried and yelled at everyone. They tried to stop me and convince me to stay, and I just went off! Don't mess with Katie on steroids!

I can sit in bed and rot all day at home, and at least I can be with my kids. I truly believe they just want the insurance money. So now I need to find an occupational therapist or hand specialist to come to my house so that I can go work on an outpatient basis. My kids need my attention really badly, so I'm going to spend the weekend with just us.

Xo Katie

## 8/17/13

I am so happy to be home, but I actually wish I was somewhere working to get better. I feel useless at home and am literally bumping into walls.

Xo Katie

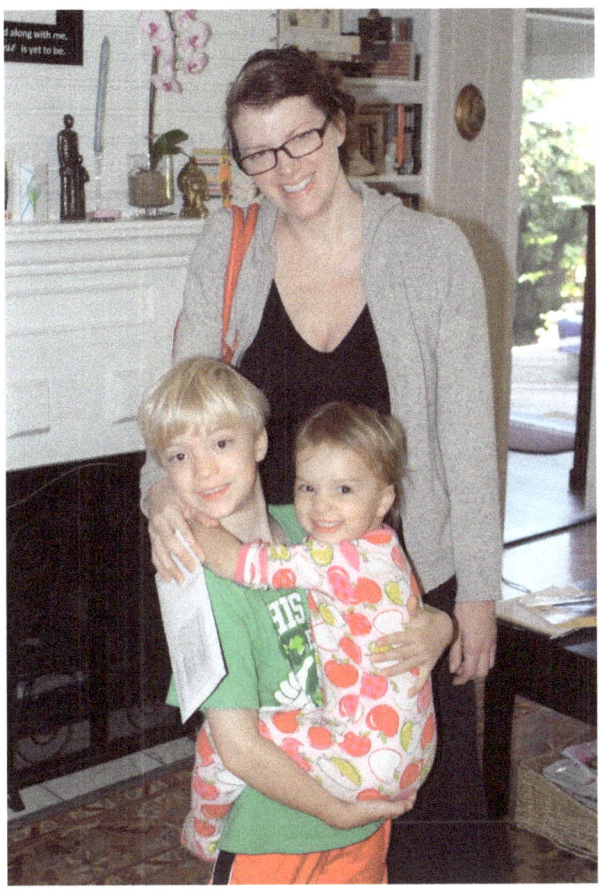

We are all happy I'm home

## 8/19/13

Doctor's appointment today. The final pathology report was misleading; it actually shows the tumor as a grade four, which would be a glioblastoma multiforme, the most dangerous, aggressive kind of tumor. The confusion lies in the fact that the person who looks at the tumor is seeing rapidly dividing and dying cells, which is a sign of an aggressive tumor, but he didn't know that I had undergone radiation and chemo, which causes necrosis, which is rapidly dying cells.

So they are grading it as a three still because they did find a small percentage of dividing cells, three-five percent, which is a very small amount, and they are happy about that.

As a grade three we could choose to do more chemo, but because there is only five-ten percent of the tumor left and it is not really doing anything, they said we could just wait and watch it. That is my choice. I honestly need a break from any kind of treatment or procedures. I want to rest, heal, and enjoy my seizure-free life. I got my stitches out today, and it was so painful. It feels like I had a facelift because of the tight, pulling feeling on the top and side of my head, and pulling out the stitches hurt a lot. Scalp skin is so thick.

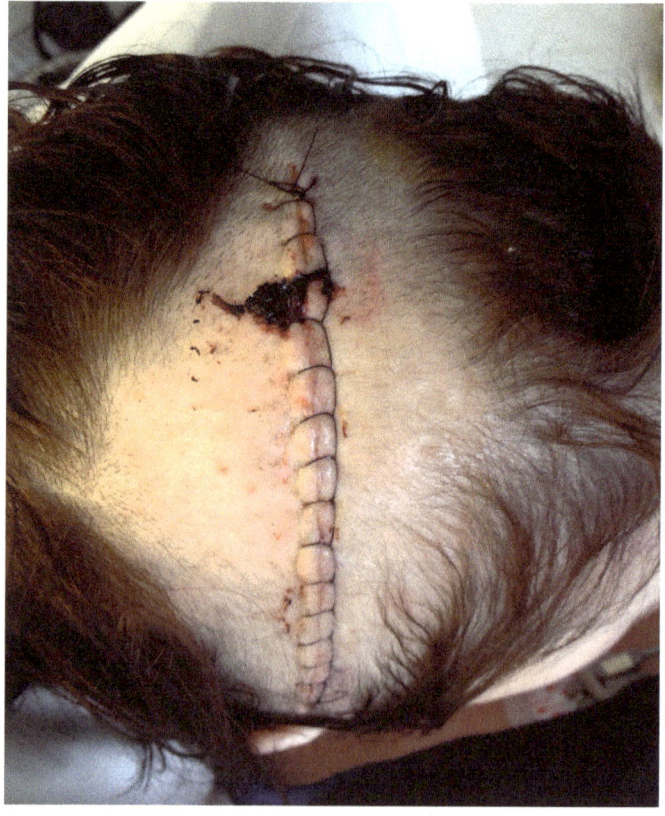

Ouchy

I remember after my first surgery this feeling like I was on another planet. I didn't notice it as much in the hospital or rehab because you kind of expect to not feel normal, but now that I'm home, it feels really strange. When I walk it's like the house is spinning or tilted. I feel dizzy and am constantly stubbing my toes and slamming my left arm into door knobs and door frames. What I don't know is whether it's from all the anesthesia, steroids, and painkillers or whether it's from having a large chunk of my brain removed. My leg is strong but I can tell it's not 100 percent okay because I have to consciously remind myself to bend my knee so I don't trip on stuff like a crack in the sidewalk. My face is still weak. My talking has improved, but my smile isn't straight yet. My hand is the weakest still. I can move my arm but can barely open my fingers. My thumb and pointer are also numb. I am starting a new rehab tomorrow. I want to work hard.

Xo Katie

## 8/20/13

I had a great day at my new rehab. It's so much better. They have the electromagnetic muscle stimulator, and they had me get a one-pound weight to do some exercises at home. I like the people and it's clean and close by. They are going to make a daytime splint that will keep my fingers open and extended, and I have my nighttime splint from rehab to keep my hand in an open and relaxed position. I am trying to use my hand more throughout the day, but it's hard to remember because it's basically just a paperweight right now, or a "stabilizer."

I rode my exercise bike for a few minutes but then got a headache and had to stop. I'm still wrestling with a fear of seizures. I haven't had any, but the fear that one will hit out of nowhere is always there.

Xo Katie

## 8/22/13

My fingers opened this morning!

## 8/24/13

This morning we did what I would consider our first "normal" activity as a family. We went to IHOP with just the four of us; then we went to Big 5 and bought Lucky some roller skates. It was nice, so nice. Even though it still hasn't sunk in all the way, I am starting to actually feel the relief and the weight of the world slowly lifted off my shoulders.
Xo Katie

## 8/26/13

I had a busy day today. First, hand therapy at 9:00 a.m. My therapist was very excited about the progress I had made over the weekend. I can now open my fingers on a regular basis. It's still clumsy, and my hand shakes violently, but I can do it at will.
Xo Katie

## 8/28/13

I am in a foul mood. I am so frustrated that I can't use my hand. The progress seems so miniscule, even though I am working so hard. Then I get a comment from Micah such as, "Are you even trying to use your hand?" Fuck me. No one understands how hard it is to even try to butter a piece of toast. First, I have to put my weak hand on the scalding piece of toast to hold it down; then I butter as much as I can before I start buttering my fingers while trying to push down so the plate doesn't fall off the counter. My thumb and index finger are still numb, so they are useless. I actually have to be careful not to injure myself as I could easily cut myself without even knowing it. I try to do the best I can, but everything is a struggle, so it's easier to just try to do things one-handed. It took me 15 minutes to zip up my hoodie yesterday. I got so frustrated I had to walk away for a while. I know it's temporary, yada yada yada. But when this happened last year, it was one of the lowest points in my life.

Want to hear something weird? I laugh differently now, I cry differently, I have a hard time sneezing, and when I yawn, my left arm goes up in the air and shakes. My brain has changed, and now I am different. I don't recognize the sound of my own crying. It's more like an animal wailing; it's so strange and painful to hear.

None of this is over for me, not by a long shot. I still have no freedom, no independence, no space. I want to drive so badly. I want to crank my music up, MY music, blast the AC, listen to whatever I want and just drive. I want to go shopping without someone telling me they don't like that or I don't need that. It's so degrading.

I thought when I was pregnant that I had never looked so awful with my acne, greasy hair, and extra 40 pounds. Now I would kill to look like that.

People avert their eyes when they look at me. I feel invisible. But I can always count on children to tell the truth. At Haven's Mommy and Me gymnastics class, a two-year-old came up to me and said, "Do you have a little bit of hair?" I said, "Yes, I have a little bit of hair."

It doesn't matter to me what other people think; it only matters what I think, and this is not me. While I was in rehab, in a wheelchair with a six-inch-long gash across a huge bald spot, a lopsided face, and short, curly brown hair, a friend came to visit me and she said, "Now this is the Katie I can relate to." How messed up is that? Why are women so insecure? Why do women enjoy seeing other women down? I've never understood the type of person who would be happy to see me in this condition. It's sad, more sad than being in the state I'm in.

Xo Katie

## 9/9/13

Strange day today. We had an appointment with Dr. Liau, my surgeon. The meeting left Micah and me scratching our heads. Regarding the pathology report, it showed necrosis, as we knew. What she explained is that necrosis can look like squiggly lines or stars. Squiggly lines would indicate that the dying cells are grade-four cancer, and star shapes indicate regular old necrosis. My tumor only had 35 percent, but they were the squiggly line type. Otherwise known as glioblastoma multiforme, grade-four cancer. So the radiation killed off the grade-four cells. Thank God! Normally if it were a GBM they would expect to see 30-50 percent of the tumor be squiggly lines. My low percentage is a good sign, but I asked if most of my tumor could be a low grade with only a small part a GBM, and she said it was possible. She kept saying that the pathology, necrosis, and diagnosis were up for interpretation. Different pathologists could interpret it in different ways. She felt there was no rush but that we should follow up with some chemo just in case.

This news confused me because we thought it was a grade three all along. This new news depressed me. My chart would forever label me as a grade-four cancer patient. The only upside to this is that it makes me more eligible for clinical trials. Unfortunately, for a lot of the trials, you can't have been radiated or have had chemo before. Thanks again, Dr. X!

There is a chance that what we saw on the MRI right after surgery was swelling and that my next MRI in October might show that she actually removed all of it. We will see. She was also pleased that I haven't had any seizures. She said the first month is the most likely time, then after three months the odds go down even more. I made it through the first month, good news!

Even with all the good news, I couldn't help but feel depressed all day. I feel like there is never any relief for me. Now I have to worry about this grade four BS. I just want some relief. The oncologist wasn't concerned, and next we will show it to my Cedars oncologist and see what he says. I need his opinion. I NEED to be able to forget about this for a while. I can't believe that in 2012 we thought it was grade two with only some grade three cells and now we are told that it was grade three with 35% grade four all along. I'm glad I didn't know that it was glioblastoma multiforme because I would have been so terrified that I think my whole attitude would have been so different. I would have felt doomed. I need a break.

Xo Katie

## 9/12/13

Yesterday my friend Nicole called and reminded me that it was the one-year anniversary of the day I collapsed at Hugo's restaurant. She was the one who caught me and cared for me, so it was a bond we shared on that day. I had forgotten. I guess that's a good sign. I obviously had not forgotten the incident and have thought about it many, many times, but this year I was more focused on remembering the tragedy of 9/11/2001, as I always am at this time of year. It's a perfect example of how things can always be worse and how lucky we really are.

Xo Katie

P.S. I forgot to mention that on the 11th I drove myself to Starbucks, the nail salon, and Target—all by myself. It couldn't have been more opposite than the way I spent it last year, in the emergency room.

Xo Katie

### 9/14/13

I had a great day shopping with my buddy Krista, got home late, tried to nap but only got about 30 minutes. When I woke up I had a seizure. Haven and I were cuddling in bed eating popcorn when my pinky and ring finger on the left hand started twitching. I didn't think much of it at first, maybe muscle fatigue; then the whole hand started shaking and clawing. It moved up my arm and started convulsing. I yelled for Micah, who was thankfully close by, and handed him my Ativan bottle. I was so freaked out because the doctor had just told us that it was great we had made it through the first month without a seizure. I had Micah give me four Ativan, oy, because I was so taken by surprise and terrified it might escalate into something bigger. We paged the oncologist, and he said it was most likely just healing and that he wasn't worried about it at all. I guess I have to curtail my driving again. I'm so frustrated. I started crying because I just can't take the roller coaster anymore. I need predictability. Will this ever end?

Xo Katie

### 9/15/13

A little part of my spirit died last night. I can't take this anymore. I'm so depressed. WTF? Now all of the plans I had for fall and winter have a dark cloud over them. Will they happen at all? I wanted this to be my happy ending. I swear to God, a person can only take so much. When will it end?

Xo Katie

### 9/16/13

I'm feeling a lot better; my mood has lifted. I actually had another seizure on the way to school this morning(I wasn't driving), but all I felt was the numbness creeping up my arm and into my chest, back, and face. There were no convulsions, so I didn't mention it right away. I just rode it out.

Xo Katie

## 9/19/13

Well, it's official, school has started. Haven is sick. On the upside I haven't had a seizure in two days, and I drove myself to rehab. Hopefully that's it. I can't wait until October. We are already decorating for Halloween!

Xo Katie

## 9/22/13

I have been frustrated and depressed at my lack of abilities. This deficit was what I dreaded the most. So many things I still can't do for myself. I know it seems silly but you really can't appreciate something until it's gone, and how hard it is to depend on other people to do the simplest things. I can't believe it may be months until I will be able to resume normal activities. The other night I was making vegetable soup for the kids, and I was chopping carrots. I was proud of myself but at the same time, because I can't feel a few fingers, the thought went through my head that if I saw one of my fingers roll across the cutting board, I would be really upset.

Xo Katie

## 9/24/13

Some Lucky-isms from this morning: "Can I wake up Haven? She's so cute," then hugging her. "It's so nice when they first wake up. They're so warm."

Xo Katie

## 9/25/13

Well, you haven't really made it until someone writes a song inspired by you! Singer/songwriter Gary Numan (most famous for writing and singing "Cars" and many others) has a song on his new album inspired by me (his kids go to our school, and our families are friends). It's called "My Last Day." My plight seems to have touched a nerve and gotten him thinking, like most people, about not being around to watch his kids grow up. He and his wife, Gemma, wouldn't tell me about the song until after my surgery. I guess it's depressing, and they wanted to make sure that surgery went well first! Here's what he said about it in an interview:

"We have a friend in LA who was diagnosed with brain cancer and was told she could die at any time. And I was incredibly impressed with her attitude and strength towards that, but it made me think about if you were told you only had one day to live what would you regret? So the song is mostly about my children, regretting not seeing them grow up. The happy side of what's quite a grim story is that she had a risky operation and they took out 95 percent of the tumor and has a very long life ahead of her. It was an incredible story and we were part of it, in a way."

-Gary Numan

Combined with Lissa Rankin's TED Talk where she talks about my surgery and meeting me, this may be the only 15 minutes of fame I ever get!

Xo Katie

## 10/1/13

On Monday I have an MRI scheduled as well as an appointment at UCLA. We will be looking to see if there is any tumor left or if it was just swelling that we saw on the MRI the day after surgery. We will also check to see if anything has changed, and we will discuss any further treatment.

I was outside on my hammock tonight listening to my music and thinking about the last year and a half. I can't believe what I've been through. For the first time I thought of myself as a brave person, a person who doesn't quit. I knew that this thing was never going to get me, but I never knew quite how I would beat it.

I don't think I'm brave because of the pain I've gone through but because of the choices I've made. Deciding to go see Dr. Liau and have a second surgery was probably the bravest thing I've ever done. The books I've read have inspired me and changed the way I look at the world and my life. I can say now that I have very little fear. I don't think about dying or whether I will be here to see my children grow up. I do still have panic attacks sometimes when I think about seizures. Today I was lying on my side in my bed going through the mail, and when I stood up my hand started tingling and there was a pins and needles feeling. I called for Micah and told him something was happening. At that moment I realized that my arm had fallen asleep, and the pins and needles feeling was the blood returning to the hand, a normal feeling. There was nothing wrong with me. My hand had fallen asleep!

Xo Katie

## 10/3/13

I've been going through my medical records and discovered that certain key parts have been omitted, such as the meeting with Dr. X where he goes over the results of my functional MRI (where he says he can take out 95 percent) as well as the meeting after the surgery where he recommends radiation and chemo. Suspicious. It looks like I will have to call his office. I've had all of my records from UCLA sent over to Dr. Rudnick. He wanted to look at everything and then Micah and I will pay him a visit. Once we are there I'll ask him if he has the missing records. If he doesn't, then I will visit Dr. X's office.

Xo Katie

## 10/6/13

I'm finally off my ice cream bender, back on the wagon now. It's strange how for the last 18 months I have craved turkey sandwiches so badly. I have probably had over 200 turkey sandwiches since my first surgery. I don't know why. I really haven't had any other cravings, maybe brownies, but I try to keep that under control. I do miss soda but I'm doing okay without it, and I miss milk sometimes, especially with my brownies! Ha!

Xo Katie

## 10/7/13

I had my MRI today at 10:30 a.m. and finally left the hospital at three! The doctor was way backed up, and we waited almost two hours to see him to discuss the results.

Basically all of the visible tumor is GONE. She got it all out! OMG! I can't believe it. What they see now is the empty cavity (it has collapsed some) along with some scar tissue around it. But, and this is a big BUT, they will not say the tumor is gone because for sure there are tumor cells they cannot see. For sure. In their opinion it is not a matter of IF it comes back, but when.

Obviously I have bought myself some time, but they have seen people whose tumors start growing back after two weeks! They don't expect this of my tumor because of my rockin' gene mutation IDH1. But they don't want to take any chances, so they want me to finish the four more rounds of chemo (CCNU). They believe this will suppress the cells that are left from growing.

To be blunt, I am buying time. My oncologist assured me that there are medications specifically for people with gliomas with the IDH1 mutation that are right around the corner from being used on humans. God willing by the time I need anything like that, there will be a cure. I'm hoping for 10 years or more. The worst part is that I will always be looking over my shoulder, waiting for that next MRI so I can breathe for a few weeks. At least I'll be breathing.

And I am seizure free! A huge blessing, and I can drive, windows down, with the wind on my scalp! Phew!

Xo Katie

## 10/15/13

I had an appointment today with Dr. Rudnick, my Cedars oncologist. We brought Haven with us as it was a school holiday. When we walked into the room, she said, "Where's your bed?" Kind of sad that that is what she's used to.

The doctor was very happy with my MRI. After reading the pathology report, he also thought that there were some cells that had become grade-four, although he was quick to say that a grade four with IDH1 is not the same as a grade-four without it, plus, they got that all out. My final question for him was did he think my prognosis had changed? Would I live longer? Long enough to see my children grow up? And he said, "ABSOLUTELY, AB-SO-LUTE-LY!" So that was a great way to end the meeting!

Xo Katie

## 10/15/13

A paraphrase from the show *Breaking Bad* when Walter's family finds out his cancer is in remission. His wife says, "You think there's going to be this relief, this light at the end of the tunnel. But there's just more tunnel." Exactly.

Xo Katie

## 10/17/13

A quote from Dr. Liau regarding my visit and questions I had from my visit with Dr. Rudnick.

"Hi Katie,

I agree with Dr. Rudnick and Dr. Cloughesy that I removed everything that was safe to remove. There is an area of residual T2 abnormality on the MRI scan within your motor cortex, but having been in your brain, I think much of this is gliosis (scar tissue) from your previous radiation and chemo, not necessarily residual tumor. I do think that there is some amount of residual tumor, but personally think it is more in the five-ten percent range (not 30 percent as Dr. Rudnick suggests). Regardless, I don't think that I could have safely removed any more, so I do believe that you had a maximal resection. We do have tumor tissue stored frozen for you, but you are not currently eligible for our Phase three DCVax vaccine trial (because you had prior radiation and chemotherapy)."

Good news, I guess. I sometimes feel that they are talking in riddles, like I just fell down the rabbit hole. I guess I'm Tweedledum. Who to believe? Who to trust? It's only my life we're talking about. Maybe I'll wake up like Alice in Wonderland and it will only have been a bad dream. Did they get it all or not?

I particularly like where she says, "Having been in your brain." That's so funny and bizarre at the same time. While lots of people are on my mind, not many are in it.

P.S. I drove Lucky to school last week, only on side streets, but it was glorious nonetheless. I have a bad cold but am going to see our friend Gary Numan perform at the Hollywood Forever cemetery tonight. Excited.

Xo Katie

## 10/19/13

We went to Gary Numan's concert, and it was awesome. The very last song was the song he wrote that he said was inspired by me called "My Last Day." It was so awesome. His wife, Gemma, came and sat down next to me, put her arms around me, and I started bawling. But it was great and we got to hang out with them afterward.

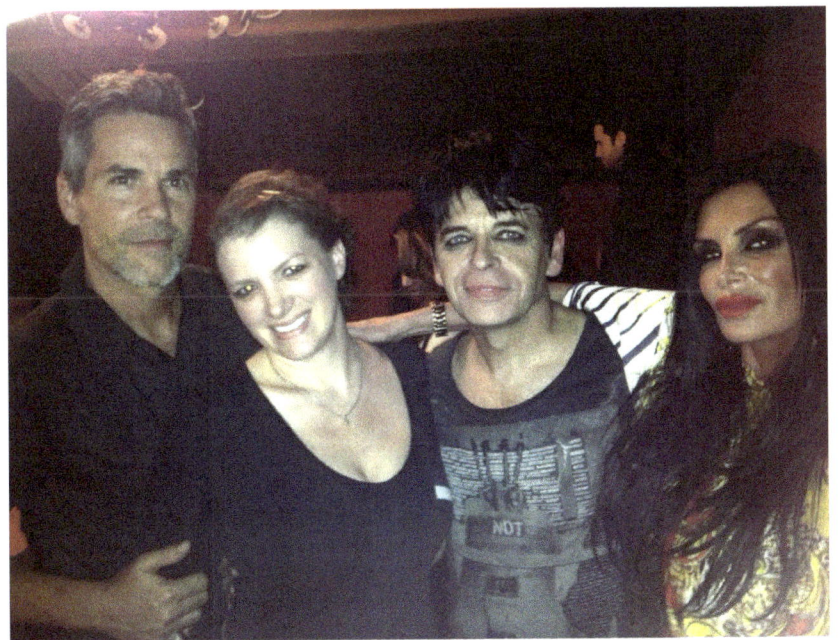

Micah, me, Gary and Gemma

I was exhausted the next day and it was so busy, I got stressed out. As I was trying desperately to unscrew a cap from a sippy cup for about 20 minutes, getting so frustrated that I absolutely could not do it, I noticed my hand and fingers becoming increasingly tired and unable to open. As I tried to pry my hand open, I thought, *I wonder if this is some kind of seizure*, and instantly my hand clawed and I started convulsing.

I quickly went to my bedroom, where I knew my purse was, and told Lucky, "I'm having a seizure." He ran to my side and I said, "Get my medicine."

He grabbed my medicine bag out of my purse, and as I was sitting on the floor holding my arm to keep it from flailing, he gave me an Ativan and said, "Should I call Dad?" He had long ago memorized the phone number. He can't work my cell, so he grabbed the house phone that we never use, brought it to me, sat on the floor next to me with his hand on my arm, and dialed Micah.

He said, "Mom's having a seizure!" As he listened to his dad's instructions, he wiped tears from his eyes. He hung up the phone and told me that Micah was calling a neighbor. I told him to go unlock the front door and keep an eye on Haven. He stood in my bedroom doorway with one eye on me and one eye on the front door as Haven yelled, "Get me my dessert!" By then the convulsing had stopped, but I couldn't move my arm or hand. I sat on the floor a while, waiting for help to arrive. My whole left side was numb and tingling. I told Lucky he could go get Haven some dessert. Meanwhile she had come in and put her hand on me and said, "Now you can go to the doctor again!" in a cheerful voice. Lucky got her some ice cream, and I got up and made my way to the couch. Micah called and said he had been calling everyone in the neighborhood, but nobody was answering and he was all the way downtown. He finally reached our neighbor Joanna, and she literally ran to our house; she came in huffing and puffing, looking panic-stricken. The numbness traveled up to my face then started to retreat. It took at least 20 minutes.

Meanwhile, Lucky was cuddled up on the couch with me as I comforted him, telling him I was okay and that I was so proud of him, that he did everything right.

I felt the need to explain to him that this happened because I was too tired, because I had promised him I wasn't going to have any more seizures. I said I was fine, even though I felt anything but fine.

When I kissed Lucky good night, I told him he was my hero.

Xo Katie

## 10/24/13

As a family last Sunday we went to the Sherman Oaks street fair. I would say fair is an appropriate adjective; mainly we were all still sick, so the kids were grumpy. The kids went on one ride similar to the teacups, but they didn't let adults on (?), so when it went spinning, Haven spun right off the seat. That was it for rides. At one booth this young guy leaned toward Micah and said, "What happened to her?" It was actually refreshing because most people either look away or just pretend they don't notice. For some reason Micah felt the need to whisper, "She has a brain tumor," as if the kids don't know. Then an older guy felt the need to put his arm around me, and the young guy said, "Oh yeah, I used to have a boss that died of a brain tumor." Not quite the most appropriate thing to say, but oh well. After a lot of "stay strongs" and hugs, we were able to move on.

Last night I had my first dream where I had brain cancer. In the dream I take off my hat and show my head to someone and tell them I have brain cancer. It wasn't upsetting; it was just the only dream I can remember where I actually included it.

Xo Katie

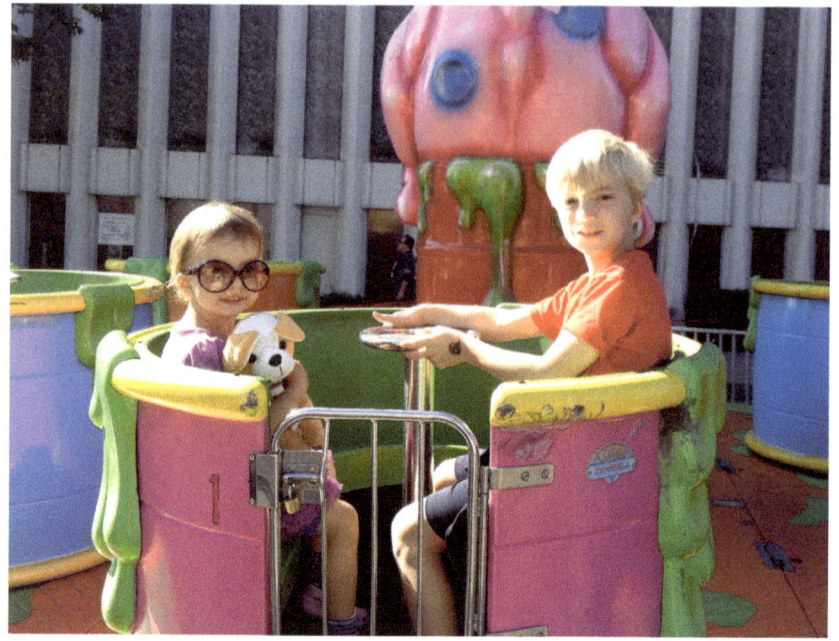

Right before Haven flew off the seat

## 10/30/13

Today I was wishing that I could have more children, and it made me cry because I always wished that I could have a big family. Unfortunately, there are too many reasons why I can't/shouldn't. Technically I could, but I won't for many reasons. I'm tired. But it's hard to give up on a dream.

I started walking today to get ready for a 5K "race" I'm walking in; it's a charity event raising money for cancer. I haven't done any kind of exercise since my surgery, and I only have less than two weeks to get ready.

I walked about a mile today. It was hard and I'm nervous about overexerting myself because being tired and being hot are seizure triggers for me.

Xo Katie

## 11/1/13

I am going to lighten my hair soon. My incision is healed and I feel like the bald spot won't be as shockingly visible if the contrast isn't as great. I want a light brown/golden color, like Haven's. It can only help.
Xo Katie

## 11/3/13

I walked two miles today! Surprisingly, what hurts the most is my back. I doubt I have any core strength. The last 18 months I haven't exercised much, before that I had a newborn, and before that I was pregnant. That's been my last four years. Hopefully this is the beginning of getting my body back.
Xo Katie

## 11/4/13

I was told once that it can take up to three years for the brain to fully heal, and if you think about how long it takes to heal from other types of surgeries or broken bones, then it makes perfect sense that I would still be healing, and that my brain would be pissed off.
Xo Katie

## 11/6/13

The minute you can't find any joy in living, you start dying.
My grandmother said, "86 is a good year to die." She had a stroke that year and died three days before her 87th birthday.
Some people may feel hurt or offended by this, but I think the soul decides when it is ready to move on. You'd be surprised how

much you fight for it when you feel the choice is out of your control. But it is always in your control; that's the hard part to remember.

Xo Katie

## 11/8/13

New hair color. I'm trying to start looking like myself again. The bald spot is tricky, though.

Xo Katie

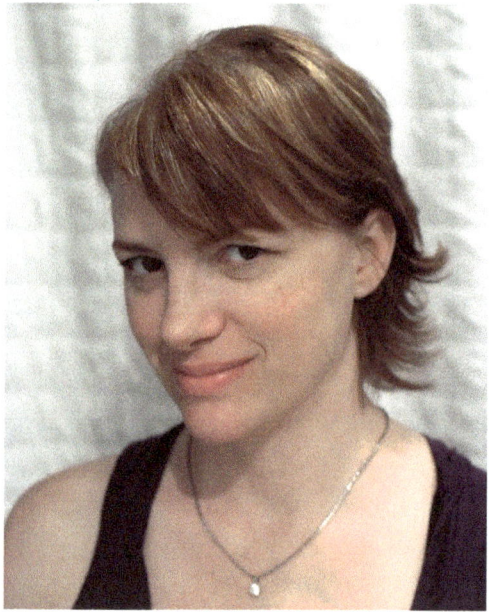

First haircut and color

## 11/10/13

Hi. I finished my first 5K charity race for brain cancer today! My whole body hurts, but I'm so happy I did it. There is no chance that I could have done this at this time last year. That's a big deal to me.

Xo Katie

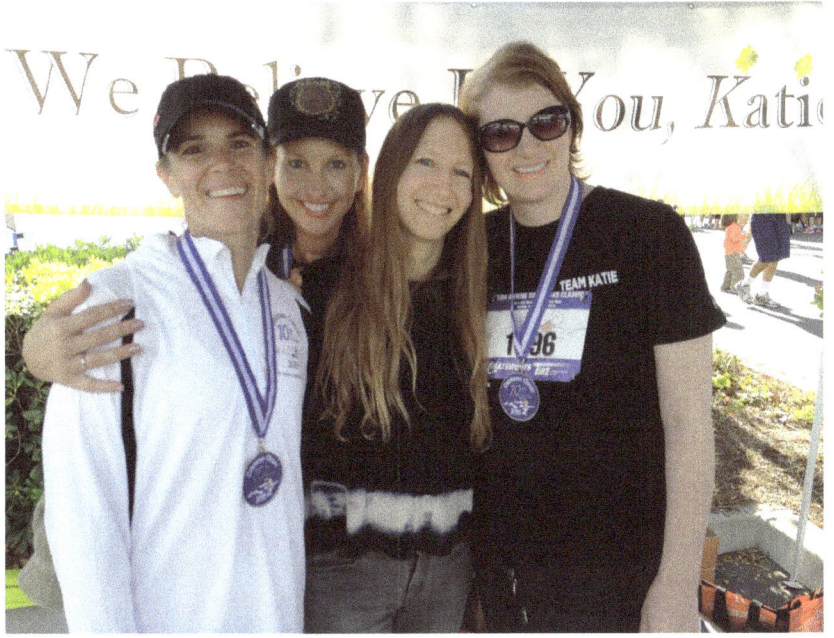

At the 5K with Krista and some high school friends, Mara and Kristen

## 11/12/13

I have an MRI on December second. Am I nervous? You bet. Xo Katie

## 11/21/13

I've been a little consumed lately. This becomes a crazy time for me and doesn't slow down until after Haven's birthday in February when I get a short break until Easter. Somewhere in there I would like to go somewhere close by where there is snow. Obviously we didn't make it last year, and the year before was a disaster. I like for my kids to see snow once a year. Haven doesn't even know what it is.

I have made a decision, and my doctors don't even know yet that I am not going to continue with any more chemo for now. I have an

MRI on December second, and if everything is stable, I'm not going to do anything. I feel that my body has literally rejected chemo twice, once with a horrible allergic reaction and then with a drop in my platelet count that has only resolved itself recently. I trust what my body is telling me, that I don't need that shit. I really wish I had never done radiation either; it has been the source of all of my problems. If only I could have had Dr. Liau as my first surgeon, but alas, I do believe there is a reason for everything. I cannot undo what has already been done, but I can start from this point on by trusting my instincts.

Xo Katie

## 11/22/13

I keep learning and evolving in this process of keeping cancer away. The only difference between people who haven't gotten a cancer diagnosis and those who have is their immune system. I don't think this is disputed. The way to keep from dying of cancer and the way to never get cancer is to strengthen your immune system. Every cell has a life span. It is created, it doubles, then it dies. It's called apoptosis. When the cell doubles but does not die, then continues to multiply out of control because your immune system isn't attacking it, you get a tumor.

It is allowed to do this because the immune system is weak. It can be weak for many reasons, such as ingesting toxins (cigarettes, artificial sweeteners, radiation, plastics...), being depleted of vitamins and minerals, being overweight, stress. You don't get cancer because of a chemotherapy deficit.

Today I went through my pantry and got rid of half of the food in there, some of it I had just purchased. Anything that contained canola, palm, or soy oil, anything that contained any soy or any corn that didn't say Non-GMO. That was most of the food in there. I am also not keeping anything that has more than 12 grams of sugar per serving. I am trying out hemp milk and coconut creamer.

As you can see, I am serious about keeping cancer away from myself and my family. No one really has the motivation until they have to. I am highly motivated. It's been a gradual process for me, which I think is fine. I don't know if anyone could make all of these changes overnight, I didn't. My first steps were to eliminate diet and regular sodas, sugar and milk, and I started juicing. That's all I did for 18 months, and it was hard. I miss those things. But since deciding not to do chemo, I realize I need to do more to boost my immune system.

Xo Katie

## 11/24/13

Today my post is going to be about my boy Lucky because today is his birthday. Eight years ago it was Thanksgiving, and I gave birth to a six-pound, 14 oz turkey! I love and adore him so much. He's an amazing, funny, kind, and loving kid.

I love you, my sweet boy!

Xo Katie

## 11/27/13

I was thinking about all of the things I am thankful for this year. Everyone who has continued to support me and my family, my friends, new and old, family and strangers who have taken us under their wings. I am thankful for my health and for the fact that I have taken control of my future. I feel good and haven't had a seizure since November 12th. Thanks to all of the support, I am not feeling stressed, which is usually a big part of my life right about now. I am looking forward to creating our Christmas cards, visiting Santa,

and wrapping presents. I'm almost done with my shopping thanks to some wonderful friends. I'm making a turkey tomorrow, mashed cauliflower, peas, and gravy, and I made homemade pumpkin pies today. Going to try homemade whipped cream tomorrow.
Xo Katie

## 11/30/13

We had a very lovely Thanksgiving, one of the best. Everything went smoothly, and Haven slept through the whole thing. Lucky didn't eat anything of course, except my pumpkin pie with homemade whipped cream. I swear I will never go back to a can! All those chemicals, yuck. We've been eating leftovers for days. God, I love mashed potatoes and gravy. I can't wait until they're gone. We are truly thankful. Monday is my MRI day at 7:30 a.m. followed by a doctor's appointment at 9:00 a.m.
Xo Katie

## 12/1/13

I canceled my MRI tomorrow so that Haven could attend her first Advent Spiral at school. I vowed that she would get to do everything that Lucky did and not miss out because she is the second child, and especially not miss out because I have been sick. So, the MRI can wait as I had no one to drive her to school in our absence. Today has been a miserable day. I have cried so much that my eyes are almost swollen shut. Sometimes I wish that I was an old, old woman so that I would have already seen my children grow up, maybe even a grandchild or two, and I could just close my eyes, go to sleep, and never wake up. That's how I feel on days like this. Seems that no matter how hard I try to make things perfect and wonderful for everyone, I am always letting someone down. I kill myself trying to make the holidays special for all of my family, I even enjoy it all, but it never gets appreciated. And that would be fine. I don't need a pat on the back or compliments. I just need to not feel judged or that I've let someone down in some minor way when I bust my ass for days to please everyone. I think, no I know, that people forget I have BRAIN CANCER and that my life has had to adapt accordingly. I guess I will never be the perfect daughter, daughter-in-law, mother, wife, aunt, sister, niece, cousin, or friend. I have LIMITATIONS! Anything I have left goes to my children and then to my husband. I wish that people could just spend a day in my shoes, in my body, in my mind, and see what it feels like to be physically limited and desperately trying to save your life. There are so many things I am not able to do that I would love to do. I would love to take my kids to the snow, to Hawaii, or even just to the aquarium. But right now my day is broken into two parts: before my nap and after my nap. When you are on three different seizure medications that make you sleepy and when you have seizures if you don't get rest, then your time is limited. I realized the other day that I need to take vitamin D because I never leave the frickin' house. So if you are one of the people above and you feel I have let you down, then join the club. I can't please all of the people all of the time, so get in line. By the way, I have been disappointed and let down too. A lot.

Xo Katie

## 12/3/13

I'm sorry, sort of, about my rant. I've never been the kind of person who lets things roll off their back, but I'm trying. I get hurt easily and it doesn't heal quickly. If I want to live, I feel like I need to overcome this somewhat because otherwise it eats at me. Everyone tells me the same thing, but it's who I am. How do I overcome who I am? I did have a better day today, and Micah took our Christmas card photo, another thing to scratch off my list. The advent calendars are on the mantel, and the elf is on the shelf. Another 22 days of waking up in a cold sweat wondering if I moved that damn elf.

Xo Katie

## 12/7/13

We got our tree yesterday, and it's starting to feel like Christmas. Going to spend the day tomorrow decorating inside and out. Tonight we all went to the Winter Faire at the kids' school. I love a chance to chat with friends that I normally don't have time to hang out with. At 5:00 p.m. we all lit votive candles, they turned the lights off, and we sang Christmas songs. It's really lovely. I'm a little sad that I may have lost another friend because they don't understand how to have empathy. They're dropping like flies, but I'm still up because I have made so many new, wonderful friends who treat me with kindness and love.

It's so true that you find out who your friends really are when the shit hits the fan. Thank you to all my old and new friends who have stuck around and continue to support me. A new good friend said to me, "People forget. You look better and act well, so they forget." So true. I will live with this, most likely in some way or another, for the rest of my life. There are after-effects and brain damage that will never go away. My mouth is still crooked, and my hand doesn't work. I had to ask Micah to take my earrings out for me, my head still has a big bald spot, and I still have seizures. I forget words and stutter sometimes, but nobody knows any of this because I hide it well. I'm not looking for sympathy. I just don't need anyone telling me I'm a slacker or pretending like none of this exists. I've worked my ass off to be a healthier, stronger, and joyful person. My life has done a 180, and I yearn to help other people do the same. You don't know who you are until you've stripped away ALL of your dignity and ego, to be totally dependent on others, what an opportunity! Not many people get an opportunity like that to discover themselves, and then be able to come back from it better than before. It's been a hell of a ride. I know a handful of people who are reading this who know exactly what I'm talking about.

Xo Katie

### 12/10/13

Yesterday I had my MRI and doctor's appointment. Good news, everything looks good. The cavity is collapsing even more and getting smaller. This was at UCLA and Dr. Cloughesy was happy with the way things looked. He said that if the tumor was growing back, the cavity would have gotten bigger. He was also fine with the fact that I was choosing, for now, not to do any chemo. There was nothing negative about the scan, so that was a huge weight off our shoulders. I can relax for the next six or seven weeks until my next scan in two months!

Xo Katie

### 12/17/13

I had a blessed day today. Everything was perfect. I haven't had a day like that in a very long time. Thank you, God.

Xo Katie

### 12/18/13

I woke up to Haven calling for me and quickly realized not only hadn't we moved the elf, but I hadn't filled the advent boxes. I jabbed Micah in the side and said, "We didn't do the elf or the boxes!" I usually don't see Micah move that fast, but I swear we are a slave to our kids! He went to the kitchen to grab the elf, and I immediately saw Lucky walking down the hall toward me and the kitchen. The house is small, and he would have seen Micah instantly, so I grabbed him and pressed his face into my stomach in a big hug. He looked up at me like I was crazy. I never do that first thing in the morning. As he was rubbing his eyes, he said, "What are you doing?" So of course I started making small talk! Now he knew I was nuts! As soon as the coast was clear, Micah took over the distraction so I could fill the boxes. It was a close one for sure. We still laugh about it.

Xo Katie

## 12/22/13

For the last few days I have been shaken off my foundation a bit. I realized that there are some people out there, people close to me, who think I'm going to die. They act differently. Even my plumber, who I've known for twenty years, gives me that look. In the course of an average day or week, I never, or hardly ever, think about dying or having had cancer. I've always said I don't want to be a member of that club. I just go about my days knowing I have limitations but not really thinking about why they are there. I'm not in denial by any means. I have always known down to my core that I would survive this, whether people think I'm crazy or not. I have total conviction, but when I realize that someone believes I'm probably not going to survive, it actually makes me doubt myself, as if they know something I don't or maybe I'm being naïve. Now, I don't really believe this, but it does have an impact on me.

Xo Katie

## 12/24/13

Wrapping, check. Stockings, check. Cookies, milk, and carrots, check. Advent boxes, check. Putting away the damn elf, check! 2013 has been a year of ups and downs, but unlike 2012 it has been mostly ups :) We have been so blessed and we hope it just continues to get better. Bless you all for your undying support, have a wonderful holiday, and now I will let Micah rub my aching back.

Xo Katie

## 12/27/13

We had a really nice Christmas. When I was six my parents divorced, so all holidays were divided amongst the parents and grandparents as well. As a result it felt like I spent the holidays driving all day. When I grew up I dreamt of staying home all day in my PJ's and never leaving the house, so that's what Micah and I have done since Lucky was born. If anyone wants to see us, they come here. It's great. Haven was so overwhelmed, it took three days until her last present was opened. Both kids were very happy and so was the family. It was a great day. Meanwhile, my OCD is kicking in, and I am ready to get the house back in order. Today or tomorrow Christmas is going bye bye.

Xo Katie

## 12/28/13

For Christmas Micah bought me a book that I hadn't heard of before, an interesting and nice surprise. It's called *Rise and Shine: The Extraordinary Story of One Man's Journey from Near Death to Full Recovery*, about a guy and his wife who were in a devastating car crash where his wife died and he suffered catastrophic injuries and brain damage. Ironically he lives here in Sherman Oaks and was hit in Hancock Park on a street that my friend lives on. Anyway, I digress. I am telling you about it because I am 70 pages in, and he is coming out of an induced coma and just finds out about his wife. He says this: "As I wept, there came the inevitable question of why this happened to Marcy and me, what we did to deserve this. But does anyone ever, at the end of a normal day, look up and wonder why no disaster befell them? And if you don't fill with wonder as the sun sets on all those good days, there's no reason to question the tragic one, the day on which each IF relentlessly piles on and crushes hope." I don't know why this struck me as so poignant and so true. It's only after the disaster strikes that you look back and wish you had cherished the good days more. We all do it—we bury our heads in the sand and hope nothing ever happens to us. We look at others and think, *Oh my God, I don't know how I would cope if that happened to me.* And then it does, and your strength and will are tested. I know from the title this book has a happy ending, and he overcomes his massive brain injuries, even though it takes years, but defies what the "experts" think he can accomplish. I am glad Micah thought to buy this for me.

A while back when I was seeing the Cedars neuro-oncologist, he told me to read about triumph over adversity stories, so that has been my focus.

Xo Katie

## 12/29/13

What's happened in the last two months is that I have learned how to compensate with my right hand so that you can barely notice that I'm not using my left. I am only typing with my right. I use my left to do things like grip a bottle, but I use my right to turn the lid. I can barely turn a doorknob with my left. I use my teeth to zip zippers, and I've gotten good at buttoning buttons with one hand. When we went to dinner for Micah's birthday, I had to ask him to cut my steak. My poor vegetarian friend Gemma cut it for me and fed me bites! The problem is that I can't do my daughter's hair. I want to cry thinking about it. You need two hands to make a ponytail. I used to be a speed braider, and I can't do it at all now; even if I could, I can't manage the rubber band. One of the things I looked forward to my whole life was having a little girl and doing her hair. I even had one of those gigantic Barbie heads as a kid so I could style her hair. I know this seems like such a minor thing considering, but it's all the minor things put together that make life worth living.

Xo Katie

## 12/30/13

I'm so weepy lately. I think the holidays were a distraction for me. I want my old life back. The fact is that I'm just impersonating someone who's normal.

## 12/30/13

This is a feeling that comes up once in a while and then passes. I don't think it will ever just go away; I have post-traumatic stress disorder. Most days I appear fine and put on a happy face, and mostly I am happy and grateful, but I also have the right to grieve and mourn what I've lost. The best thing to say to me is "You're right, it sucks!" That's all. Micah has learned after being with me for 14 years not to try to "fix" me, but just to empathize and be a source of support. I don't want pity or pep talks. This blog is simply here for me to say whatever is on my mind and in my heart with no filter. Which means I may not be "happy, strong Katie" all the time.

Xo Katie

## 1/1/14

Happy New Year! I love the hope that comes with a new year. Even though today is just the day after yesterday, and days, weeks, months, and years are just things humans invented, it always feels new and full of promise. Yesterday was a hard day. We had some fun with friends in the evening, but we weren't in good moods. Today was a really good day. We took the kids to Toys 'R' Us this morning to use some gift cards they got for Christmas. Lucky had a particular Lego set in mind that he wanted, and I picked out some fun things for Haven. Then on the way home, we went through a Baskin Robbins drive-thru, the only one I know of, in Burbank. It was after 11:00 a.m., so that was lunch! That was a special treat we've never done before.

## 1/4/14

Sore throat :( How many hours until school starts?

## 1/12/14

Yesterday I fulfilled something on my bucket list. It seems small and silly, but I've always wanted to learn how to play chess. I was intimidated by it and thought it was too complicated. My dad wanted Lucky to learn, so he thought he would teach me and then I could teach Lucky. He bought me a chess set, came over, and showed me how all the pieces move, and the whole time Lucky was watching and studying. Within minutes he knew all of the names and was remembering all the different ways they could move. My dad and I played a couple of games, and when he left, Lucky and I played. I can't believe how good he is; we both learned at the same time, and he consistently beats me. He has also beat Micah, who used to play as a kid. I love how smart and interested he is. I'm so happy I learned and that we can play together. As we say in chess, check!
Xo Katie

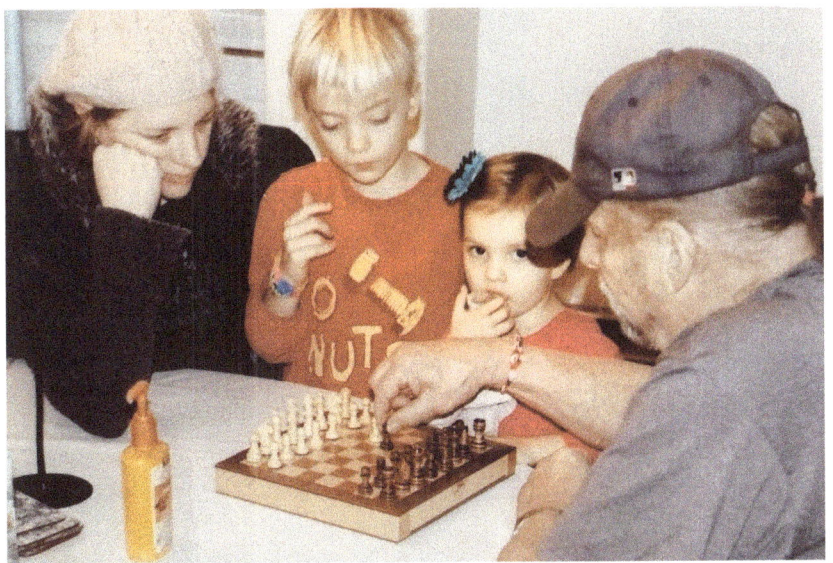

Learning to play chess with my dad.

## 1/15/14

Up at midnight while my boy christens his brand-new loft bed with vomit. Yay!

## 1/16/14

Not a great night. Poor Lucky was throwing up until 1:00 a.m. Micah did three loads of laundry and slept on the floor with Lucky. Haven called for me at 5:00 a.m., and Micah just left for work for the whole day. I barely slept thinking of all the possible scenarios. One of my worst fears is getting a stomach bug, only because if I can't keep down my medicine, I would most likely go to the hospital for IV meds. Then next I worried all night about Haven throwing up in her bed. Every sound she made woke me up; a little cough here and there woke me up. UGH, I hate stomach bugs!

Xo Katie

## 1/17/14

Lucky is fine now. He went to school today and has his appetite back. So far (knock on wood) no one else has gotten it.

In the next month or two, I plan on getting breast reduction surgery. I've been wanting to do it since Lucky was done nursing, but I knew I wanted more children, so I thought I should wait. Some women's shrink but mine kept getting bigger and bigger. Then when I got diagnosed, I thought I'd have to be crazy to do any elective surgery, and it seemed like such a low priority. I've waited eight years, and I suffer every day. I have terrible neck and back pain, I can't exercise without wearing two sports bras so tight I can hardly breathe, and I even sleep in a bra every night. I can't wear tank tops, sundresses, or anything strapless. I'm tired of it. I feel so matronly. We are all on borrowed time, and I want to fully enjoy that time whether it's one day or 10 years without regretting not doing something nice for myself. I want to wear a bikini!

Xo Katie

## 1/21/14

I had a consultation today with a plastic surgeon. I'm waiting to hear if my insurance will cover it. I had a glorious day yesterday. Micah took the kids to Riverside to see his parents, and I stayed home to work on our taxes (that's not the glorious part; it's actually my least favorite job in the world), but the house was SO quiet! I am never actually in my own house by myself—ever! I rode my exercise bike, made a huge pot of vegetable soup, lay outside on the hammock, and while I worked I watched *All Is Lost*, the Robert Redford movie that has no dialogue! Total peace and quiet. A rare day. I recently discovered that I can feel a screw protruding from my skull. There are multiple screws holding the baseball-size piece of my skull on, but I can actually feel this one poking out. I was thinking that maybe the swelling has finally just gone down enough for me to feel it. It doesn't really hurt unless I push on it, but it explains why it's more uncomfortable to sleep on that side. I wonder if it's worth having it removed once my skull mends. We'll see how it goes.

Xo Katie

## 1/28/14

So...yesterday wasn't the greatest day. It started with a seizure right as Micah and Lucky were about to head out the door for school. Haven was staying home with me because of a runny nose. I had about a seven-second warning where a feeling just came over me. I sat on the floor of my room and yelled for Micah. He came with my Ativan, and Lucky and Haven sat down next to me. Lucky asked me if it was "a big one," and when I told him it wasn't, he stroked my arm and kept repeating, "You're okay, you're okay," and smiling at me. Haven did her best to comfort me by pushing on my leg (haha). What compassionate people they are already; they are amazing little people. I always feel the need to hold my hand tightly to keep it from flailing around and to keep my nails from digging into my palm. Once the convulsions end, then the numbness begins where it travels up my arm and into my face and torso. That lasts about 10-15 minutes.

People, even myself sometimes, forget that my hand is fine; it's my brain that is "broken," and I think it's exhausted. Which is a little disconcerting because it means there could be more seizures, and the small relaxation I was feeling is gone again.

Lack of funds causes a ton of stress, and Micah and I have been at each other's throats. Just being honest. Then I got a call from my dad, who was in the ER in Arrowhead, which is an hour and a half away. We will see what comes of that, but I was worried. I wrote this

exact post before I went to bed, and then my computer crashed. I lost the whole post. I went to bed so pissed off. What a day. Great from beginning to end. So I started writing again this morning because I really needed to vent. Hoping for a better day.
Xo Katie

## 1/29/14

I am sick :( It happens every time I get stressed, like clockwork. UGH.
Xo Katie

## 2/1/14

I'm still really sick. I had to cancel all of our plans this weekend, including a party tonight for all of the parents of kids in the nursery and kindergarten. I'm bummed. Last night I could literally feel the cold moving into my voice box and chest. I woke up and couldn't speak at all; then after a while I could whisper, and now I can speak, but I don't recognize my own voice. I heard once, I think it was a Buddhist thing, that if you lose your voice, it's because you are tired of talking, and if you get an earache, it's because you are tired of listening. Wow.

There were definitely calls I didn't want to have to make this week, so I really believe it! Yesterday I felt so crappy that I bought myself some Haagen-Dazs ice cream. Totally off my diet but damn was it good! Have a nice weekend,
Xo Katie

## 2/3/14

I just had my MRI and am waiting in the exam room to get my results, a nerve-racking 30-120 minutes, depending. Here are my tips if you ever need an MRI. Don't drink a lot beforehand. There is not much worse than being strapped inside a machine for an hour and told not to move and having to pee really badly. But do drink a lot after if you had contrast dye injected—gotta flush that crap out of your system. Dress in sweats and a sports bra for you ladies; that way you don't have to change into a flimsy gown. They keep it frigid in there. No metal on your body whatsoever, and don't forget about the doohickies around your sweatpants string or your bra straps. Today I wore sweatpants, a sports bra, a long, pullover shirt, socks, and slip-on shoes. Oh and a sweater. Take off all your jewelry at home, and do NOT bring in a phone or any credit cards; they will be wiped clean of all info. It's a giant magnet! Ironically the screws in my head are cool because they are titanium and my IUD is copper, so those are okay. Wish me luck today. I'll keep you posted.

Xo Katie

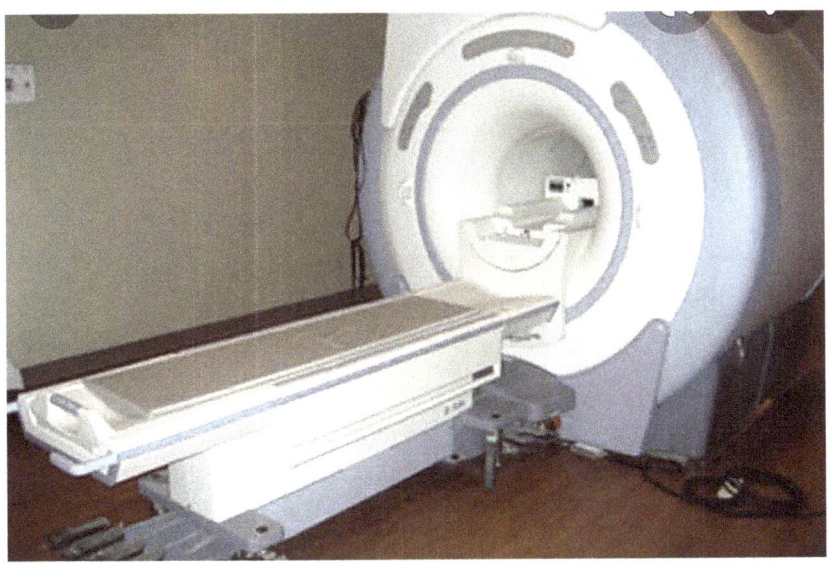

A typical MRI machine

## 2/3/14

All good news!
No growth, two more months of breathing relatively easy. Thank you, God.
Xo Katie

## 2/6/14

Well, God certainly knew what I needed when she brought Haven to me. Not even three years old, and she now wakes up, gets herself dressed, with socks, and poured herself a bowl of cereal with soy milk this morning. AND she still doesn't climb out of her crib! When she wakes up Lucky goes in to get her; he's up at 5:00 a.m. Then she takes care of business. I'm not kidding when I say that Lucky still wanted us to dress him when he was four and five. It was always "You doooo it!" With Haven it's always "I want to do it MYSELF." Such an independent little creature. There are no coincidences. When Lucky was born he was a needy baby and child, and I had the time, energy, and motivation to attend to him. Haven has been independent and so smart and happy since birth, and I needed that, although I didn't know it at the time. I could not have handled another high-maintenance baby. Sometimes I feel a little like she's getting the short end of the stick, but I do believe she would be this way anyway. I don't think she'd want me doting all over her. I think I miss it more than she does. It is nice to be able to stay in bed, though!
Xo Katie

## 2/11/14

Totally exhausted. Went to hand therapy, where I spent one hour trying to move my thumb up and down only using the joint nearest to my hand, keeping the other joints straight. It requires me to tense my whole body. That's all we did. My spasticity was bad today. I need to stretch more. After that I spent an hour of completely wasted time shopping at Ralphs. Their organic sections are pathetic. They are only good for paper towels and cat food, very frustrating. I get grumpy when I don't get my green juice every day. I ordered Haven's birthday cake yesterday. It's going to be special and beautiful. It made me very happy. I can't help but remember what happened last year on Valentine's Day.

Her cake will have pink and purple edible butterflies all around it. She's a scrapper, but also a girlie girl and I am so thrilled and having too much fun.

Xo Katie

## 2/12/14

This whole week has been stressful for me. I got sick AGAIN and have been having flashbacks to one year ago. I just want to get through Haven's birthday and then I can relax.

Xo Katie

## 2/14/14

Three years ago today, I was starting labor, hoping my daughter would be born on Valentine's Day to carry on the tradition of holiday birthdays (I'm July 4th, my dad is St. Patrick's Day, and Lucky is Thanksgiving). Now I'm glad she wasn't; now she can have her own special day. Looking forward to celebrating her birthday tomorrow. I adore her so much.

Xo Katie

## 2/15/14

Thank you, everyone! The day went off perfectly, and Haven was over the moon! More importantly I was conscious for the whole thing! A great day.
Xo Katie

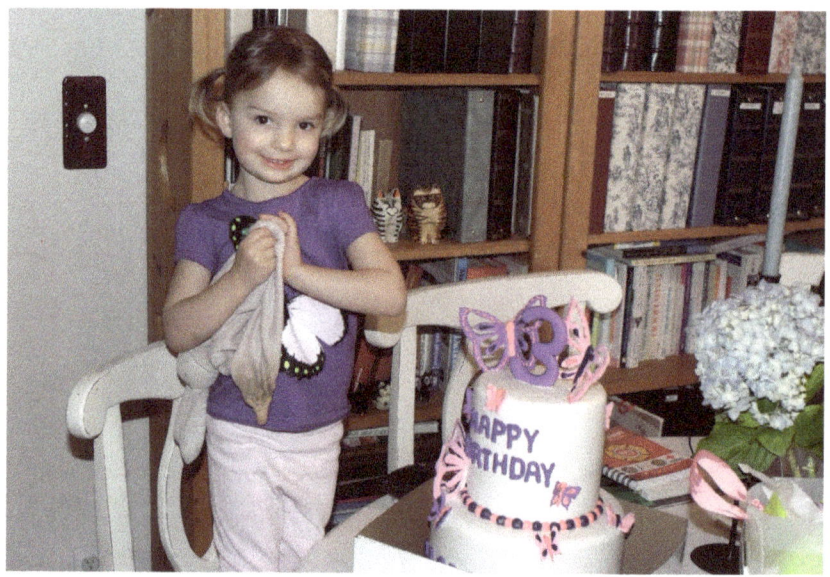

Haven turning three with her butterfly cake

## 2/23/14

I am in a mood. I am feeling so overwhelmed lately. The kids have been on vacation for nine days for Presidents'"Day", and I am at my wits' end. Except for today I don't think I have been alone for one minute in nine days. I love my family very much, but since my first surgery, I have been very sensitive to noise and lights, and the kids have been at each other the whole week. I need, require, and crave solace and quiet. In these last two weeks, I have done everything for Valentine's Day for the kids, planned and executed Haven's birthday, and packed, unpacked, packed, and unpacked again for a trip we took to the mountains, all while being sick. Both kids and I have been dealing with various forms of illness for weeks. Haven and I have major sinus issues, she has been coughing all night, which means no sleep for anyone, and tonight Lucky was crying and saying his ears hurt. We had a great Valentine's Day, birthday, and trip, but I'm exhausted.

I have had insomnia lately. I don't know if it's because of the weaning off the Klonopin process or what, but I can't turn off my mind. It makes me sad that I have spent most of my life, since 11 years old, babysitting and being a nanny, raising other people's kids (one for six years, one for eight years), and now that I have my own, everything I always wanted, I don't have the energy or tolerance that I had with those other children. I honestly am so happy that school starts tomorrow, and I feel guilty about that. I need a vacation from my vacation. Am I insane? Will I ever feel normal again? Will I ever be carefree? Tonight Lucky asked me to lie down with him until he fell asleep. I gently rubbed his back and I started thinking about how we have a Daddy/Daughter dance at our school but no Mother/Son dance. It seems unfair to the parents who have no daughters and the mothers who would like to spend a special night with their sons. Then I started crying wondering if I would ever dance with my son at his wedding.

Xo Katie

## 2/24/14

What I thought was a screw coming out of my head is actually a metal plate, two or three actually. I had no idea I had plates in my head. They do hurt when I rub my head or sleep on my side, now that the swelling has gone down. The doctor said I could have them removed, but I'm not anywhere near ready for that—yet.

Xo Katie

## 2/25/14

This is about Klonopin. I looked it up because I've been feeling crazy these last few days. UGH.

"Benzodiazepine withdrawal syndrome—often abbreviated to benzo withdrawal—is the cluster of symptoms that emerge when a person who has taken benzodiazepines and has developed a physical dependence undergoes dosage reduction or discontinuation. It is characterized by often severe sleep disturbance, irritability, increased tension and anxiety, panic attacks, hand tremor, sweating, difficulty with concentration, confusion and cognitive difficulty, memory problems, dry retching and nausea, weight loss, palpitations, headache, muscular pain and stiffness, a host of perceptual changes, hallucinations, seizures, psychosis, and suicide. Further, these symptoms are notable for the manner in which they wax and wane and vary in severity from day to day or week by week instead of steadily decreasing in a straightforward linear manner. It is a potentially serious condition, and is complex and often protracted in time course."

Fantastic.

Xo Katie

## 2/26/14

I found out yesterday that a friend has cancer. I don't think she's ready to talk about it, so I thought I'd share what I've learned here and maybe she'll read it. In a nutshell:

1. Don't panic. You're not going to die today, tomorrow, next week, or next month. This thought comforted me when I would panic. You're still here. Breathe.
2. Don't make any decisions based on panic or fear; they won't be good choices. Think things through, and do your research.

3. Be very wary of charlatans who claim they can cure you. No energy healer, Chinese herbs, ionic foot baths, or dirt from Brazil is going to heal you.
4. If you have something that can be cut off or cut out, then do it; a lot of people do not have that option. You will live longer. I was blessed to have an operable tumor. There are certain parts of your body that are not necessary for survival. Your children need you. That doesn't mean it doesn't suck ass, though.
5. Combine "alternative" or "complementary" treatments like nutrition, acupuncture, and massage with traditional treatment.
6. Radically change your diet. Take your nutrition seriously! No or very little sugar (that includes alcohol), no or very little dairy, and very little meat. No caffeine. Adopt a plant-based diet. Add avocado, coconut oil, nuts, and tons of greens. It will keep the cancer from coming back. This is your new job. These are only my recommendations from my research and experience. I'm obviously not a doctor or nutritionist.
7. Read only inspirational books. Don't read "cancer" books. Confusing and depressing. I can recommend great books.
8. You are not a national statistic. We live in Los Angeles with access to some of the best doctors in the world.
9. Stay away from websites. You have NO expiration date! People outlive their prognosis every day. I read brain cancer survivor stories only!
10. Mourn and grieve, and let yourself really feel it. Scream, cry, and yell—it's okay.
11. Learn how to ask for help; it's hard but you will need it.
12. Keep a bubble around your children, and only tell them what they need to know. My kids have seen way more than I hoped they would, but they are okay.
   Even better, it has built character and compassion.

13. Doctors will treat you like a child and tell you nothing. Come with a list of questions and demand answers, and ask them about what to expect. It's better to know about things that will probably not happen than to be surprised when they do.
14. Friends and family want to help, but they may not always know what to do or say. Some will say stupid stuff, most won't. You may lose some friends, but you will gain many new ones.
15. I worried a lot about being here for my kids. I wrote my will, planned out my funeral, and wrote letters to my kids about what I wanted for their futures. I wrote to my husband. I actually felt better doing this. Now, instead of it weighing on me, I don't have to think about it anymore. If you think this would make you feel better, then do it. Get it out of the way, then out of your mind. Actually, everyone should do it. It doesn't mean you're giving up; it will just bring you peace.
16. Last but not least. Bring as much peace and joy into your life as you can. It will boost your immune system!

Love to all and anyone struggling with health issues.
Xo Katie

**In response to: What can friends and family do to help someone newly diagnosed?**
Hi Cara,
Thank you for asking. This is a great question.
Here is my advice on how to be a good friend to someone with cancer, or any health issue:

1. Never tell them it's a blessing or a gift. I wouldn't give it to you, so it's no gift. Don't say, "Everything happens for a reason" or "God has a plan." Even if there are positives that come out of it, I would give anything to have the last two

years back. Anything. Just to be carefree and have the use of my body back.

The best thing my friend Robyn said to me was "This is SO FUCKED UP! ARE YOU KIDDING ME?" "I'm so sorry" is nice, but It doesn't really capture the true horror of the situation. Pity doesn't help, so don't come at me with a sad face or tears. It makes me feel like you think I have one foot in the grave. Just say, "This is terrible. This sucks!" Really.

2. Don't say, "If you need anything, give me a call." We won't. Just do it. Accepting help is harder than you think. If you see a need, fill it. Don't ask first.
3. Cards and flowers are nice, but gift cards to restaurants so Micah could take the kids out to eat were really helpful.
4. Sign-up sheets or websites for food drops were great and very appreciated.
5. Playdate sign-ups were great, but saying, "Just drop the kids off anytime" isn't. I don't know whose kids would be okay being dropped off with virtual strangers, but mine weren't. Coming over to play with the kids is good, but don't expect to be entertained by the sick person.
6. We get bombarded with books and advice; wait until the dust settles.
7. Make them laugh. A friend sent me DVDs of *Modern Family*, and it was a great distraction.
8. Talking about the illness can be cathartic, but it can turn stressful and scary too. Follow their lead, and don't ask too many questions all at once.
9. Small things like going through stacks of mail can feel overwhelming; come over and help organize. Order can be comforting; chaos is stressful. Tackle one project at a time.
10. Don't forget the spouse! Have friends take them out for a much-needed break. They need to unload and grieve too.

11. A lot of people would say, "Oh, I know a friend with the same thing. You should call them." I always did out of desperation for camaraderie, but sometimes the stories were depressing. Be careful who you recommend.

This is a good place to start. Thank you for asking. I hope it doesn't sound too harsh.
Xo Katie

## 3/4/14

They say that after you have a child, you wear your heart on the outside of your body. Meaning you are extra emotional and extremely vulnerable.

After brain surgery, I feel like I wear my brain on the outside of my body. I am extremely sensitive to lights, emotions, and especially sounds. A car honking or a loud knock on the door feels like I've been hit with a taser gun. A volt of electricity goes straight up my spine and into my head. My adrenaline surges and fear takes over, all in a fraction of a second. It's a horrible feeling because, once again, it brings on that "I'm going to have a seizure" feeling.

I bring this up because it happens almost every day. Tonight Micah and I went out on a rare date to see a movie. It's a thriller, so there was a lot of adrenaline going through me a lot of the time. By the end I almost couldn't take it anymore. I was overwhelmed. I left feeling tense and exhausted, not thrilled. I worry that now I won't even be able to handle the bumper cars at the fair, or the teacups at Disneyland. Anything that makes my brain feel altered in any way makes me feel really bad. I haven't had a sip of alcohol in two years for that reason. Being a passenger in a car is hard for me because I feel out of control, and I keep trying to use that imaginary brake! I'm tense the whole time.

Life, for me, feels more precarious than ever. I want so desperately to live fearlessly, but I find myself sometimes more afraid than ever. I realize, in a way that most people can't, that life can change on a dime.

Xo Katie

## 3/9/14

Oh my God, I can't take this heat. I have never liked the heat, I despise summer, especially living in the valley with no pool, but now when I get hot, I actually feel like I'm going to throw up and pass out. Maybe it's the drugs, or maybe I am just more sensitive, but I don't think I'll be going out much this summer unless it's from one air-conditioned building to another. It's hard because Micah doesn't like the air conditioner; it's one of those things we can never agree on. Even in winter, I need the car air conditioner blowing on me. I think I should move to Seattle. I love the rain.

I was sent this via email; it's an interesting quote.

"Don't fear transformation; transform fear. Change is absolute. Nothing ever stays the same. Suppressing or denying this absolute fact is a recipe for personal disaster. Only cowards suppress their fear. Only cowards deny change. Subsume cowardice by assuming a heroic posture toward life. Realize that fear is natural, accept it for what it is, and then transform it into courage. This is emotional alchemy at its best. Nobody is perfect. We all have fears. Change for the better should never be a goal of perfect conception but advancement from misconception to ever more refined misconception." (Unknown)

So there :)

Xo Katie

## 3/11/14

I have been able to put Haven's hair in a ponytail three times without help! It's the little things. I'm easy to please.
Xo Katie

## 3/12/14

Today was a crappy day, not something I want to talk about, but it was hard. At one point I found myself lying on Lucky's rug while he was at school, and I was curled up and wailing like an animal. This was a sound I had never heard come out of my throat before. I suppose I am allowed this once a year.

I have every reason to be happy, things are good as far as I know, but the stress of everything never goes away. It takes a toll. We struggle with how to live in this new existence.
Xo Katie

## 3/15/14

I have a problem with my hand in that it tends to want to clench into a fist all the time. It's the default setting in your brain when there is damage. Just like with a stroke, you will often see the person with one hand clenched against the chest. It's like when you put your finger in a newborn's hand, and they grab hold of it but can't let go. The difference is that I hurt myself by stabbing myself with my fingernails. The reflex is so strong, even when my nails are super short, they dig into my palm. Since August I have been wearing a plastic splint at night that forces my hand open and keeps it there all night. It worked great in the beginning, but as my hand has gotten stronger, so has the clenching, and now my fingers are able to pop out of the straps, and it wakes me up all night.

The reflex is especially strong when I yawn or stretch. My PT calls it "tone" or spasticity. So after months of fiddling with this thing and it not working, I finally have a new, smaller splint. Only two fingers need to be strapped in because my hand can't clench unless all of the fingers can. Isn't that weird?

So with Micah and his CPAP mask and mouthguard for snoring and grinding and me with my hand splint, if you were to walk in on us sleeping, it would look like we fell asleep during some weird S&M scene :)

XO Katie

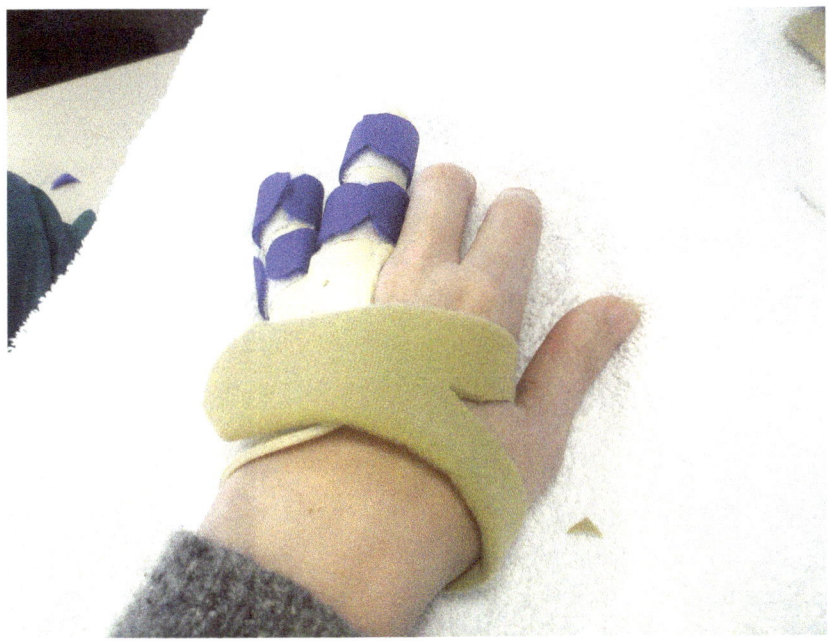

New splint

## 3/18/14

I had the most frustrating day at rehab today. Ironically, I can control a 2,000-pound vehicle, but I can't push the button to roll my window down.

The earthquake on Monday was really scary. The epicenter was only two or three miles from my house. The adrenaline surge as we flew out of bed was awful. My brain did not like that. That rush of adrenaline feels very much like a panic attack and the feeling during a seizure. Everybody else was back to normal in a few minutes, but it took me over an hour to calm down.

Xo Katie

## 3/25/14

I am having my breast reduction surgery on April third, but only if my MRI is good, so there's a lot riding on it.

I know you might be thinking I'm crazy to have surgery that might be considered unnecessary, but it is necessary for me to have the full life that I want to have. To me, it's a symbol of the fact that I am optimistic about my future and the fact that I know I will have a future. It will make you feel better to know that both of my neurologists have signed off on it, saying it is completely safe for me to do this. That makes me feel really good because I know they wouldn't say it's okay if they didn't think I was going to live long enough to enjoy it! My plastic surgeon required a letter saying it was okay, and he said he got a really nice reply from Dr. Rudnick.

Yesterday I got my medicinal marijuana prescription or "recommendation," and I got a good recommendation for a dispensary that has high CBD, low THC strains.

When I went to the "doctor" to get my prescription, I filled out a form, and when he looked at it, he got a look of horror on his face and said, "Really?" I doubt they get too many cases of brain cancer there or any other legitimate ailments. I got a discount :) I'm not sure how I expect people to react, but it always upsets me when someone acts horrified. I want to say, "It's okay, really, I'm going to be fine,"

but I can't change the effect those words have on people. I actually feel lucky most times because the reality is that brain cancer is such a deadly disease that it gets a ton of research money and has lots of clinical trials available. I'm lucky to have a slower-growing tumor but still have access to all that research. And also, except for the surgery, I have never had much pain. I've had miserable side effects, but they don't usually involve much pain. I do have PTSD and seizures, but I know people who are suffering much more than I am, and I don't know how they get through the day. Also, my cancer can't spread to other parts of my body; that's why it's "graded" instead of "staged." For example, stage-four cancer means it has spread throughout your body, whereas grade-four brain cancer means it's an extremely aggressive form of brain cancer. It can't spread to other parts of your body. Other cancers like melanoma can spread to the brain, but a brain tumor that starts in the brain (a primary tumor) can't travel outside of the brain, which gives me tremendous peace of mind. If I had to worry about that too, it would be awful. See, I'm lucky. Get that look off your face!
:)
Xo Katie

## 3/31/14

Waiting to get my MRI results. Good thoughts.

### Later...

Everything is good! MRI looks good! The cavity is smaller and no other change! Yeah! Two more months of freedom from worry and got the green light for the cannabis oil.
Xo Katie

*Welcome To* KATIE'S BRAIN

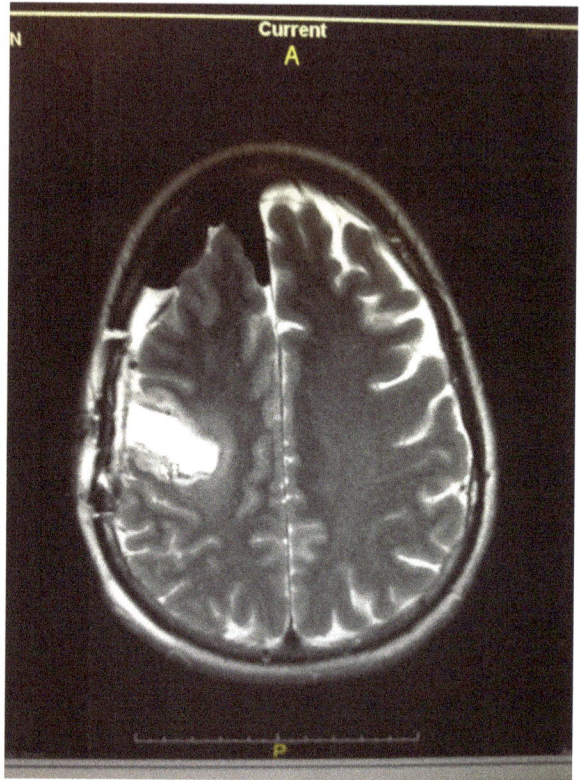

The white is the cavity filled with fluid

## 4/2/14

How can I live my life surrounded by love and serenity when it seems like there is always someone out there who is set on destroying my peace of mind? Don't people understand that my life depends on me focusing my energy on maintaining my health and keeping the joy in my life? I cannot afford to live in a state of constant stress. But people don't change unless they are motivated to do so, and most people aren't. So I repeatedly have to deal with these issues over and over and over again. It's exhausting. I am far too sensitive. I care too much about what others think. To save my life I have to start being true to myself and let the shit just hit the fan. I am trying really hard to not let it affect me, but it continually creeps in. I am learning. It's 42 years of living one way, of being bullied constantly, and now I am standing up to the bullies, and they don't know what's hit them. They don't recognize this new person, they don't like this new person, but this is who I am from now on. Like it or not. I only have to live for myself, my children, and Micah. I hope I make them proud.

Xo Katie

## 4/3/14

Hi. I started exercising this week. Two years ago when I was diagnosed, I radically changed my diet and lost the 15 pounds of baby weight I had been hanging on to. After my surgeries when I was on steroids, I would fall off the wagon and eat brownies for three weeks straight. Once I was off the steroids, I got back on my diet, and once the holidays were over, I ramped it up even more by cutting off anything not organic and not Non-GMO. This limits the restaurants I can go to drastically. I stick to it except for the occasional meals out with my family. But it's not always easy to find organic, Non-GMO, vegan food wherever you go.

Xo Katie

## 4/4/14

I'm reading a good book recommended by a friend, one of many books on my to-do list. It's called *Break Out* by Joel Osteen. I don't consider myself a religious person, more of a spiritual person, but I'm not put off by all of the Bible quotes because it's not done in a preachy way at all. It's all about how we need to raise our expectations of what God is capable of in our lives if we have faith that anything is possible. If we think that the possibilities are limited or that we will

always be in need or never have enough, then that is what we will experience. If I think that I will never be well, then I won't, but if I believe that God is capable of keeping me well and that I deserve to be well, then I will be. It's about believing and having faith that anything is possible and that all it takes is one thing to make everything turn around. I am only a quarter of the way through, but it is very inspiring. I was reading to Haven the other night and came across a favorite prayer by one of my favorite children's authors, Margaret Wise Brown: "Dear Father, hear and bless thy beasts and singing birds, and guard with tenderness small things that have no words."
Xo Katie

## 4/13/14

What a beautiful day today, a perfect California day, not too hot and not too cold, breezy but not windy. Perfect. I had to go for a walk tonight so I could soak in the great weather. When I walk for exercise now, I practice my balance and try to create new synapses in my brain by crossing my feet one in front of the other as if walking on an imaginary line, like a sobriety test (not that I've ever done that). It really challenges my brain because I have to concentrate on my feet and also cross the midline of my body, which is good for my brain. I practice crossing my midline in occupational therapy all the time. I've had an issue with balance and proprioception (knowing where my body is in space) since my surgery. It is getting better with practice and time. Months ago I was stubbing my toes on furniture multiple times a day and bumping into walls when I would turn to go into a room, but only my left shoulder. I also have to be careful and conscious to lift my left foot so I don't trip over a crack in the sidewalk. I'd like to ride my bicycle, but I'm not sure my balance is ready. I had another great night's sleep; must have been the weedo.
Xo Katie

## 4/17/14

I am so confused and tired of all the food debates and cancer diet information. Every time I think I've got it down and am doing the best I can, I find out that something I have been eating is bad for me. I don't drink milk anymore; we are an organic, Non-GMO soy milk or almond milk family. Now I find out that many of the milk substitutes have something called carrageenan in it. Well, it's a carcinogen. It causes cancer. So now I'm back to reading labels and swapping brands. Did you know that anything roasted (nuts, coffee, some teas, chicken, turkey, etc.), smoked, pickled, or salted is a carcinogen? How about celery? Has carcinogens in it. Jeeeez! What is safe to eat?

I actually got into an online debate/argument with someone over the fact that I eat peanut butter. You know that mold grows on the peanuts when they sit in a hot silo waiting to be turned into peanut butter, even organic peanut butter with no added oils or sugar. UGH! The more I research the more depressed I feel because I think I could be doing better. What else am I eating that is making me sick and I don't even know it? Should I be on a raw food diet? The paleo? The ketogenic? Gerson diet? Coffee enemas anyone? At what point do we just say, "You know what, I can't obsess about this anymore. I'm doing the best I can"? It's so scary when your actual life depends on it; it's not about losing weight or jumping on some fad.
Xo Katie

## 4/21/14

Hi. We had a really nice Easter. I hope you all did too. I always put a lot of pressure on myself because I want it to be perfect, the way I remember holidays as a child. I figure that I had my turn, and now I want it to be special and magical for my kids for as long as they still believe.

Xo Katie

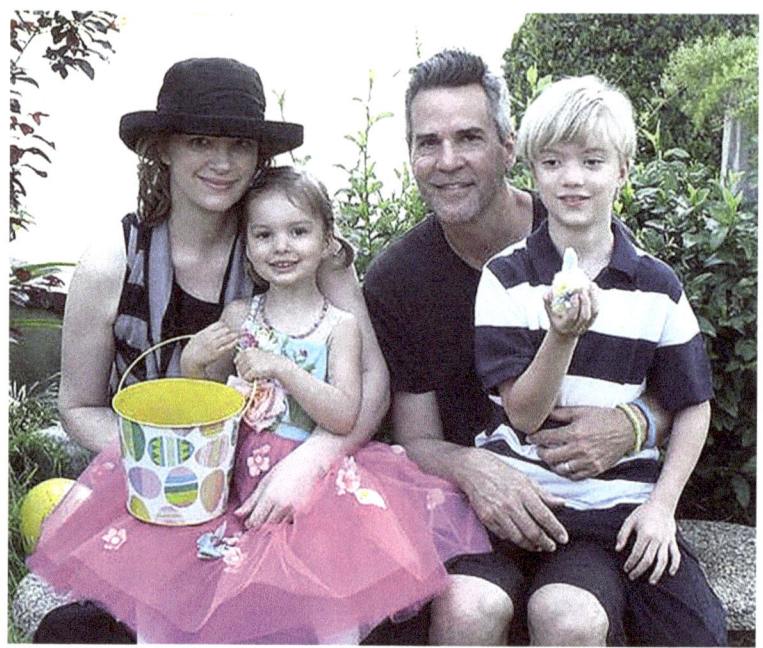

Easter with the Smiths

## Later...

Right after I posted I got on my exercise bike, and in one minute I had a seizure. It started as a tingling feeling coming over my head; then my face on the left became completely numb, and I felt it twitching, even though Micah said he couldn't see it moving. It felt like bugs under my skin. My left eye and half of my tongue went numb. Just like at the dentist. Then I felt my index finger tingling and then my other fingers tingling then going numb. Soon it was my whole hand. My face stopped twitching but was still numb for a long time. Then the numbness started going up my arm and stopped at the elbow. It just stopped, but I still feel residual weirdness. This was very different from the usual convulsing of my left arm and head. I am grateful for that because my hand still works, and all of my hard work in therapy is not lost! I am hoping that it means my CBD tincture is working, and without it, it would have been a typical seizure.

I'd like to eventually start making the oil myself so that I can actually have the full-fledged super strong oil. It is apparently so strong, you have to start out with a dose the size of one grain of rice and work your way up to one gram, the amount in a small, skinny syringe. I believe that once I start taking that, I will have no more seizures. I think my brain is trying to heal from the surgery. I was told it could take a year or more, and that won't be until August.

Xo Katie

## 4/22/14

Good news, my hand seems better today than it has been, and even my face seems more symmetrical. I really think I'm healing.

Xo Katie

## 4/22/14

Once again I have disappointed someone. I was under the illusion that Easter had gone smoothly and that everyone had enjoyed a wonderful day, but I was wrong. Apparently someone felt slighted because I didn't pay them enough attention, a grown adult, and was upset with me. Please give me a fucking break. Now what was a beautiful day for me is forever tainted. When I was first diagnosed and made an announcement that I was no longer going to be a "people pleaser" as my job now was to take care of myself and I could no longer be responsible for other people's happiness, I was met with "That's fine, we don't want you to take care of us." "We never asked you to be responsible for our happiness." But that's a lie. It is expected of me. I have been blamed for either doing too much or not enough. Mostly not enough. I don't call enough, I don't say the things I'm expected to say, or I don't say them when I'm expected to say them. I didn't send a card for some random holiday. I cannot win. As far as I'm concerned, the holidays are for the kids, and I spend months preparing for the birthdays, Christmas, and Easter so that I can get pleasure by watching them get pleasure. I put pressure on myself, but I enjoy that. It's what I live for. No one is making me do it. I love it. I want it to be magical. If I die my kids will know how special the holidays are to me and how important family is to me.

The holidays were the happiest moments of my childhood, and I want to carry that on to my children. I need to find the joy in living wherever I can get it. None of us know if this will be the last holiday we get to spend with our family, so why can't everyone just enjoy it? I'm doing the absolute best I can. I can say that knowing it's the God's honest truth. If people can't appreciate that fact, then I'm sorry. Let's see you do better, even without my handicaps!

Xo Katie

## 4/30/14

There was an article in *People* magazine about how they are injecting the polio virus directly into grade four brain tumors, and it is working to shrink them. The plus side to having a grade three/four tumor is that it opens up my options for clinical trials that I wouldn't qualify for if I was only a stage three. Luckily I don't need it now or hopefully in the future, but it's nice to know it's there if I do!

I am going to apologize in advance because this post is going to be all over the place. I walked out on my hand therapy session yesterday. I was completely frustrated not only by my lack of ability but also by the therapist, who I usually like but who kind of dropped me halfway through my session to work on someone else, then gave me busy work that I wasn't able to do. I felt myself get angry and frustrated and started to cry, so I just got up and walked out. I can sit and do nothing at home. I don't need to pay someone to piss me off. I can get that at home! I feel in general that I have not progressed very much but that I'm actually just adapting to being handicapped. I can do a little more because I've figured out ways to get around having to use my hand. Nobody even notices that I'm not using it.

The thoughts about my possible demise come up multiple times a day. Again, I don't talk about it, but I don't operate on autopilot anymore. The freedom of just going about your life not thinking, *Will I be here this time next year?* is gone. I never thought I'd feel this way at 44, maybe at 84, but not now. For now, I just push the thoughts away because I am doing well. I have to believe I will continue to do so.

Xo Katie

## 5/4/14

I'm having my breast reduction surgery tomorrow, at 7:30 a.m. I'm not really nervous, but saying good night to the kids tonight was hard. I feel guilty doing something that's in any way risky, especially when I don't have to. It feels selfish, but I need to do this for myself. I deserve it. Prayers, please.

Xo Katie

## 5/5/14

I'm high as a kite, but everything went smoothly! I can see my feet! Thank you, God.

Xo Katie

## 5/6/14

I'm so happy I did this and that it's over. Thank you for all the support, pun intended.
Xo Katie

## 5/8/14

I'm doing much better. During my downtime, I have been working on my blog, on transferring these posts, thousands of them, onto a new document. I hope to inspire and educate other cancer patients.

In the process, I am going back to the beginning and reading, editing, and adding more details to the earlier posts. While reading these I become very emotional. I cannot believe what I have been through, just in the first six months! I find myself feeling very sad and very sorry for that girl. It seems like a very long time ago, not two years ago. Even as little as one year ago, I didn't know if I would ever be able to lead a normal life, go out to a restaurant, see a movie, dance, drive... I was having eight seizures a day, needing care 24 hours a day. I look at where I am now, the surgery I just had, the life I have back, and I can't believe it. I was dying, there is no doubt about it. A year ago I had inoperable brain cancer and I was dying. I never chose to believe that, but I know my doctors did. Now I have renewed hope. I have my life back. Thank you for your continued support throughout this nightmare.
Xo Katie

## 5/12/14

I hope everyone had a lovely Mother's Day. Mine was nice. Maybe the nicest I've had. We celebrated with Micah's parents on Saturday, and I'm going to celebrate with my mom when I'm healed, so yesterday was just us. I requested breakfast in bed, and it was very nice. The kids woke me up, and I had my porridge (plain oatmeal) with berries and my chai tea. We just relaxed all morning, ate lunch, and went out for ice cream, my favorite food that I only allow myself once or twice a month. Haven and I had a nap; then we all went to a local county fair. I really wanted to take Haven there since I've taken Lucky many times. We read books about fairs, but she didn't really know what that meant. Don't worry, I didn't go on any rides, and she wasn't tall enough to go on much, even in the little kids' section. Next year will be really fun! We left after an hour and a half, and it was perfect. I love, love, love these milestones and being able to participate in them. I get sad sometimes thinking that the only way she will remember any of this is through photos and videos. I know it's true because I always have to remind Lucky when he gets jealous that everything I do with her, and for her, I also did with him, and that he never had to share my attention as she does. I'll ask him, "Do you remember when we went to the snow" (or beach, or fair, or whatever) and he'll say no. And when I think, *What's the point of it all?* I remind myself that even if they don't remember the activity, it's still shaping their personalities, their hearts, and their minds. When do they start remembering all of the things you do together? I have a dear friend who lost both of her parents in an airplane crash when she was three. When I got diagnosed I grilled her about what she remembered about her parents. I don't know if it's a blessing or a curse that they don't remember much at that age. I don't think about dying as much as I did last year, but this fear of my kids not remembering me haunts me. I know it worried Micah as well because he would bring out the camera more and make sure to get pictures of me with the kids. Anyway, just more of my ramblings, my inner thoughts.

Xo Katie

*Welcome To* KATIE'S BRAIN

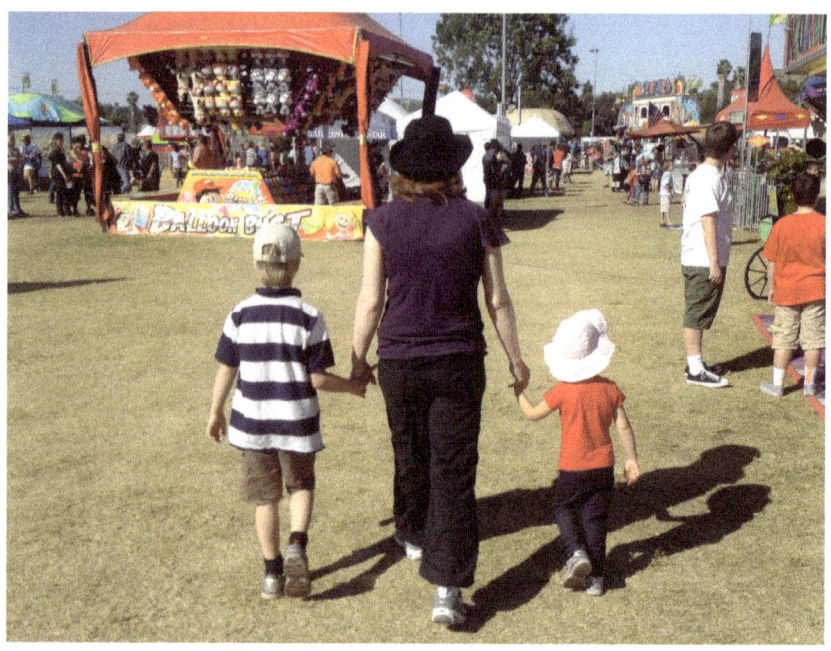

At the fair with my babies, I'm holding Lucky's hand with my left hand. That's all I need!

## 5/15/14

I have been spending hours working on my old blog posts. (How come no one told me I couldn't spell? I guess there's no point in kicking me while I'm down!) At the time I was writing them, a lot of people were saying I should turn it into a book, but I was deranged out of my mind, just trying to get through each day. It's been hard for me to read, but I look back at all of my epiphanies and I can see how much I've evolved in such a short time. In three days it will be two years since I was diagnosed. It feels like so much longer. I've metamorphosed into a new person, a person I'm proud of. You can ask Micah, things don't stress me out anymore. Whereas I would stew and stress over things before, now I just trust that all is as it should be. I finally have my priorities straight, and it only took almost 45 years! I'm interested to start re-reading the 2013 posts. It's almost like I'm reading about someone else. Little bits of that person come out from time to time, like when my bandages were coming off this week I started to have a panic attack. I had to stop and breathe deeply for a while. That would've never happened before my diagnosis, but I have to come to terms with the fact that my brain is forever altered. It's a small price to pay, that and my hand.

Xo Katie

## 5/20/14

Two days and two years ago, I was diagnosed with a brain tumor. It feels like an eternity. I looked in the mirror last night and told Micah that I was starting to recognize myself for the first time since my first pregnancy 10 years ago. Oh, there I am! No steroid water retention and moon face, no giant, droopy boobs, no steroid acne or palsy in my face, no droopy eye or crooked mouth. No short, curly black hair. My short, curly blonde hair with a permanent bald spot is the only visual reminder. The lack of function in my hand is the biggest reminder for me. I am happy I walked out of my hand therapy.

Yesterday I had an evaluation at UCLA's outpatient rehab. The therapist I was assigned to finally got that it wasn't an issue with my hand but with my brain. Thank you! She is going to try to get a neuro therapist working with me.

Off topic, when I was first diagnosed, I felt so sad that my kids, especially Lucky, had to be subjected to my illness. I worried that he would be damaged for life, traumatized. But now I see that people who lead charmed lives with no negative experiences are lacking that undefinable depth, that internal struggle to overcome odds, and the ability to empathize. My surgeon, Linda Liau, lost her mother to a brain tumor, and that's why she became a neuro-surgeon. She obviously can empathize and is driven to help based on her own experiences. I don't want my kids' lives to be perfect. I want them to be happy, but I want them to have depth and character so they can help others. I want them to read this blog someday so they can know all that I've gone through, and how I fought my way out and never gave up. I can't think of any more important lesson than that.

Xo Katie

## 5/23/14

I awoke this morning after a pretty good sleep. Micah got up with the kids, and a few minutes later I felt my hand tighten up. I called out for him, but he didn't hear me. Now my arm was raised up against my ear and was convulsing and rigid at the same time. I yelled for Micah two more times loudly, and he finally heard me. I was flat on my back, so I couldn't reach my own meds. I said "Ativan" and Micah grabbed a bottle off my end table and put one in my mouth which I chewed up quickly. Unfortunately, it was Valium left over from my latest surgery. He quickly grabbed another bottle and put an Ativan in my mouth. Both kids then jumped up onto the bed next to me. Lucky grabbed my arm and started slowly kissing it up and down. He said, "Remember, Mom, to take deep breaths and that everything is okay." Haven said, "What's happening? Did you have a bad dream, Mommy?" I was able to tell them that I was fine, but the seizure continued. Soon they got bored with it—God love 'em—and went back to the living room. Still, it continued. Micah stayed with me until it finally stopped. I'm so proud of my children. I guess I don't have to worry about their character :)

Xo Katie

## 5/27/14

I have my MRI today at 9:30. I'm not as nervous as the last time and then I worry that because I'm not worried, then something will be wrong. I have had terrible insomnia every single night for the last week. It used to be just a couple of nights a week, but now it's every night. We were thinking that I might be still detoxing from Klonopin because it's not just that I can't sleep; it's also like I'm getting little electric shocks to my muscles, and I get super restless and can't stop moving. It's an extremely uncomfortable feeling and also unnatural, so it must be drug-induced. I started taking the super-strong cannabis oil three days ago. The first two nights it hit me like a ton of bricks. I got very sleepy within 10 minutes, but last night, probably because I had napped, it didn't make me sleepy at all. I lay there awake for 45 minutes and had to take some Valium to stop the buzzing and zapping in my muscles. I will ask the doctor about it today.

Xo Katie

## 5/27/14

My scan was perfect, as perfect as it can be. The doctor says the shadow that exists is a "residual tumor" that is doing nothing, and the radiation could still be at work but will only attack a cell that has divided, a cancer cell. So the fact that it is still there means it's not dividing. It is maybe even a bit smaller, which he will attribute to radiation, but I think it's the oil. He has also agreed to move my scans to once every three months instead of two! Another month of freedom. He said I could definitely still be detoxing from Klonopin and that my symptoms of insomnia and muscle twitching are common. Unfortunately, he couldn't say how long it will last, just that it's a really hard drug to get off of. It seems like 90 percent of my problems have been from medications and treatments, not the cancer itself. Besides the weakness I had in my hand originally, I had no symptoms of any illness. I never felt sick. Surgery and "treatments" made me feel sick. The irony.

Xo Katie

## Welcome to KATIE'S BRAIN

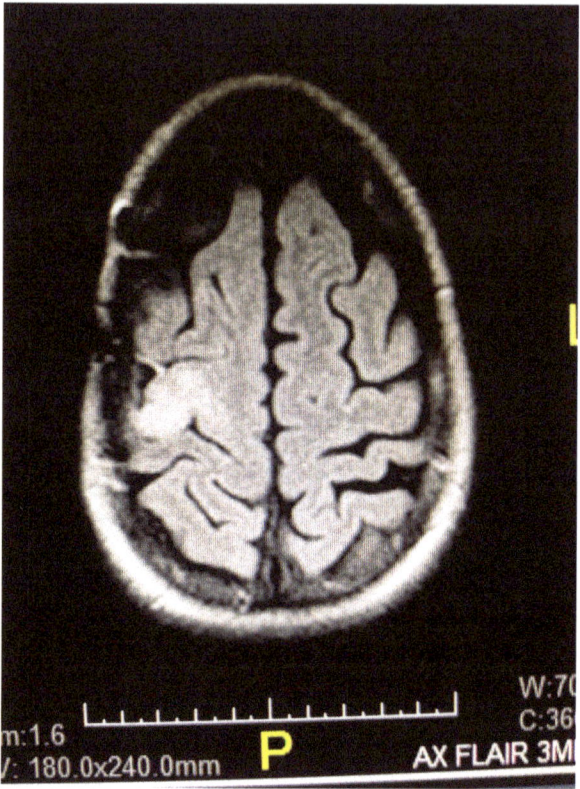

The white part is scar tissue or residual tumor that's dead.

## 6/6/14

Last night I ended up in the ER. I think I overdid it with the oil. I've been doing it every night for two weeks, starting with half a grain of rice size and now I'm up to a pea size. I also take a gram of tincture and I smoke. I haven't had any problems. I've actually been sleeping better.

The night started out normal, but I woke up at 1:45 a.m. freaking out. I was hot and sweaty, and when I stood up, I got faint and felt like I might throw up. I first thought I might have the stomach flu, so I actually smoked some more because it usually helps me fall back to sleep and can be good for nausea, but when I lay back in bed I started hallucinating, feeling like I was having a seizure but also a panic attack. It was like a really bad acid trip. I tried really hard to talk myself out of it, but I couldn't. I woke Micah up and told him something was wrong. He tried to calm me, but it progressively got worse. Sometimes the shaking would stop; then it would suddenly get worse. I couldn't look at him in the face. He kept saying, "Look at me, look in my eyes," but I couldn't! I don't know why. I felt like I was psychotic, like I might hit someone. Every muscle in my body was contracted, which resembled a seizure, and my left hand was shaking the most and was unusable, which is always a seizure. My mouth literally stopped producing saliva. It was like the desert. I felt like my tongue was swelling and made Micah check (it wasn't). I took a Valium and debated about calling 911. The Valium didn't help so I told Micah to call. I was taken to the hospital. My mouth was so incredibly dry, I couldn't even swallow. I was begging for water, but they wouldn't give me any.

Once again, Lucky saw me taken away in an ambulance. They said it wasn't a seizure but panic and they gave me Ativan. After about an hour the twitching was almost gone and I was calm enough to leave, so I went home. It was about 4:30 a.m. Every panic attack I've ever had has either been during a seizure or something that just comes out of nowhere and disappears within seconds. This was unlike anything I've ever experienced before. Usually, a seizure will cause me to panic, but this time the panic caused what felt like a seizure. I couldn't use my left hand at all, my face was twitching, my throat felt like it was closing, my jaws were locked shut, my teeth were rattling, and my whole body shook uncontrollably. It was extremely scary. I'm not 100 percent sure why this happened. Some of the people in the Cannabis Oil Facebook group I'm in say that this has happened to them, most likely from taking too much too fast. I'm really hung over from all the meds. Talk soon,

Xo Katie

## 6/7/14

Today is my and Micah's 11th anniversary. Unfortunately, it will pass without any fanfare or celebration. No sitters available and with all of the drama, we didn't even get cards for each other. After everything we've been through, I have wanted to renew our vows for three years now. I went from wanting a big party where all my girlfriends and I could wear our wedding dresses again (because no one ever gets to) to renewing our vows in some cheesy Vegas chapel with Elvis presiding. So I have seriously downgraded my dream. No one has honored their vows more than we have, especially Micah. In good times and bad, for richer or poorer, in sickness and in health. Our marriage has been tested over and over again since our second year with four miscarriages and eight surgeries just to have Lucky and Haven. Just when we thought we were done with medical problems and my dreams had come true—blamo! The worst of the worst. All of our hopes and dreams, and kids, were pushed aside. Even though sometimes we can't stand to even look at each other, we love each other with all our hearts, and we know someday we will be rewarded when all our dreams will come true. I love you, Boo Boo.
Xo Katie

## 6/7/14

My life is a series of cruel jokes. Song of the day:
**"Send in the Clowns" by Judy Collins**
Xo Katie

## 6/8/14

I know that comparatively, I have it easier than most of the world's population, but in my little world, my life seems so fucking hard. I'm having a hard time finding enough joy in my life to sustain me. Besides my children, I don't really know what I'm fighting for. More pain, heartache, stress, sorrow? I feel like I am living in some psychedelic parallel universe, and I just want to go home. When you get an illness like this, people always want to know if you would go back and change it, take it away. 100 percent yes. I would rather forget everything I've learned and even the people I've helped, because I am losing myself. I will continue to fight to stay alive because I don't want to leave my children, but some days I wish I was never born at all.

Xo Katie

## 6/13/14

Friday the 13th, appropriate for today's post because I need to vent. This last week Lucky's teacher pulled Micah aside and told him that Lucky had been talking to the other kids about when I was taken by the paramedics in the night. The teacher took him aside and talked to him, and she said he was crying. I got so sad. He's been through so much. I decided to talk to him privately. I asked him if he was worried about me, and he said yes. After a long talk I think I was able to quiet his fears, but I have been depressed.

My panic has been so bad since last week and my hospital episode. Yesterday I had to walk out of the school assembly due to a panic attack. Later today I am seeing John, my hypnotherapist, to try to help me with my panic attacks. I am also depressed that I have no help for my hand and arm. I would give up one of my legs to have my hand back. I'm dead serious.

I had an evaluation two weeks ago at UCLA, and they were supposed to refer me to a neuro-physical therapist, but they never got back to me and aren't returning my calls. My hand is definitely worse, and it's very stressful. I don't know what else to do. Two friends recommended acupuncture, but the only one I know doesn't take insurance. I guess I'll look for someone else. The zapping and pinging I talked about previously is apparently restless leg syndrome. I never knew how truly awful it is. I don't know if it's worse for me or not, but whenever my leg or my whole body jerks, I think it's a seizure, so I have that fear on top of the annoying sensations and inability to sleep. I'm hoping it's still the result of the Klonopin withdrawal.

Thanks for letting me vent. It's been an especially stressful week.
Xo Katie

## 6/23/14

Today I had my new hand therapy at UCLA and then an appointment at Cedars Sinai to see my original oncologist, who wanted to see my most recent MRI. He thought it looked good. There was one area that was enhancing a bit, and he wants to keep an eye on it, but he's happy to see me in three months and then in six months if everything looks good. I asked him about a couple of things. My memory is sketchy. I wanted to email a friend yesterday but couldn't remember her name. I tend to stumble over words when I talk too fast and stutter a bit, and my vision has deteriorated some. Also I have hyperreflexia in my arm and hand, meaning that if I or someone else pats me on the hand, it jumps off the table. If I get startled, it feels as though I was hit with a stun gun. Very uncomfortable to say the least. Unfortunately, he said that the hyperreflexia probably wouldn't go away. He was optimistic, though, that my hand strength could get better, with a lot of work.

Finally I want to say that I am so grateful for my group of friends. I've been lucky to spend time with a lot of friends in the last week, and I am so happy to have all of them. My whole life I have only ever had one or two close friends at a time, and they never really knew each other. In a group I was always the shy outsider(hard to believe now!). I never felt included in a group. Now I am proud to say I have a wonderful group of friends who all know each other, and I am no longer feeling like an outsider. I am blessed. In addition I have other long-term friends who I love and trust and who I know have only my best interests at heart. I love you all and I hope you all know I would do anything for you.

Xo Katie

## 7/3/14

My birthday is tomorrow, the fourth of July. I will be 45. Normally that number would be pretty depressing, but I am so grateful for every year I get to be on this planet. My friend Renee called me the other day and told me that a friend of hers and her husband's was just diagnosed with a grade-four glioblastoma and it's inoperable. She asked if I would call and speak to him. His name is Sean and yesterday I spent time at his house with his wife, Maria, and her mother. They also have a three-year-old son. I brought an arsenal of information with me, probably overwhelming them :). I couldn't talk fast enough about all of the things I wanted him to do. I think it was good for him to see me and talk to me because he couldn't believe how well I seem. I told him about some of my side effects from surgery and radiation: stuttering, memory problems, my hand, etc., and he said, "You are so sharp! I would never know that!" I felt good, like I was talking to one of my clients (I had been a parenting coach). I told him things that the doctors never told me. It felt so good. I want to help him so badly. With Sean I have a chance to make a real difference, even if it just buys him time with his wife and son or helps him live with some hope and a positive attitude.

I have been reading a book called *Radical Remission* by Kelly A. Turner. She's a PhD in oncology, and she studies cancer patients. The book is about people who recovered from cancer with either no traditional treatment or after traditional treatment had failed. She went on a quest to research these "spontaneous remission" patients and what they did to be able to recover when all other hope was lost. She discovered, after interviewing thousands of people, that all of them had nine things in common, sort of a formula that worked for all of them. As I read this book, I realized that I, too, have done all of these things over the course of the last two years. Not to keep you in suspense, I will tell you the nine things, but you have to read the book to get the details.

1. Radically changing your diet—usually to a plant-based, low-sugar diet
2. Taking control of your health
3. Following your intuition
4. Using herbs and supplements
5. Releasing suppressed emotions
6. Increasing positive emotions
7. Embracing social support
8. Deepening your spiritual connection
9. Having strong reasons for living

Yesterday Sean asked me, "When did you start to feel like you had cancer?" I answered, "I have never felt like I had cancer."
Xo Katie

## 7/5/14

I had a nice birthday. We took the kids to our friend Andrea's parents' house that overlooks the Rose Bowl. The kids had a blast, and we had fun catching up with friends. Tomorrow my parents and in-laws are coming to celebrate with me. I feel guilty because I have been eating way too much sugar and carbs this weekend, but it's only once a year! It's hard to let the nagging voice in my head not beat me up for it. I have a brain tumor friend, Jessica, and she admits that she has developed an eating disorder where she actually obsesses too much on eating the "right" foods for cancer, so much so that the anxiety that comes with it is making her sick. I don't want to be that bad, but you almost can't help falling into that trap when you feel that your life depends on it.

Xo Katie

## 7/8/14

As I started falling asleep last night, I felt that familiar extension and tightening of my fingers. I yelled out to Micah, who jumped up and turned on the light. By that time my arm was in full convulsion. It was jumping so hard, I held it down with my right hand. For a full two to three minutes, this went on until my arm hurt so badly. It's similar to when you get a cramp in your calf muscle or the bottom of your foot. It's a muscle contraction that just seems to go on and on. I vocalized it to "stop, stop," but it had to run its course. I took deep breaths and tried hard not to panic. I don't want to just take an Ativan because it won't help for 15 minutes, and I will be drugged the next day, hung over.

Xo Katie

## 7/9/14

I went to physical therapy today. My therapist seemed to think that my seizure was caused by my Empi machine, the unit that electrically stimulates my muscles to open my hand. She went on to say that she wouldn't have recommended that I use this machine, that the jury is still out on whether it is helpful or detrimental to brain cancer patients. It made me feel better. Thinking back I can't remember if my more recent seizures were on the same days when I used the

Empi. I know the one in May wasn't, but I won't be using it anymore. She said that my extension is good on its own, so it's not even really useful anyway. It was useful right after my surgery when I couldn't open my hand at all, but I don't need it now. I think the shoulder strengthening exercises are helping my hand. We'll see.

Xo Katie

## 7/12/14

I had a very mild seizure today, an exhausting weekend so far. It started with my left eye going into convulsions—a very strange feeling. They were so strong, I almost couldn't see, and then my nose and my left cheek went numb. Then it just stopped after about two minutes. Bizarre. I was too tired and worn out from too many busy days. It's like that scene in *Steel Magnolias* when Sally Field pleads with Julia Roberts and says, "There are limits to what you can do!" See, I think I'm normal, just like everybody else because I want to be, but then my body has to remind me that there are limits to what I can do.

Xo Katie

## 7/26/14

I haven't written in a while, not because I haven't had anything to say but just because I've been so busy. Summertime with young kids is more work than the rest of the year. They require so much. Lucky asked me if he could have a baby brother, and Haven wants a "big sister"! Anytime I get sad about not being able to have more kids, all I need to do is spend a whole day with the two I have and then I'm grateful I only have two. If I was thirty and healthy, it would be a different story. I'd love to have a bigger family. In my next life.

I had an interesting experience today. I went swimming. Now,

I've sat in a pool since my last surgery, but I haven't swam, or is it swum? I really don't want to be the mom who never swims with her kids or just dog paddles to not get her hair wet. I really enjoy swimming, but I get nervous now. My big fear has been about having a seizure in the pool and drowning. I don't think I'll ever feel safe swimming by myself again. Since I hadn't gone swimming since my surgery (I've been in a pool but always where I could stand on the bottom), I realized that swimming with my weak arm is a challenge. I was doing pretty well and then Haven wanted me to jump in with her while holding hands. I haven't jumped into a pool since I don't know when. Haven was so excited to have me in the water with her that I couldn't turn her down. We jumped in together, and though I was nervous about taking her down too far with me (she wears a swim vest), it went fine. Then I swam to the edge and attempted to climb out—wasn't going to happen. By the way, when I would hold onto the sides, my left hand would claw up. I really need to stretch a lot to keep it loose, and I hadn't done that. So next I went to the part in the deep end where there are built-in steps and metal rails to help you out. I put my feet in the steps and my hands on the rails, but my hand clawed up and my arm wasn't strong enough to pull me up. I looked at my hand, and I couldn't open my fingers to get a better grip; they were cramped up. I called out for Micah because I was stuck. He helped me out, and I got my towel and sat in the sun. I felt terrible, traumatized. The realization that I couldn't get myself out of the pool hit me really hard. I started crying. My friend came to comfort me, and I tried to hide my tears from the kids, but I broke down. It was/is so depressing to constantly be reminded that I am not normal anymore. I feel robbed. The only way I get out of my funk is to think of people who have it much worse than I do; there are plenty and I know it. I am the lucky one. To prove it to myself, I decided I would jump into the pool again—in the deep end. I hate being afraid and I like to teach my kids to face their fears. So I did it. Those few seconds where you sink as far as you are going to sink before you can start swimming up again are very scary for me. Would I have the strength to swim back up? But I did it. Then I proceeded to swim to those steps again. I got a good grip and I pulled myself out, damn it! And that's all I have to say about that. **Song of the day: "Don't Give Up" by Peter Gabriel.**

Xo Katie

# 8/2/14

The drama continues. For some as yet undetermined reason, my mouth felt like it had been burned with acid this past week. It started on Sunday, when I would wake in the night with what felt like a really dry feeling in my mouth. I assumed it was the cannabis oil, but it got progressively worse and then at some point I noticed that I had sores and spots on the back of my throat, then my tongue and the roof of my mouth. The next day my lips on the inside were so red, it looked like they were bleeding, even though they weren't. It got so bad, I couldn't eat anything. I could only drink shakes and smoothies. I stopped my oil, my vitamins, anything acidic, anything salty. My tongue was raw on top, on the sides, and underneath. I didn't know what kind of doctor I should go to or who to call. I thought it was an allergic reaction. I finally called my dentist and described it over the phone. He didn't think it was an allergic reaction because it would be on the outside too. He said it could be a virus (my kids had had coxsackie virus or hand, foot, and mouth disease a few weeks before, but it had passed the incubation period). He also said it could be a stress response. If you read my last post, it was a definite possibility. He told me to get a gel at the pharmacy for canker sores, but when I used it, it felt like it was burning me because what I had was more than a canker sore. I was completely raw. I made an appointment with my ear, nose, and throat doctor and saw him yesterday. He also ruled out an allergic reaction. He suspected a virus, and mentioned stress response. He brought up something else I had read about—vitamin deficiency. Sometimes you can take one vitamin or mineral, and it will prevent one of your other supplements from being absorbed properly; he said it was common with B-12, iron, zinc, B1, B2, B3, and magnesium. Eating a lot of soy and other nuts and seeds, which I do, can also cause vitamins and minerals to not get absorbed. So he ended up testing me for some viruses and vitamin deficiencies, but we won't get the results for a few days. In the meantime I have been swishing with Benadryl liquid, which helps with the inflammatory response, and it seems to be healing. If the results come back negative, I may never know what caused this awful nightmare. It's so hard not to get completely beat down by all this shit.

Xo Katie

## 8/5/14

I've been spending quite a bit of time looking at old photos. It's so funny how I look at those photos and think, *Wow, I would do anything to look like that again.* Yet, at the time, I probably was thinking, *Ugh, I look awful. I hate my hair. I hate my teeth. I wish I was thinner.* How ironic and sad. Maybe 10 years from now, I will look back at photos of myself now and think, *I didn't look as bad as I thought.* It's a funny thing when you have brain cancer, if you are standing, walking, and talking, people always say, "You look so amazing!" Ha! What they really mean is "You look so amazing *for someone who has brain cancer*!" "You've lost weight; *you were so puffy before*," "Your hair is so long *except for that big bald spot*." It's hard to take a compliment seriously. I know how I look.

I had to move my MRI up because I have been having panic attacks all day, every day. Driving has been really bad. I always drive in the slow lane because I'm constantly on the verge of pulling over;

then I talk myself out of it and carry on. It's a horrible feeling. The other night I had a panic attack just sitting on my couch. I had to get up and try to distract myself. I walked into my kids' rooms to watch them sleep, but that only helped for a second. My heart was racing, adrenaline surging. I felt my hand cramping, so I went to my bedroom and told Micah what was happening and asked him to talk to me. With his help I was finally able to calm down, but it was bad. I'm freaking out about this MRI, so I decided to get it over with sooner. Now it's on the 15th, but I can't see my doctor until the 25th so I'm hoping I can talk over the phone and he can tell me everything's alright. My mouth is better but still feels a little raw after I eat. I don't have any test results yet.

Xo Katie

## 8/12/14

I just found out I have very low iron counts and very low vitamin D. Now at least I know why I'm always so frickin' tired yet have insomnia and muscle cramps. Also causes hair loss (great), weight gain, and depression! Vitamin B results aren't back yet. The low iron can cause burning in the mouth. I hardly eat any meat and I never go in the sun because I can't handle the heat, so no wonder those are the things that are low. I'm going to seriously supplement, and we'll see how it goes. On a happier note I got to fulfill a big dream by going to see Paul McCartney last weekend at Dodgers Stadium. And even better is that I got to take Micah and the kids! It was truly one of the best nights of my life. When he first came out on stage, the woman sitting in front of us and I both started crying! I was overwhelmed with happiness. To see one of the actual Beatles play live, it was amazing. To hear him play "Hey Jude" and have 50,000 people singing along to the "Na na na na na na na" part with their phones lit up in the air was the highlight of the night. Unforgettable, and another thing off

my bucket list. It's also so great that Lucky and Haven can say their first concert was with Paul McCartney. Still glowing,
  Xo Katie

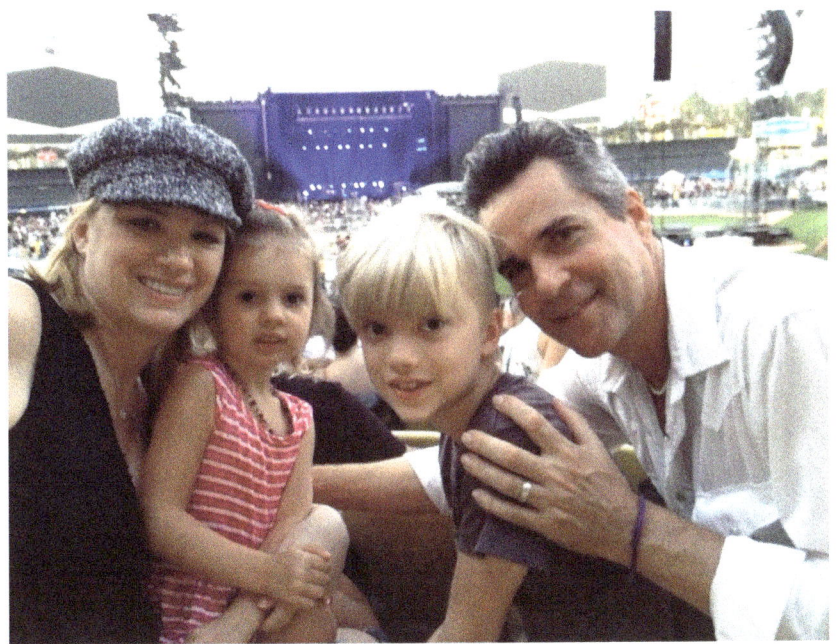

At the Paul McCartney concert

## 8/16/14

An email from my doctor today: "Scan looks good, no evidence of any tumor growth." Woohoo! I had my MRI at 9:45 last night at UCLA. I was hoping I would hear something from my doctor but also worried that I might not hear anything until Monday. He knew how panicked I was, because I told him, so it was very cool that he let me know this afternoon. We are going on a vacation, sort of. Let's face it, with little kids is it ever really a vacation? At least I can relax and enjoy this break without worrying about my health.
  Xo Katie

*Welcome To* KATIE'S BRAIN

## 8/17/14

I spoke too soon, ended up calling the paramedics yesterday and going to the hospital at almost midnight, at which point I couldn't walk or move my arm and could barely speak. I had been in full body tremors and spasms for three hours. My leg on the left was cramping so badly that even when the spasms stopped, you could still see the muscle moving under my skin. My hand and arm were crammed into a claw, and I couldn't open it. I had a washcloth stuffed in my mouth for fear of breaking my teeth. Micah and I rode it out as long as we could; he gave me four Ativan, but it wasn't helping. Finally we called it at about midnight and called 911. I don't understand how they can simply call it a panic attack when it's clearly brought on by my cannabis oil. I can't speak, and every time I hear someone speak, it gets worse. I get super hot, and my blood pressure and pulse are through the roof. I hallucinate. Thoughts are racing in my head a million times a minute. I can't focus. The things that help me calm down are actually more morbid thoughts, like *I need to relax or my heart will explode* or telling myself, *It's just a bad trip; you took too much, Lucky's going to see me taken away again. What if I die now and my spirit leaves my body, and I'm watching all this from above the room? Pull yourself together or you're going to die.* When the ambulance and fire department came, they saw the shape I was in and called the paramedics. I couldn't look anybody in the face, the shaking started again, wet washcloth never left my mouth because I knew from the last time that they wouldn't give me any water. Four Ativan in and no improvement. We didn't know what else to do. We knew that the only thing they would do for me was give me more medicine, but home felt unsafe. The anxiety I've been feeling lately with this last MRI and then taking a double dose of oil (not intentionally) sent me into a tizzy to say the least. When the paramedics came, Micah said they kind of rolled their eyes and said something like, "We see this all

the time. She's just really high." By the time we got to the emergency room and settled in, I was starting to calm down and then the actual "high" part kicked in, and I started laughing. When I saw a doctor walking around in full green scrubs I said, "He's the Jolly Green Giant" and burst into hysterics! Micah was not as amused as I was.
Xo Katie

### 8/19/14

Thanks, everyone, for your support. On vacation and feeling better panic wise, but I caught Lucky's chest cold and am feeling pretty crappy today so far. It didn't help that I went on a waterslide yesterday and forgot to hold my breath at the end and swallowed a huge mouthful of pee-filled water. These kid activities have a learning curve for sure. I haven't been on a waterslide for 30 years, but in true Katie fashion I did it again and held my breath! I scared Micah the first time I went down; he didn't know whether to laugh or call 911! Why is it that I sink like a stone now? Because I had my boobs reduced?
Xo Katie

### 8/31/14

I need help. I really need help. I'm in a very bad place right now. My panic attacks are almost constant unless I'm busy and distracted, and I am in a deep depression. I feel I might be having a nervous breakdown. My mind plays tricks on me, and I feel it's possible that I could snap and do something crazy. I feel crazy. For two years I have completely held it together and been so strong throughout this whole nightmare, and now that I am doing well, I am losing my mind. All the stress I kept at bay has taken hold of me. I can have hours of feeling perfectly fine, and then I will start crying at the drop of a hat. I start panicking, my mind goes to bad places, and I spiral from there. I need Valium to sleep, and anytime I have time to think, I think bad thoughts. I frequently have bad panic attacks while driving and feel like I need to pull off the road. Even writing this is hard. Last week I was home alone with the kids asleep because Micah was at a friend's party. I was fine until about 11:00 p.m. and then I started freaking out. I called him to come home, but he was about 40 minutes away, so I called Betsy across the street, who Micah had asked to keep her phone on. She came over and we sat on my front stoop until Micah got home. I had already taken an Ativan, which didn't help me. I told my neuro-oncologist about this, and he contacted UCLA's social worker who supposedly is going to contact their psychiatrist who will allegedly call me. That's a lot of "what-ifs." If I don't hear from them soon, I will have to make some calls myself because I can't live like this. I know I need medication because this started when I got off my ant-ianxiety pill, Klonopin, and it's just slowly getting worse, much worse. Now I am depressed as well. Last night I went into Haven's room because sometimes watching her sleep can calm me down, but tonight I started thinking that I don't know what I am capable of. Could I kill her in her sleep? Am I that crazy? I was in there a while, and when I came out, I said to Micah, "If I go into the kids' rooms, you need to check on me because I'm feeling crazy, and I don't know what I am capable of. Don't leave me in there alone for that long."

In the beginning I needed a lot of help from my friends, and I need you again. I need to be busy, to have things to look forward to, to have joy, to be with people who make me laugh or who have been in this position. Please help me. I hide my panic attacks pretty well, so you may never know that I'm having one. Micah doesn't know until I tell him. I just need this help until I get some medication. Thank you in advance.

Xo Katie

## 9/1/14

Thank you for all of your messages. I think I have responded to most of you privately, and if I haven't, I will.

For those of you who can't understand this kind of panic or depression, I remembered hearing about Brooke Shields and her severe postpartum depression and how severe cases can turn into psychosis. How she would be driving and think, *I could just turn and drive my car straight into that brick wall.* She didn't, but those are the kind of tricks my mind thinks of too. Obviously I don't want to die, my panic is partially related to my fear of dying, but that's the crazy part. Yesterday I thought I was going to have to be committed. My fear of seizures brings on panic, the panic can actually bring on a seizure, so my fears are really about having panic attacks and the panic bringing on a seizure. I feel damaged from the last two years and what they have done not just to my body, but more importantly to my mind. This is a dark time. Last night I read from one of my favorite books by Joel Osteen. It comforted me. He says you have to "play through the pain," that "even though you're hurting, you have to stay in the game" like an injured football player. I am in pain but I'm going to stay in the game. It comforts me to know that others have experienced the same thing, or similar things. I appreciate the comments. Thank you.
Xo Katie

## 9/2/14

I'm doing a little better today. I talked to our friend Dan, the neurologist who helped me get diagnosed. We had a long "consult," and he gave me great advice. He strongly feels that my seizure med Keppra is causing my anxiety, and he feels I don't need to be on it since I'm not having those big "epileptic" seizures anymore, and I

especially don't need the huge dose that I'm on. We agreed that when I am more stable, I will wean off the Keppra but stay on the Vimpat, my other seizure med. Dan is going to prescribe me Celexa as an antidepressant, so I will have that hopefully by tomorrow, and a mild anti-anxiety drug to take as needed. I actually feel so much calmer already, just knowing there is a plan and that relief is hopefully around the corner. Since he knows my oncologist at UCLA, he will talk to him as well. Again I want to thank everyone who has commented or messaged me privately.
Xo Katie

## 9/10/14

I haven't been writing much; it's been too hard. I'm still struggling to get hold of my anxiety. I am now on Celexa for depression, although I am only taking half the dose because of how sensitive I am to medication, so it may take longer to get the full effect. I do find that I am crying less. I was up to three or four times a day just breaking down. I broke down at the kids' school and talked with two friends for a while who could both relate in different ways, and it helped just to feel understood. My friend Gemma kept telling me that I wasn't crazy, even though I felt like I was losing my mind. She said my anxiety was justified; therefore, I wasn't crazy. If I just had anxiety for no reason, then I might be crazy, but with all I've been through, it's a wonder I have held it together for this long. I actually feel a bit guilty because I feel like I've been this role model, touted for being so strong, and now I'm letting you all down. It's weird. I am slowly decreasing my seizure drug Keppra from my mega dose of 4,000 milligrams a day to 2,500. I do feel like I'm having some side effects like extreme sleepiness, headaches, etc., but it's hard to know if it's from the Celexa, the Keppra, or the Xanax I take daily to control my anxiety. I have only been taking a quarter of the Xanax because it works so well for me, and I am such a lightweight with drugs. I'm in a vicious cycle right now: I'm afraid to go off the seizure med because I might have a seizure, but my anxiety may be caused by the seizure med itself! UGH! I'm also afraid that all this stress and adrenaline may cause my tumor to grow back, and that makes me stress more! I really need to focus on bringing the joy back into my life. It's the only thing that can help reverse all of this stress and anxiety. In the last two days I have witnessed two big milestones with Haven, and that brings me joy. She is no longer in a crib (she got her big girl bed). It looks so beautiful and she loves it! She is also now 100 percent potty trained as of this week, phew! Finally, two great milestones that I am here to see and also bittersweet that my baby is growing up. Whenever I start to feel down about my kids growing up, it's so easy to turn it around to be grateful to see them grow up.

Xo Katie

## 9/22/14

"What would you change if you knew you were to die in a week or in six months? Well, considering you might, why not make those changes now. This is no rehearsal. The time is now. If you are not living in joy, loving what you are doing and with people you love, why not?" I like this quote very much. I am trying so hard to live this way; it's an important message for everyone.

My anxiety has improved, mainly because I had an epiphany about where the core root of my fear was coming from. One day while I was in the kitchen watching Micah wash the dishes (don't be jealous), I was just in my own head and realized that I was feeling like I wasn't doing enough to keep my tumor from coming back. I wasn't being the "perfect cancer patient." I constantly compared myself to other people with brain tumors who are doing all kinds of things that I wasn't doing. Looking back, when I was first diagnosed, the only feeling of peace I got was that I could DO things that would cure myself. I consulted with nutritionists, saw energy healers and Chinese medicine doctors, read tons of books, etc. It gave me a feeling of control in an uncontrollable situation. I took 40 supplements a day, was super rigid with my diet, took strange concoctions, drank strange teas, bought a rebounder, used a dry brush to improve my lymph system, and more, and this made me feel calmer. When the supplements made me feel sick to my stomach and didn't do what they were purported to do (reduce swelling for example), I became disheartened by the idea and backed off for a while. When the second surgery became an option, I stopped all the other stuff.

After my surgery I was immediately put on the strongest anti-anxiety medication, Klonopin. They didn't ask me and told me it was also an antiseizure. I didn't ask questions. For the last year my focus was on healing from the surgery and doing rehab. I didn't worry much about the tumor. I was just relieved they had gotten most of it out. Then two things happened. To recap, my doctor and I decided to wean me off Klonopin. It is very addictive and makes me sleep two to three hours during the day. The second thing is that I discovered cannabis oil. By May of this year I was completely weaned off the Klonopin. I was nervous and had withdrawal symptoms but seemed okay. The research I had done on cannabis oil led me to believe that it is a miracle for cancer patients—this was my magic bullet. It was all I needed to keep the tumor from growing back. I started on it right away. Everything was going well, even though I could feel my anxiety slowly returning now that I wasn't on any anti-anxiety meds. One night I took too much oil and had a major freakout and landed in the ER. After that I wasn't the same. My anxiety was back, but I still believed in the oil, so after a break I started on it again. I did fine for a while; then one night I took too much again, and the same thing happened. Now I had to stop. I took an indefinite break. I don't even smoke pot anymore, I'm afraid of it. I think that was in July, and I haven't taken any since.

In August I was to have another MRI. It would also be the one year anniversary of my surgery. One night I read something on Facebook about a mother with the same tumor I had, and it was about a fundraiser for her. It erroneously said that these tumors usually return within one year of surgery. As soon as I read that, I had a seizure. Since it was my one year anniversary, I became riddled with panic. It had also been three months since my last MRI, the longest I had gone between them. I was in a constant state of fear. I actually moved my MRI sooner by a couple of weeks thinking that I couldn't wait any longer. I needed to know. When the results came back fine, I was surprised that I wasn't more relieved. The panic remained.

This is when I really started to lose my mind. I became horribly depressed and so crazy panicked all the time. I thought I was having a nervous breakdown and that I might need to be committed because I was afraid of what I might do. I went on antidepressants, and on the advice of my friend Dan, the neurologist, I started weaning off my seizure med Keppra, as one of its side effects is anxiety and suicidal thoughts.

When I had my epiphany, I realized that because I had stopped the oil, I had also lost what I thought was my only hope for survival. I had nothing now.

I had been putting pressure on myself to start doing it again, but I was afraid. Whether the oil works or not, I had lost my placebo effect too. Within minutes of this realization, I felt my anxiety dissipate. Just knowing what it was gave me relief. I told myself that I was doing enough, that I was healthier than I had ever been, and that I was no different from anybody else by this point. I started putting Post-It's all over my house that said things like "You are doing enough," "You are doing a great job," "You are healthy and happy." If we all have cancer in our bodies and it's just a matter of keeping it from growing, then I am no different from any of you.

I take a few vitamins and drink my green juice every day, and I sometimes have ice cream. My anxiety is not 100 percent gone, it comes back at night, but usually the days are good, and I don't need to take anything. I will keep trying to find that peace and cut myself a break. I want to live in this moment and not worry about what hasn't happened yet.

Xo Katie

## 9/27/14

I'm feeling much better and haven't taken any anxiety meds for four days.

Micah and I went to see my oncologist at Cedars Sinai for my every-once-in-a-while check-in. We keep up that relationship for many reasons: it's always good to get a second opinion; he prescribes my seizure meds because it's impossible to get anyone at UCLA on the phone, plus I know he cares about me; he's proven that by sending me to UCLA; and he's funny. We went over all the recent developments, and I asked a bunch of questions. I expressed my fears about not doing enough, and he said, "Are you insane?" He confirmed for me that what I'm doing is enough and that a lot of the other stuff is just a way to scam people out of money. He did say he has a bunch of patients doing cannabis oil, but it's very common to do too much. I also asked him if my tumor came back, would it always come back as more aggressive, and he said no. If it came back, it could be a low grade that we wouldn't even have to treat right away. He said he has an 80 year-old with a grade-four tumor who is doing fine, and he has also seen a grade two patient die within a year. I had always thought that if the tumor came back, I would need another surgery right away, and that scared me to pieces. I don't ever want to go through brain surgery again; two times was enough.

We also talked about the fact that immunotherapy treatments

(where they take your tumor and manipulate it to actually fight and kill new tumors) are showing to be very effective, and new things are right around the corner. When I asked him if it is common for tumors to come back within one year of treatment, he told me to "stop reading" and that it was nonsense. He said they look at the past behavior, like the fact that it hasn't come back, and that it was a slow-growing tumor to begin with. He agreed with the lowering of my Keppra and warned me against getting hooked on Xanax. No problem there. I hate drugs of any kind. Overall we left there feeling very positive, and that has helped my anxiety a lot.

Xo Katie

## 10/20/14

Hi. It's been a while. Sometimes that can be a good thing because it usually means things are status quo over here. Our house is massively decorated for Halloween, and costumes are ready. Micah and I have been very actively working on our Halloween book for kids that we wrote last year, but unfortunately, we won't make it for this Halloween because the illustrations are very time-consuming. I work very closely with our illustrator, and I am a perfectionist. We put up a website if you want a preview: https://www.Sweetsthewitch.com.

My anxiety has greatly decreased, thanks to Celexa. I saw my new psychiatrist last week, and she felt that I was doing everything right as far as medications go and referred me to a psychologist who I'm waiting to call me so I can start some "behavior modification"; apparently I am distracting myself from the anxiety as opposed to dealing with it, which I am able to do most effectively during the day. When night time comes, I don't have enough distractions, so my anxiety creeps back. It's still not as bad as it was, though, but only because of the medication. She did diagnose me with traumatic stress disorder—not post-traumatic stress because the stress is ongoing. My kids and Micah are great, and that is wonderful. We are ready to celebrate a fantastic Halloween.

Xo Katie

# 11/11/14

I haven't written in a while, sometimes because I don't have much to say or I get busy, or I just want to avoid thinking about my health, or sometimes I have so much to say that I get overwhelmed. I have an MRI tomorrow afternoon. I've been on Celexa now for about two months. I started on a very small dose because I'm such a lightweight, but I have gradually increased to 40 milligrams, which is still a small dose. The good news is that my mental health is vastly better; the bad news is that almost instantly after I started taking it, my left side became significantly weaker. My hand took the biggest hit, becoming more clawlike and shaking a lot, but also my left leg is noticeably weaker. I fall trying to get out of a chair, bump into walls, trip, stub my toes... It's upsetting, but it's something I have to put up with for my sanity. It's really hard because I was getting so much better.

Since July I have been dealing with a major problem with my salivary glands. As my mouth became dryer, my lips would burn, my tongue would get little cuts every time I ate, and my gums would get sores all over. Eating was excruciating. I tried eliminating anything I regularly ate or drank, even my chewing gum and my toothpaste. I saw three doctors and dentists, including a head and neck surgeon. No one could tell me what it was. My salivary glands worked and had no tumors or stones. It wasn't from the radiation either.

I became so frustrated and sorry for myself. I felt doomed to suffer all my life. I did hours and hours of research online and slowly started adding things into my supplement regime that I felt might be lacking. A lot of vitamin and mineral deficiencies can cause dry mouth. All the doctors either blamed my meds or radiation or stress, but no one mentioned or ever asked what or how I ate. If they had they would have known that I have been on a very restrictive diet. First I added vitamin D3 because I don't go in the sun or drink milk or fortified juices. Then I added iron, magnesium, calcium, and zinc. Those cured my restless leg syndrome. Then I realized some important things. I had been told by my cancer nutritionist that I should eliminate iodine from my diet because people with brain tumors do better with an underactive thyroid. We switched our salt from iodized to pink Himalayan sea salt with no iodine. I don't eat seaweed or seafood, so I don't get any iodine at all, so I added a kelp iodine supplement. I also badly needed B12, which I wasn't getting from my other supplements.

When I went to see my psychiatrist for the first time, she asked me a lot about my history, including medical. Just by chance I brought up my many miscarriages. I told her all of the crazy things I found out were wrong with me during our struggle to have kids, including having a genetic DNA mutation called homozygous MTHFR, which causes a clotting problem. Along with this mutation comes an inability to absorb enough folic acid (get yourself checked for this! One in five people have it!). When I mentioned the mutation to her, she said, "I was just about to ask you that." Really? How random is that? She said that the homozygous MTHFR can cause depression. I had no idea. No one ever told me that. She told me it was important for me to take a large dose of methylated folate. I added that. Ironically, deficiencies of folic acid, iodine, and B12 can all cause dry mouth.

Very long story, short response—I am cured! No more dry mouth, sores, or cuts. I was malnourished! Instead of succumbing to taking salivary production pills, or switching my seizure pills, or thinking that this was for the rest of my life, I cured myself. I have slowly been adding things back into my diet that I was afraid to eat, like my favorite tea or decaf coffee, popcorn, and even the cannabis oil, and

I am still fine! I feel so happy about it. I emailed the head and neck surgeon who kept telling me it was probably radiation that had damaged my salivary glands (two years later!), and told him I had cured myself with nutrition and that he might want to start asking people what they were eating, and he actually emailed me back with a thank you! Anyway, this post is long enough. Wish me luck tomorrow!
Xo Katie

## 11/12/14

Another clean MRI! So grateful!
Xo Katie

## 12/17/2014

I haven't written in a while. It's just too hard for me.

Over the course of the last two or three months, I have not been doing any physical therapy because my anti-anxiety medication makes any progress I make disappear. I took a long break, and now I find my hand so weak that I can barely do anything with it.

One day I did what I was told I should do, which is to put my right hand behind my back and only use the weak left hand to do everything. The problems with that are many! No one ever uses their non-dominant hand to brush their teeth, put makeup on, cook food, etc., let alone open a jar or carry something heavy or fold clothes. It's impossible. When you take into consideration that I have zero fine motor skills and only about 50 percent gross motor skills in that hand, it adds up to one frustrating mess. Regardless, I did the best I could and just picked up toys and straightened up. A few hours later I had a seizure out of nowhere. I suspected that it may have been caused by the unusual amount of left hand activity, but I couldn't be sure. Whatever the cause, I didn't want it to happen again, so I haven't done that since.

Then last week I decided to do some fine motor work on my hand, just picking up fat pegs and putting them into holes. Within an hour of that, I had another seizure out of nowhere. After that I felt sure that the work I was doing was irritating my brain in some way, maybe by making new connections or by reactivating the connections that were previously there but had now atrophied. I have been scared to do any therapy since.

My doctors have advised me to continue to exercise but to take some medication ahead of time to ward off any impending seizure that may result. The problem is that the medication makes me sleepy, so it's something I really have to plan out. There's also the possibility that it won't work and I'd have a seizure anyway. Most people don't realize the impact that even a small seizure has on me. I was explaining this to my new therapist yesterday. If it was just about my arm shaking for a few minutes, it would be fine, but there is so much more to it. In the past, granted it was when I still had a tumor, I had seizures that lasted from 10-20 minutes. That fear that a small seizure could escalate into something bigger is always there.

When I have a seizure, I start to panic because I feel like I can't get any air. As a result I start to hyperventilate, which makes it even worse. You wouldn't guess it and no one really talks about it, but seizures hurt. At least mine do. Everyone is different and seizures are unique, but I know that most people who don't lose consciousness, like me, have some pain involved. I feel as though I'm being electrocuted. All the muscles on my left side cramp up, including my throat and face, and jerk and shake or twitch. It can be an effort to talk, or it can be impossible at times. My left leg will buckle out from under me. There is a very uncomfortable sensation of electricity, and once the jerking stops, I still feel the twitching under my skin for up to five minutes. Then my arm, hand, and face go completely dead, like my arm doesn't even belong to me and I just spent the day at the dentist.

It's very disconcerting to say the least. That can last 30 minutes, and the feeling comes back slowly. The worst thing, though, is that for the next two weeks after a seizure, the nerves in my arm constantly feel as if I'm going to have another seizure at any minute. It becomes a muscle memory, and I panic and have constant anxiety throughout the day, every day.

This affects my whole life. So...it's not just a matter of "Can't you just relax through it? You're not going to die; just ride it out." I wish it were that easy. I'm trying to deal with this and live my life as best I can. Writing about it can sometimes bring on anxiety, so I have to wait until I feel like I'm in a good place to do it. It's good that I don't lose consciousness because I could fall and hurt myself, but at times I wish that I could just black out and then wake up and not remember a thing. The fact that I'm awake means that I feel the pain, I feel the fear, I hear people talking about me as if I can't hear, and I relive it over and over.

I know I talk about seizures a lot here, and it's repetitive, but it's because the actual brain cancer has not been as bad or elicited as much fear as the epilepsy. That's a big statement.

Xo Katie

## 1/15/15

Happy New Year! What a great date today: 11515. I prefer even numbers, but the odd-number years have always been the best for me. Born in 1969, graduated high school in 1987, I met Micah in 1989, and we started dating for the second time 10 years later in 1999. I graduated college, got married, and bought a house in 2003; Lucky was born in 2005; Haven was born in 2011, and my successful surgery was in 2013.

I have great excitement for what this year will bring. I know you never hear me say this, but I actually feel great!

Aside from a mild sinus infection, I feel really good. This is going to be a really good year for me and my family—I can feel it. I have an MRI coming up in February, but I'm not overly worried about it. I feel the same, even better, and I'm so in touch with my body that I would notice any significant changes. I am trying to get an appointment to see my hand therapist again; it's been a couple of months. My arm and hand are extremely weak, and it's going to take some time to get them back to where they were before I started on the Celexa. It's really caused a disconnect between my brain and my hand. I can look at my hand and tell my fingers to open, but they just won't move. But if I stretch my arm out, I can open my hand no problem. My fingers aren't straight, but they will open. It's very weird.

I've been seeing my therapist (for my anxiety), and it really helps. It's not so much what she's doing, but just going there and being able to unload my grief is priceless. I never really realize how much I am holding in until I go there and start talking; then the floodgates open, and I'm good for another week. I had to go out and buy waterproof mascara just for those appointments! I asked her, "When will I be able to talk about this without breaking down?" She said, "When you've told the story so many times that it starts to feel like someone else's story. That could be 1,000 times or 10,000 times, but it will happen."

Anyway, hope you all have a fantastic year!

Xo Katie

## 2/14/15

Happy Valentine's Day! Four years ago today I went into labor, and on 2/15/11 I had my beautiful baby girl, Haven. I feel so blessed. A friend of mine who has a brain tumor, and was diagnosed at age 28, is having to grieve the loss of not being able to have children.

She's worried it would make her tumor grow. I feel blessed that I wasn't diagnosed until after I had my kids because I may not have had them knowing what I know now. I don't know if I could bring a child into the world knowing that I may not live to be their mother for long. I don't know if that's something I could recover from.

I just started my occupational therapy again. It's been since October and I definitely need it. I have also signed up for physical therapy because I have had one too many falls. I'm starting to actually hurt myself. I've actually fallen while sitting down! How do you do that? I just started leaning to the left and couldn't stop, and I couldn't use my left arm to catch myself or brace my fall. I feel like an idiot! I fall going upstairs (that takes a special skill!) and downstairs, but mostly while trying to stand up. I need serious help with my balance. I feel like one of those people who should be wearing a helmet all the time. The other day Micah and I were at CVS drugstore, and I was squatting to look at something on the lowest shelf and I fell over. I was like a turtle on its back with my legs in the air, and Micah yelled out, "Cleanup on aisle five!" We started laughing so hard, and so did the other man in the aisle! Anyway, I'll keep you posted on my progress. Happy birthday to my beautiful Haven!

Xo Katie

## 3/3/15

I had a troubling conversation with Lucky the other night where he came to me crying and said he was nervous and scared and wanted to sleep in our bed. This from a kid who has slept with us a total of one time when he was nine months old—and sick. He asked me what would happen if Micah and I both died at the same time. He couldn't tell me where this thought originated from, but he had spent the previous night at a close friend's house, and I asked him if he missed us. Through tears he said yes. He still pushed me to tell him what would happen if we died, and I explained that he would live with his guardians, who he knows and loves, and that he could still go to the same school, etc., but that the chances of that happening were incredibly small. I asked him if he was scared about us being gone, or what would happen to him. He cried again and said, "Both." I tried not to cry as this brought up all of my worst fears. I had the same fears as a child and never felt safe, and I was desperately sad that he was having to think about this scenario.

His response was "How would they know?"

"What do you mean?"

"How would they know?"

"Do you mean how would they know we had died?"

"Yes."

Good question, how would they know? I had to think about it. Flustered, I rattled off the chain of events that would likely happen: grandparents being called, etc., as well as the fact that his guardians knew of the plan, and it had been all worked out and discussed. This reassured him somewhat, but more questions came. "What if we are all together and get in an accident and you and Daddy die? What would happen to me and Haven?" I said that someone would call for help and the police, fire trucks, and ambulances would come. "Oh, okay." My poor little boy wanted facts; he wanted to know there was a plan. I told him about all of the people who loved him and that he would always be taken care of, where he would live, and even about our life insurance. I wanted him to know he wouldn't be out on the streets like the homeless people we see everyday. My heart broke for him. Again I told him that this was so unlikely to happen, that he didn't know anyone whose parents had died, and how rare it was. I had to comfort him; he would learn the truth soon enough. I told him how Micah and I have both of our parents, and we are old! That made him feel better. I don't really know where this came from.

Something he overheard? Read? Or from my illness. I think this is part of something called the nine-year change that they talk about in Waldorf schools. It's when children anywhere between eight and 11 have a sort of existential crisis. They are not living in the fantasy land they have enjoyed up until now. Reality is sinking in and they are becoming grounded. They are looking for the answers that we all want. Why are we here? Where did we come from? And what happens when we die?

He did sleep with us that night, and I liked having his little arms wrapped around me. I liked watching him sleep and how beautiful he looked, his breath on me. Since I got diagnosed there have been two Katies: the one who hates the fact that my kids are growing up so fast, and the other Katie, who wishes they were already grown. Why would I want that? Because it would be such a relief for me to know that I had been there to watch them grow up and that I was there for them. It's a sad way to think, and I don't dwell on it often, but this brought that feeling up in me again.

Xo Katie

## 3/25/15

I got an email from a fellow brain tumor survivor who is studying what all her fellow survivors are doing, and this was my response. I thought you might be interested.

"Hi Jess, I want to say I'm great, and I am—if you don't look at all of the deficits and anxiety/panic attacks and the very occasional seizure. I feel good except for being tired all the time. I still drink about 12 ounces of green juice every morning, and I take fish oil, turmeric (two pills), 4,000 Vit D, methylate folate/Vit B-12, nine mg melatonin (working my way up), not sure if it's making me tired during the day, Vit A 5000iu, maitake mushroom fraction D pills, garlic pill, Biotin (for my big bald spot), iodine, mag/zinc/calcium and probiotics.

This is all in addition to my low sugar/plant-based/organic/Non-GMO diet.

My last scan in February was clean, but I don't think I can ever relax, especially because they call this a 'terminal illness.' I worry that if I do survive what the ramifications of the radiation to my brain will be."

I have started going to physical therapy for my left leg now. I have been focusing on my arm and hand so much that I pretty much forgot about my leg. It has gotten weaker because of that, and I find myself falling, dragging my foot, stumbling, and swinging my hip out, which ends up looking like I waddle. My knees have been in a lot of pain. My physical therapist recommended I start using a cane until we can improve my balance and strength. So those of you who see me regularly, don't freak out. It's just for PT. I really feel self-conscious. I especially don't want everyone to see me and think the worst. One of the reasons I am writing this is so people won't worry. It's a good thing. Haven wants one for herself now!

Xo Katie

## 1/29/2016

Long time no hear! It's been a long time since my last post! Let me start by saying the old adage of no news is good news. I'm good. I have been living my life instead of talking about it. I have been missing this blog, though. You can't really be yourself entirely on Facebook; it's too complicated with too many diverse groups of people. Here I can speak freely, and I don't care or worry about offending anyone. So In the last four or five months or so, I have felt really good (considering). I exercise, I engage and participate with my kids, who are now five and 10 (can you believe they were one and six when I started this blog!). I cook, I shop, I host for the holidays, I drive everywhere, I garden. I have accepted the fact that I will likely always have seizures, and always be mostly paralyzed in my hand. The weakness in my leg and face has improved with exercise and practice daily. I still limp and sometimes fall but rarely choke anymore. My hand is a constant frustration, but I adapt. Now that the kids are older, they can help me more. Haven takes pride in zipping up my jackets and scratching my itches for me, and Lucky carries things and opens doors. He is a great helper.

Micah and I are still a great team and are able to now share the household responsibilities more. It's taken a lot of time and work to figure out our new roles. Micah can get stuck in the role of caregiver and not know when to let me do things for myself. There are times over the years when he has been resentful of the fact that he has had the lion's share of responsibility. We are human. I get angry when I want to do something but am physically unable to do, so I get angry that he is angry. Major illness is hard on relationships. I want to be clear about that and not paint a picture that everything was always smooth sailing. Many marriages collapse under the pressure. It's not always the case that "It brought us closer together." It's a rebuilding process. It's getting used to the new Katie and how are we going to be husband and wife again? This is real life, not a movie.

As far as my health, my seizures can happen once a week or once every two months; it really depends on the circumstances. The worst circumstance is stress. A very stressful day will usually cause an evening seizure once I am relaxed. Exhaustion is another. I still nap most days, but I can go without if I need to. Anxiety is number three. It can be a subtle thing that can send me into a panic, maybe a name or just hearing about someone who has cancer. Weird things like seeing someone with a handicap like cerebral palsy, hearing about someone else with seizures, the word brain, or even just the word neurologist can set me off. I can't predict it. I see a new psychiatrist now as well as a psychologist, conveniently in the same building! I still take Celexa for depression and anxiety. I hope I won't always have to.

Xo Katie

## 3/10/16

Hi. I got another clear MRI! Yay! I still take my supplements almost every day, I exercise every day now, but I got into some bad eating habits over the holidays, and I'm now trying to get back on track. I've been thinking a lot about my relationships with people: family, friends, and acquaintances, and how they change and evolve. You really get to see who people are in a crisis situation. When I was first diagnosed, I had a nice group of friends. When the news broke my friends fell into three categories.

1. The Hero: Someone who works great in a crisis and likes to take over, organize, plan, and dictate. In a crisis these are your best friends. You need them. However, some of them only want to be the hero, they're in it for the glory, and if you're lucky enough to recover, they disappear. Some don't expect or want you to recover. You will rarely hear from these people again. I trusted them and thought they loved me. Luckily, I only had a few of those, but it stings nonetheless.
2. The No-Shows: These people just cannot handle your kind of crisis at all. Maybe it's too overwhelming; they don't know what to do or say, so they do nothing. Or maybe it just hits too close to home. "If it can happen to her, it can happen to me." It's very disappointing that they can't take themselves out of the equation, but I forgive their weakness.

3. The True Blue: These are the best, the most loyal. They can be the hero or the worker bee, but they are there for you no matter what, at any time day or night, and are genuinely happy when you are doing well. You may not see them very much, but you know that if things went south, they would be there again. I'm so lucky that most of my friends and family fall into this category! Thank you!

Xo Katie

## 1/20/22

Can you believe this year in May will be my 10 year survivor anniversary? It's hard to believe how far I have come. Obviously I am alive, but also I have not had any recurrence of the cancer, no growth at all. My neuro-oncologist, Dr. Cloughesy, cannot say whether what shows up on my MRI is dead tumor or scar tissue, and that's fine. I don't care. My life is pretty great! Lucky is now 16 and Haven will be 11! Crazy! My parents and Micah's parents are all healthy and doing well too. We are very blessed.

One of the greatest things is that about four years ago, my epilepsy doctor introduced me to a new seizure medication that had just been approved by the FDA; it's called Briviact, so we added it to my Vimpat and I haven't had a seizure since! It has literally changed my life. I can live without being in constant fear of falling or crashing my car, and I don't have panic attacks constantly. Occasionally I will have a little bit of panic or muscle memory of seizures creeping in, but I can quickly refocus onto something else. I still deal with the fact that I have paralysis on my left side. I have fallen many times and have luckily only had minor injuries, but we worry a lot about me hurting myself badly. My biggest fear is injuring my good hand, which would make me totally dependent on others for everything. My left hand hasn't changed; it's still only barely useful, but I appreciate even the little bit that I can use it. Everything helps.

In January of 2020, right before the pandemic, I made a big decision to have scalp reconstructive surgery. I had spent eight years looking at my surgery and radiation scar, the giant bald spot. It was the one thing that was still making me feel not like myself, and it was the one visual clue of what I had been through. I was over it!

I know from my past that there are charities out there to help people from all walks of life with everything you can think of, so I decided to start researching if there was someone who could help me (you know I like to research!). I came across a charity called Operation Restore. They help people who have been burned restore their hair, even burns from radiation! I filled out an application and they accepted me!

A couple of weeks later, I went to meet with a doctor, a specialist in hair restoration. He and his partner looked at my scar tissue and said they didn't think a regular hair transplant, the kind where they implant individual hairs, would work out very well. They felt that the hair wouldn't take root because the scar tissue was too thin with no fat underneath, so there was nothing for it to take hold of. Long story short, they thought it would be best for me to do a scalp transplant. This is a much more complicated procedure where an expander is surgically placed between the scalp and the skull and slowly inflated with liquid to an insane proportion until there is enough extra scalp and hair that would cover up the bald spot. Then it's deflated and the extra scalp is pulled over and sewed on. Yes, I did it! I'm insane!

## Welcome To KATIE'S BRAIN

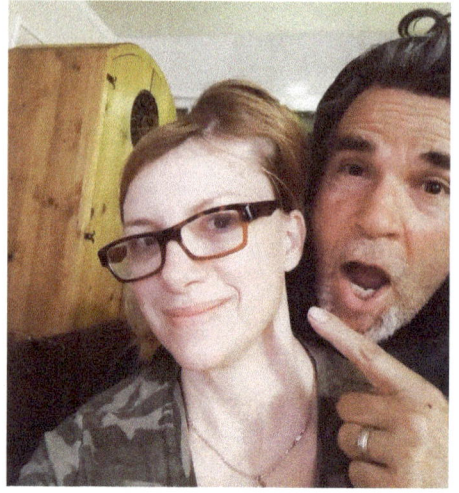

Scalp getting inflated.                    Crying from the pain.

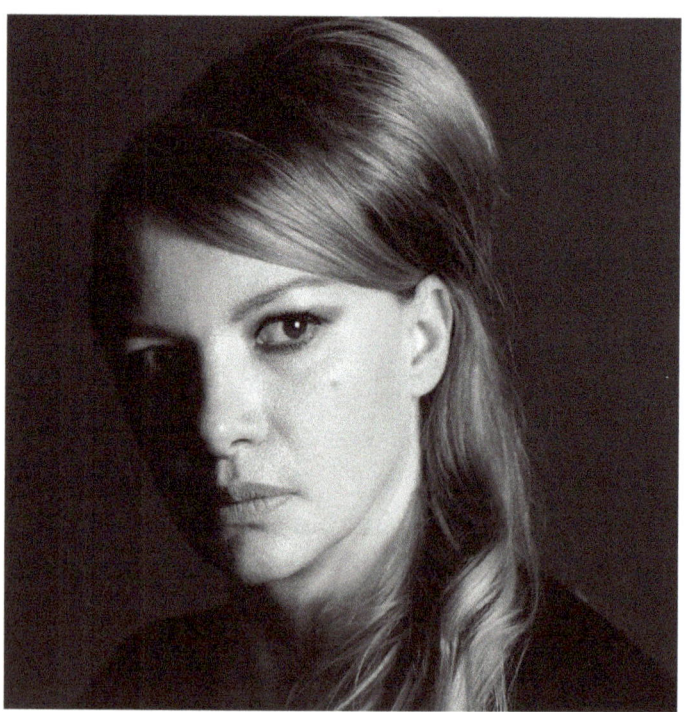

That's not a beehive hairdo; it's my skin!
Playing around with Micah's photography skills.

## KATIE KAISER SMITH

This was excruciatingly painful, and I've been through some pain in my life. I immediately regretted it the first night. I wanted it out ASAP. But you know me by now, and I got through four months of crazy pain until the port in the back of my head tore open. It was as awful as it sounds. It looked like the back of my head was giving birth to this bag of blue fluid. The expander was crowning, and it had to come out. Because it was premature they weren't able to cover the entire bald spot, and they did end up doing some individual grafts for the rest. Ultimately I am very happy because the bulk of the transplant created enough hair to hide where the grafts are thinner. You can't even tell I was ever bald there. It's amazing!

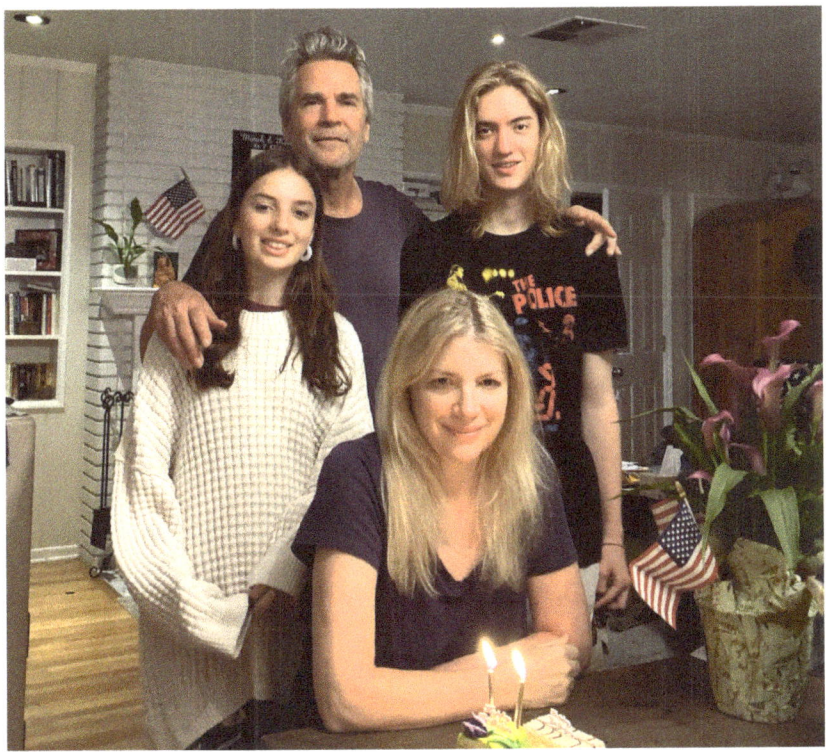

Bye bye, bald spot!

If you remember a post from the first year when I was newly diagnosed, I went to a Reiki healer, who asked me to visualize myself 10 years from then, and I said I was in Hawaii on the beach with Micah and our kids. I could picture it.

Well, next month we are all finally going to Hawaii to celebrate my 10 year survivor anniversary. I actually had tickets two years ago, but then Covid-19 hit and I had to cancel, so I think it was meant to be that we are going now, just like I imagined.

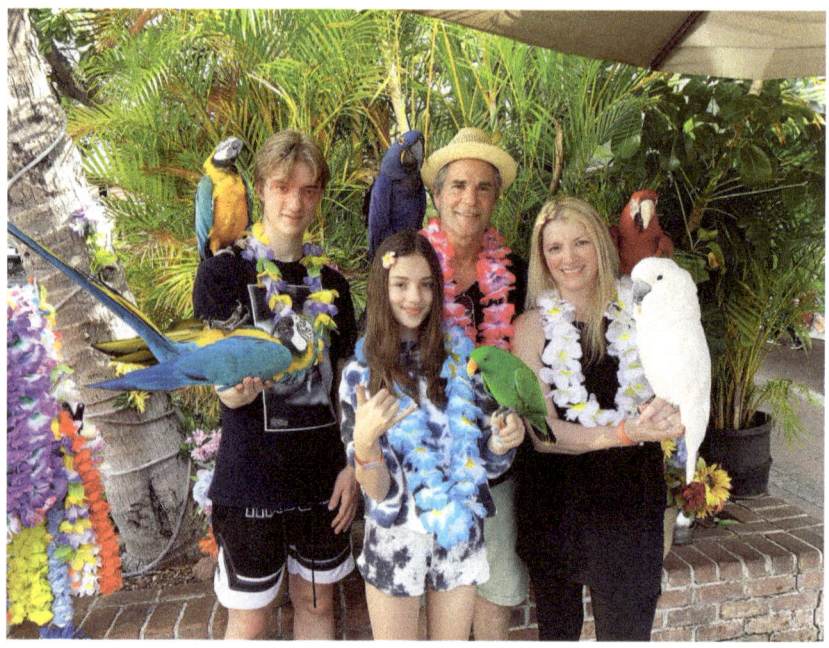

10 year survivor anniversary Hawaii trip! Lahaina, Maui

Although I didn't come out of this nightmare unscathed, I will always deal with my disabilities, epilepsy, and the fact that the tumor could return, but I am so blessed because I have had these years to see my children grow, and I know now that they will remember me. We have made lasting memories and had many great times. Micah and I are still happy and in love, and we look forward to spending the rest of our lives together with our kids and grandkids, and we did finally renew our vows in a cheesy Vegas chapel with Elvis presiding! It's finally feeling like someone else's story.

Thank you for reading.

Xo Katie

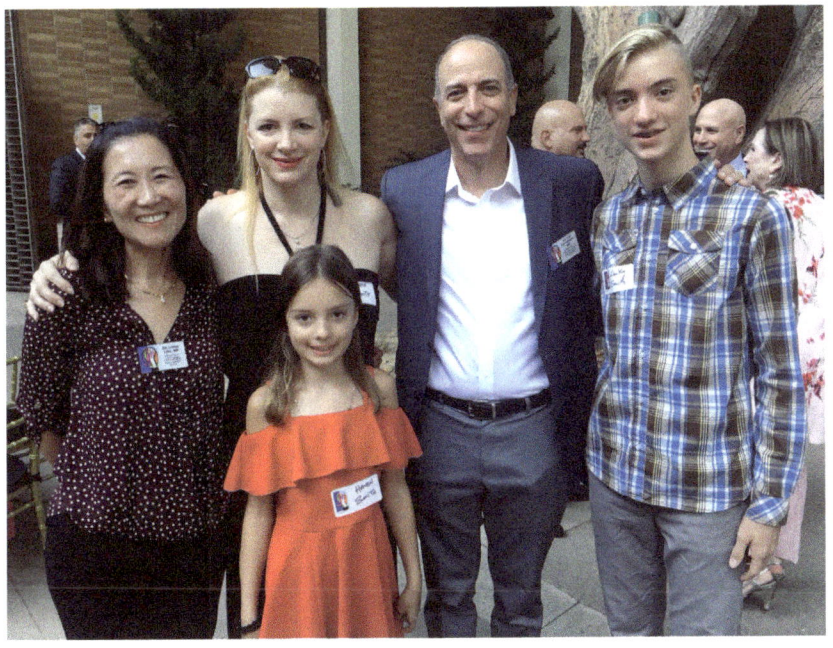

Me, Haven, and Lucky with Dr. Liau and Dr. Cloughesy—my heroes

*Welcome To* KATIE'S BRAIN

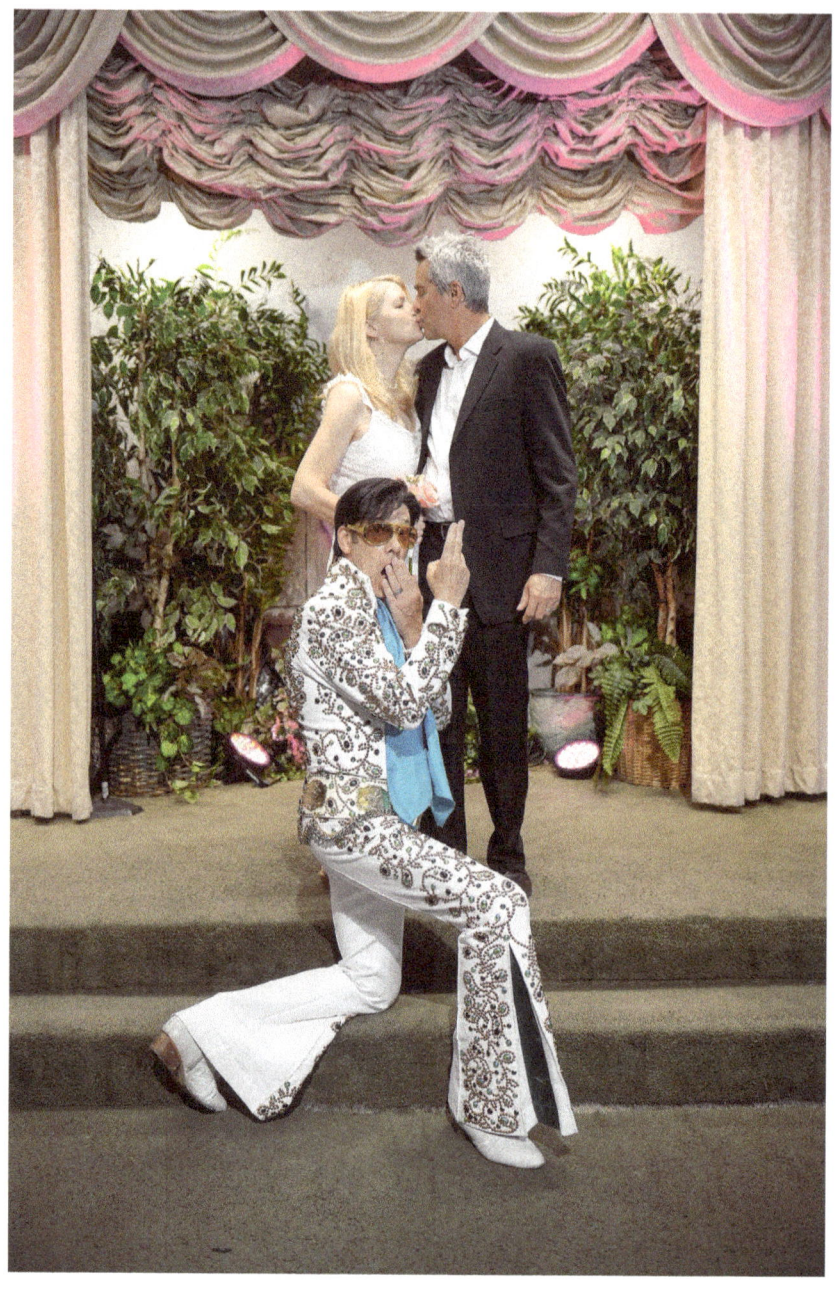

Vow renewal with Elvis!

# Conclusion

This book has taken many years to write. While the blog pretty much wrote itself, the editing process has been incredibly difficult with many stops and starts. Going back and reading my posts brought back some horrible memories, and there were many times that I needed to take a break. When I was still having seizures, it was impossible for me to read about that time in my life.

I am so grateful I had the blog because I know without it I would not have been able to remember those years and all of the details. The blog was so therapeutic for me; I was able to reveal my deepest, darkest thoughts and feelings and get such abundant support in return. I'm sad about all of the friends I made along the way who didn't survive this horrible disease and I'm thrilled for my fellow survivors.

I'm reminded of what I tell my kids: Being brave doesn't mean you aren't scared, but that you keep going in spite of the fear. Never, ever give up!

Xo Katie

Milton Keynes UK
Ingram Content Group UK Ltd.
UKHW051332070724
445092UK00006B/53